P9-EEG-566

OXFORD MEDICAL PUBLICATIONS

Exposure assessment in occupational and environmental epidemiology

WITHDRAWN

UTSA LIBRARIES

Whilst every effort has been made to ensure that the contents of this book are as complete, accurate and up to date as possible at the date of writing. Oxford University Press is not able to give any guarantee or assurance that such is the case. Readers are urged to take appropriately qualified medical advice in all cases. The information in this book is intended to be useful to the general reader, but should not be used as a means of self-diagnosis or for the prescription of medication.

Exposure Assessment in Occupational and Environmental Epidemiology

Edited by

Mark J. Nieuwenhuijsen
Imperial College
London

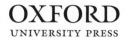

OXFORD

UNIVERSITY PRESS

Library
University of Texas
of San Antonio

OXFORD

UNIVERSITY PRESS

Great Clarendon Street, Oxford OX2 6DP

Oxford University Press is a department of the University of Oxford.
It furthers the University's objective of excellence in research, scholarship,
and education by publishing worldwide in

Oxford New York

Auckland Bangkok Buenos Aires Cape Town Chennai
Dar es Salaam Delhi Hong Kong Istanbul Karachi Kolkata
Kuala Lumpur Madrid Melbourne Mexico City Mumbai Nairobi
São Paulo Shanghai Taipei Tokyo Toronto

Oxford is a registered trade mark of Oxford University Press
in the UK and in certain other countries

Published in the United States
by Oxford University Press Inc., New York

© Oxord University Press, 2003

The moral rights of the authors have been asserted

Database right Oxford University Press (maker)

First published 2003

All rights reserved. No part of this publication may be reproduced,
stored in a retrieval system, or transmitted, in any form or by any means,
without the prior permission in writing of Oxford University Press,
or as expressly permitted by law, or under terms agreed with the appropriate
reprographics rights organization. Enquiries concerning reproduction
outside the scope of the above should be sent to the Rights Department,
Oxford University Press, at the address above

You must not circulate this book in any other binding or cover
and you must impose this same condition on any acquirer

A catalogue record for this is available from the British Library

Library of Congress Cataloging in Publication Data
Data available
ISBN 0-19-852861-2 (Pbk)

10 9 8 7 6 5 4 3 2 1

Typeset by Newgen Imaging Systems (P) Ltd., Chennai, India
Printed in Great Britain
on acid-free paper by
T.J. International Ltd., Padstow, Cornwall

Library
University of Texas
at San Antonio

Foreword

Occupational and environmental epidemiology has generated a number of important scientific discoveries resulting in successful preventive measures. The era of cholera outbreaks and dramatic air pollution episodes is over in much (but not all) of the world, with attention shifting to more subtle effects of air and water pollution, pesticide exposure, and ionizing and non-ionizing radiation, for example. Societal concern with hazards in the workplace and community, and the resulting link between epidemiological evidence and regulatory policy, has led to a demand for more refined studies to address the most subtle of effects. An important consequence of the policy relevance of research in occupational and environmental epidemiology is the development of sophisticated approaches to monitoring exposures, largely motivated by regulatory pressure. We are able to measure minute amounts of agents in the environment and often do so. Nevertheless, the assessment of human exposure to these agents remains the single most important limiting factor in the quality of evidence that epidemiology can provide.

Combining the strong public interest with potential threats to health in the environment, the associated economic and policy relevance, and extensive monitoring data should create a highly favourable situation for characterizing exposure. Why is it so difficult to assign exposure accurately in epidemiological studies? The specific challenges depend on the exposure source, agent, and pathway, but a number of recurrent reasons can be offered. (1) Exposure is rarely constant, and the temporal variation in exposure is often over shorter intervals than those of etiologic relevance, thus forcing epidemiologists to integrate in some manner. This occurs in workplaces, as job duties and locations change over time, and in the community, with daily, seasonal, and secular changes in pollutant levels. (2) The agents of interest are diverse and often consist of complex mixtures, as are frequently found for solvents, pesticides, particulate air pollution, and drinking water disinfection by-products. (3) Human behaviour alters exposure, so that human exposure is a combination of environmental exposure and where people spend time, how much they breathe, what they eat and drink, whether they exercise, and so on. (4) Responses to a given exposure are quite variable, particularly at low exposure levels. The search for susceptible subpopulations, whether defined by age, presence of chronic diseases, or genetic constitution is an acknowledgement that we are often concerned with effects too subtle to be readily seen in the population at large.

This book represents an important attempt to come to grips with the distinctive challenges and opportunities in exposure assessment for occupational and environmental epidemiology. This book addresses both the need for seeking coherence across diverse realms of application and examines exposure assessment methods used in several important substantive areas. The tools and strategies used to refine human exposure assessment to particulate air pollution or silica in mining operations may well have applicability to examining drinking water disinfection by-products or endotoxins in agricultural settings if we could only grasp the underlying strategy. An appreciation of the environmental monitoring technology and the data it produces is required, along with the ability to translate such information into human exposure estimates. Practical issues regarding the ability of individuals to accurately report exposure and behavioural determinants of exposure needs to be considered. Biological markers of exposure offer great potential, but require careful consideration of their merits relative to other approaches.

As research teams are assembled to address environmental health concerns, there is often a gap between the chemists, physicists, or toxicologists on the one hand, and the epidemiologist on the other. This gap can be filled by an expert in exposure assessment. By bringing together the critical components from engineering, statistics, toxicology, and environmental science to focus on the application to epidemiologic research, this book should provide a valuable guide to applying state of the art methods in epidemiological research and a platform from which further advances can be made.

David Savitz
Chapel Hill
North Carolina

Preface

The book brings together contributions from an international group of practioners to provide a comprehensive reference on the 'state of art' methods and applications in the field of exposure assessment for occupational and environmental epidemiological studies.

The recent and rapid expansion of occupational and environmental epidemiology and health-risk assessment looks set to continue in line with growing public, government, and media concern about occupational and environmental health issues, and a scientific need to better understand and explain the effects of occupational and environmental pollutants on human health.

Risks associated with occupational and environmental exposure are generally small, but the exposed population, and hence the population attributable risk, may be large. To detect small risks, the exposure assessment needs to be very refined. Exposure assessment is the study of the distribution and determinants of potentially hazardous agents, and includes the estimation of intensity, duration, and frequency of exposure, the variation in these indices, and their determinants. Epidemiological studies can utilize information on variation and determinants of exposure to optimize the exposure–response relations. Many methodological and practical problems arise when conducting an exposure assessment for epidemiological studies and these are addressed in the book, as is the issue of measurement error and exposure misclassification and its effect on exposure–response relationships.

The aim of this book is to develop an understanding and knowledge of exposure assessment methods and their application to substantive issues in occupational and environmental epidemiology. The emphasis is on methodological principles and good practice. It focuses on exposure assessment in both occupational and environmental epidemiology since there are many similarities but also some interesting differences. The book outlines the basic principles of exposure assessment, and examines the current status and research questions in the exposure assessment of occupational and environmental epidemiological studies of allergens, particulate matter, chlorination disinfection by-products, agricultural pesticides, and radiofrequencies.

The book will be of interest to anyone concerned with exposure assessment and epidemiology. It will be a valuable resource for undergraduate and postgraduate courses in exposure assessment, occupational hygiene, environmental science, epidemiology, toxicology, biostatistics, occupational and environmental health, health-risk assessment, and related disciplines and a useful resource of reference for policy makers and regulators.

Contents

List of abbreviations

ACGIH	American Conference of Governmental Industrial Hygienists
AHS	Agricultural Health Study
AM	Arithmetic mean
ANOVA	Analysis of variance
AUC	Area-under-the-curve
BDCM	Bromodichloromethane
CDBM	Chlorodibromomethane
CERC	Cambridge Environmental Research Consultants
CFS	Chronic fatigue syndrome
COPD	Chronic obstructive pulmonary disease
CP	Chloropicrin
CV	Coefficient of variation
DBP	Disinfection by-product
DMA	Dimethylarsinic acid
DMRB	Design Manual for Roads and Bridges
EC	Elemental carbon
EIA	Enzyme immuno assay
ELF	Extremely low frequency
EMFs	Electromagnetic fields
ETS	Environmental tobacco smoke
FA	Flour aeroallergen
FP	Fine particulate
GC-MS	Gas chromatography-mass spectrometry
GFR	Glomerular filtration
GIS	Geographical information systems
GM	Geometric mean
GPS	Global positioning systems
GSD	Geometric standard deviation
HAAs	Haloacetic acids
HANs	Haloacetonitriles
HI	Harvard impactors
HKs	Haloketones
HMW	High molecular weight
HSE	Health and Safety Executive
IARC	International Agency for Research on Cancer
ICC	Intra-class correlation coefficients
ICNIRP	International Commission on Non-Ionizing Radiation Protection
ICP-MS	Inductively coupled plasma-mass spectrometry
IEA	International Epidemiological Association

IEGMP   Independent Export Group on Mobile Phones
JEM   Job-exposure matrix
JSQ   Job-specific questionnaires
MCMC   Markov chain Monte Carlo
MLE   Maximum likelihood estimator
MMA   Monomethylarsonic acid
NAAQS   National Ambient Air Quality Standard
NMAPS   National Morbidity, Mortality, and Air Pollution Study
OC   Organic carbon
OPs   Organophosphates
OSPM   Operational Street Pollution Model
PAH   Polycyclic aromatic hydrocarbons
PBPK   Physiologically based pharmicokinetic
PEF   Peak expiratory flow
PEMs   Personal exposure monitors
PM   Particulate matter
QSAR   Quantitative structure–activity relationship
RIA   Radio immuno assay
RR   Relative risk
SAM   Stationary ambient monitoring
SAR   Specific energy absorption rate
SCEs   Sister chromatid exchanges
STEMS   Space–time exposure modelling system
TACC   Time above a critical concentration
THMs   Trihalomethanes
TINs   Triangulated irregular networks
TOC   Total or organic carbon
TSP   Total suspended particulates
VOCs   Volatile organic compounds
XRF   X-ray fluorescence

List of contributors

Wolfgang Ahrens Bremer Institute for Prevention Research and Social Medicine, University of Bremen, Linzer Str 8-10, Bremen 28359, Germany

Ben Armstrong London School of Hygiene and Tropical Medicine, 1 Keppel Street, London WC1E 7HT, UK

David Briggs Department of Epidemiology and Public Health, Imperial College School of Medicine at St Mary's, Norfolk Place, London W2 1PG, UK

Alex Burdorf Department of Public Health, Erasmus University Rotterdam, PO Box 1738, 3000 DR Rotterdam, The Netherlands

Philip Chadwick Microwave Consultants Limited, 17B Woodland Road, London E18 2EL, UK

John W. Cherrie Department of Environmental & Occupational Medicine, University of Aberdeen, c/o Institute of Occupational Medicine, 8 Roxburgh Place, Edinburgh, EH8 9SU, UK

Roy Colvile Department of Environmental Science and Technology, Imperial College of Science, Technology and Medicine, Royal School of Mines, Prince Consort Road, London SW7 2BP, UK

Mustafa Dosemeci Division of Cancer Epidemiology and Genetics, National Cancer Institute, Occupational Epidemiology Branch, 6120 Executive Blvd, EPS/8002, Rockville, MD 20852, USA

Pierre Droz Institute of Occupational Health Sciences, Lausanne University, Rue du Bugnon 19, Lausanne 1005, Switzerland

Dick Heederik Institute for Risk Assessment, Utrecht University, PO Box 80176, Utrecht 3508 TD, The Netherlands

George Loizou Exposure Modeling Section, Health and Safety Laboratories, Biomedical Services Group, Broadlane, Sheffield S3 7HQ, UK

Mark J. Nieuwenhuijsen Department of Environmental Science and Technology, Imperial College of Science, Technology and Medicine, Royal School of Mines, Prince Consort Road, London SW7 2BP, UK

Sean Semple Department of Environmental & Occupational Medicine, University of Aberdeen, c/o Institute of Occupational Medicine, 8 Roxburgh Place, Edinburgh EH8 9SU, UK

Martin Spendiff Exposure Modelling Section, Health and Safety Laboratories, Broadlane, Sheffield S3 7HQ, UK

Patricia Stewart Division of Cancer Epidemiology and Genetics, National Cancer Institute, Room 7032, Executive Boulevard, MSC 7242, Bathesda MD 20892-7335, USA

Helen H. Suh Department of Environmental Health, Harvard School of Public Health, 401 Park Drive, Room 404G, Boston, MA 02215, USA

Kay Teschke School of Occupational and Environmental Hygiene, University of British Columbia, Room 370A, 2206 East Mall, Vancouver, Canada V6T 1Z3

Martie van Tongeren Centre for Occupational and Environmental Health, School of Epidemiology and Health Sciences, The University of Manchester, 4th Floor, Humanities Building, Oxford Road, Manchester M13 9PL, UK

I Methods

1. Introduction to exposure assessment

Mark J. Nieuwenhuijsen

1.1 Introduction

Exposure is a substance or factor affecting human health, either adversely or beneficially. More precisely, in occupational and environmental epidemiology exposure to an environmental or occupational substance is generally defined as any contact between a substance in an environmental medium (e.g. water, air, soil) and the surface of the human body (e.g. skin, respiratory tract); after uptake into the body it is referred to as dose. Exposure assessment is the study of distribution and determinants of substances or factors affecting human health. It consists of three components; the design of the study, data collection, and the interpretation of the data. This chapter discusses briefly some of the basic issues, and introduces topics for the following chapters.

In occupational and environmental epidemiology, the focus is on chemical, biological, and physical substances at work or in our everyday environment respectively. In today's world risks associated with occupational and environmental exposure are generally small and therefore to detect a risk when there is truly a risk, the exposure assessment has to be very refined. This generally requires considerable effort and resources. Part of the exposure assessment process in occupational and environmental epidemiology is to optimize the exposure estimate with the aim of detecting a possible risk and/or optimizing the exposure–response relation in an epidemiological study. This can be achieved, for example, by optimizing the distribution of the variance of the exposure estimates. The main focus of this chapter will be on chemical and biological substances, but the underlying principles will apply to other exposures as well.

Although the main focus of occupational and environmental exposure assessment and epidemiology is different, associations between work place exposure and disease and environmental exposure and disease respectively, the underlying principles and methods used are often very similar. Time and location (space) play an important role. The boundaries also become less clear when the exposure of interest occurs both in the environment and in the work place and through other pathways (e.g. mercury exposure for a subject with amalgam fillings working in a chloralkali plant, living in the vicinity of the plant, and eating fish). Traditionally exposure levels in the work place tended to be higher than in the general environment and the duration of exposure was generally shorter (approximately 8 h per day vs. up to 24 h per day). The higher exposure levels were often easier to measure than the lower environmental levels and the work place provided a more defined environment in time and space than the general environment. In the work place the populations of interest are adults while outside the work place there are also other (susceptible) groups such as children and the elderly with, for example, different behavioural patterns. Work place populations tend to be healthier than the general population. The focus here is on the underlying principles and methods and therefore the areas are combined with examples from both. This book is an extension of a previously published book on exposure assessment (Armstrong *et al.* 1992), but with more focus on environmental and occupational exposure.

1.2   Epidemiological studies, designs, and need for exposure indices

A major aim of occupational and environmental epidemiological studies is to determine if there is an association or not between a particular substance of interest, the exposure, and morbidity and/or mortality. If there is an association, it is desirable to be able to show an exposure (or dose)–response relationship, that is, a relationship where the rate of disease increases as the level of exposure (or dose) increases. This will aid in the interpretation of such studies.

In recent years there has been increasing interest in the field of exposure assessment causing it to develop rapidly. We know now more than ever to what, where, and how people are exposed and improvements have been made to methods for assessing the level of exposure, its variability, and the determinants. New methods have been developed or newly applied throughout this field, including analytical, measurement, and statistical methods. This has led to a considerable improvement in exposure assessment in epidemiological studies, and therefore improvement in the epidemiological studies themselves.

In occupational and environmental epidemiology, there are different study designs to assess the association between exposure and disease. The main study designs to obtain exposure–response relationships are as follows.

(1) *Cohort study*, in which a group (i.e. cohort) of subjects are followed up over time to assess whether they develop the disease of interest or not. The subjects are classified by level of exposure (e.g. yes/no, low, medium, and high) at entry to the study, but may be re-classified at a later stage. A risk estimate (e.g. relative risk or incidence rate ratio) is obtained by comparing the disease rate in subpopulations with different levels of exposure or external controls. The study can be prospective, that is, a cohort is assembled and followed up in the future, or retrospective, that is, the assembly date of the cohort and follow up was in the past. Prospective cohort studies have the advantage that the exposure can be determined at the time of field work. Retrospective cohort studies require a reconstruction of historical exposure. They may need to go far back in time for diseases with a long latency time, which may make exposure assessment more difficult (see Chapters 7 and 8).

(2) *Cross-sectional study*, where at one point in time in a population subjects are classified by different levels of exposure (e.g. yes/no, none, low, medium, and high) and the frequency of disease is assessed for each level of exposure. A risk estimate

(e.g. prevalence ratio) is obtained by comparing the disease frequencies in subpopulations with different levels of exposure or external controls.

(3) *Case–control study*, in which the exposure of diseased subjects (cases) is compared to the exposure of (randomly selected) controls from the underlying sampling population. A risk estimate (e.g. odds ratio) is obtained by dividing the odds of exposure (in the past) for the cases by the odds of exposure (in the past) in the controls. A reconstruction of historical exposure may be required, going far back in time for diseases with a long latency time, which is often challenging. Recall bias, that is, bias where cases are more likely to recall exposure in the past compared to controls, may be a particular problem. A case–control study could be nested within a cohort study, thereby reducing the effort required for the exposure assessment, given the smaller number of subjects, or improving the exposure assessment if the same effort is maintained, but for fewer subjects than in the full cohort.

(4) *Time series study*, in which the day-to-day variability in exposure levels is correlated to the day-to-day variability in disease rate. Recently this approach has frequently been used in air pollution research, where measurements from ambient air pollution monitoring stations have been linked to daily morbidity and mortality data. A specific issue is how well the ambient monitoring station results reflect the personal exposure of subjects in the population (see Chapter 14).

Other study designs that have been used include case studies, ecological studies, and panel studies, but they are not discussed further.

All the study designs require exposure estimates or exposure indices to estimate the risk associated with the substance of interest, but they may differ depending on the study design. The design and interpretation of epidemiological studies is often dependent on the exposure assessment and therefore needs careful consideration. Quantification of the relation between exposure and adverse human health effects requires the use of exposure estimates, which are accurate, precise and biologically relevant, for the critical exposure period, and show a range of exposure levels in the population under study. Furthermore there is also a general need for the assessment of confounders, that is, substances associated with both exposure and disease that may bias the study results. Assessment of confounders should be in as much detail as the assessment of exposure indices since measurement error in confounders may also affect the health risk estimates (see Chapter 12)

1.3 Source–receptor models and exposure route and pathways

The physical course a pollutant takes from the source to a subject is often referred to as exposure pathway, while the way a substance enters the body is often referred to as exposure route. Source–receptor models include the routes and pathways of exposure and are helpful in understanding how people are exposed. In this kind of model it often becomes clear that humans create their own exposure by, for example, their activities and where they spend time, and that there is an interaction between the two. Figure 1.1 provides an example of a source–receptor model for air pollution. The source may be cars and air pollutants such as particles, carbon monoxide, and nitrogen dioxide, are

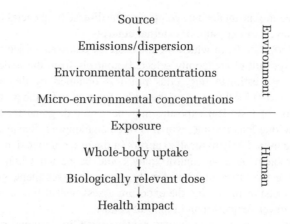

Fig. 1.1 Source–receptor model for air pollutants.

emitted from exhaust pipes. Dispersion will take place into the streets and beyond leading to environmental concentrations. Dispersion takes places into so-called micro-environments such as houses, travel routes and modes, and work places, where people come into contact with the pollutants and is now referred to as exposure. People will inhale the pollutants through the lungs leading to whole-body uptake (dose), where it may react with the lung cells or it may be distributed to other parts of the body and may react with body tissue (biologically relevant dose). The reaction with the body tissue may have an impact on health.

In this case there is only one exposure route (inhalation). There are however three possible exposure routes for substances:

- inhalation through the respiratory system,
- ingestion through the gastrointestinal system,
- absorption through the skin.

The exposure route(s) of a substance and the amount of uptake depends on, for example, the biological, chemical, and physical characteristics of the substances, location and activity of the person, and the persons themselves. Inhalation of particles through the respiratory system depends on the particle size or diameter (physical characteristic). Smaller particles are more often inhaled and penetrate deeper into the lungs. The inhalable dust fraction (particles with 50% cut-off diameter of 100 μm) is the fraction of the dust that enters the nose and mouth and is deposited anywhere in the respiratory tract. The thoracic fraction (particles with a 50% cut-off diameter of 10 μm) is the fraction that enters the thorax and is deposited within the lung airways and the gas-exchange region. The respiratory fraction (particles with a 50% cut-off diameter of 4 μm) is deposited in the gas-exchange region (alveoli) (ACGIH 2002). Furthermore, inhalation depends on the breathing rate of the subject: those doing heavy work may inhale much more air and more deeply (20 lmin^{-1} for light work vs. 60 lmin^{-1} for heavy work) (activity of person). And, people move through different micro-environments with different particle concentrations (location).

Exposure pathways   Exposure routes   Biomarker

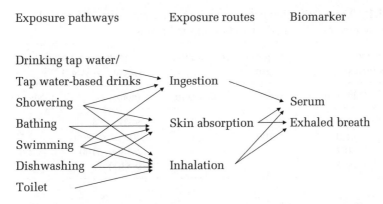

Fig. 1.2 Examples of exposure pathways, routes, and biomarkers for trihalomethanes.

Skin absorption can play an important role for uptake of substances such as solvents, pesticides, and trihalomethanes (see Chapter 9). The volatile trihalomethanes are formed when water is chlorinated and the chlorine reacts with organic matter in the water. In this context there are a number of possible exposure pathways and routes (Fig. 1.2). The main pathway of ingestion is drinking tap water or tap water-based drinks (e.g. tea, coffee, and squash). Swimming, showering, bathing, and dish washing may all result in considerable uptake through inhalation and skin absorption and, for the former three, ingestion to a minor extent. Standing or flushing water in the toilet may lead to uptake via inhalation through volatilization of the trihalomethanes. The uptake of trihalomethanes may be assessed using the concentration measured in exhaled breath or serum (see Chapters 11 and 15).

In the human body, the uptake, distribution, transformation, and excretion of substances such as trihalomethanes can be modelled using physiologically based pharmico-kinetic (PBPK) models (see Chapter 10). These models are becoming more sophisticated although they are still rarely used in occupational and environmental epidemiology. They can be used to estimate the contribution of various exposure pathways and routes to the total uptake and model the dose of a specific target organ. For example, where trihalomethanes through ingestion may mostly be metabolized rapidly in the liver and not appear in blood, uptake through inhalation and skin increases the blood levels substantially. Furthermore, metabolic polymorphism may lead to different dose estimates under similar exposure conditions and this can also be modelled. For a number of agents the level of external occupational or environmental exposure may either be reduced or increased depending on the capacity of Phase I (activation), Phase II (detoxification) and DNA-repair enzymes. In this approach, genetic susceptibility markers (e.g., CYP1A1, CYP2E1, NAT1, NAT2, GSTM1, GSTT1 or DNA repair capacity) are used as if they were internal personal protective equipment. For example, low capacity of activation enzymes (e.g., CYP1A1), and high capacity of detoxification (e.g., NAT2) and DNA repair enzymes would have higher protective functions than high capacity of activation enzymes, and low capacity of detoxification and DNA repair enzymes that may result in reducing cancer-causing doses of xenobiotics (Vineis, 1999).

Table 1.1   The relationship between various silica exposure indices and silicosis in nine North American industrial sand plants

Employment duration (years)		Exposure concentration ($\mu g \, m^{-3}$)		Cumulative exposures ($\mu g \, m^{-3} \times$ years)	
Index	Odds ratio	Index	Odds ratio	Index	Odds ratio
<16	1.0	≤100	1.0	≤700	1.0
16–22	1.0	>100	2.4	700 to ≤1800	2.5
22–27	0.7			>1800–5100	4.6
>27	2.6			>5100	5.2

1.4   Exposure dimensions

Besides the actual nature of the exposure there are also three dimensions:

- duration (e.g. in hours or days),
- concentration (e.g. in mg m^{-3} in air or mg l^{-1} in water),
- frequency (e.g. times per week).

In case of exposure through ingestion the dimensions are concentration, amount (e.g. litres), and frequency. Any of these can be used as an exposure index in an epidemiological study, but they can also be combined to obtain a new exposure index, for example, by multiplying duration and concentration to obtain an index of cumulative exposure. The choice of index depends on the health effect of interest. For substances that cause acute effects such as ammonia (irritation), the short-term concentration is generally the most relevant exposure index, while for substances that cause chronic effects such as asbestos (cancer) long-term exposure indices such as cumulative exposure may be a more appropriate exposure index.

For example, Hughes *et al.* (2001) carried out a nested case–control study to study the relationship between exposure to silica and the chronic disease silicosis in nine North American industrial sand plants. They found little association between employment duration (as proxy for exposure duration) and silicosis, some association between the concentration of silica and silicosis, but a strong association between cumulative exposure to silica and silicosis with a clear exposure–response relationship (Table 1.1).

1.5   Exposure level and variability

The concentration of exposure varies temporally and spatially. Figure 1.3 provides the exposure levels of PM$_{2.5}$ (particulate matter with a 50% cut-off diameter of 2.5 μm), expressed as the number of particles, in a house during one day. Peak exposure levels, that is, exposure levels considerably higher than the overall average, are caused by someone smoking in the house. Furthermore, the measurements show that although there appears to be a very good correlation between the PM$_{2.5}$ levels in the kitchen and the living room, the actual levels differ.

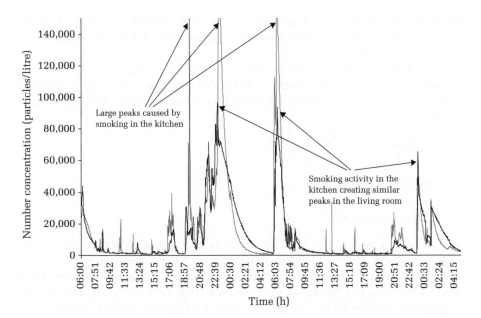

Fig. 1.3 Variation in fine particulate levels in the kitchen and living room over a day.

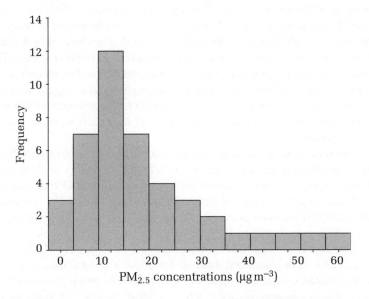

Fig. 1.4 Distribution of personal exposure measurements of $PM_{2.5}$.

Exposure data often show a lognormal distribution, that is, the distribution of the measured or model data is skewed to the right. Figure 1.4 provides an example of the distribution of approximately 50 personal exposure measurements of $PM_{2.5}$. On the *y*-axis the number of measurements is shown and on the *x*-axis the $PM_{2.5}$ concentration.

As can be seen the distribution is skewed to the right. Statistical tests can be carried out to assess if this is a lognormal distribution (e.g. Kolmogorov–Smirnov or Shapiro–Wilk tests).

The central tendency (i.e. the peak of the distribution) of a lognormal distribution is generally described by the geometric mean (GM), while the variability is described by the geometric standard deviation (GSD) (Esmen and Hammad 1977). They can be calculated as follows:

$$\mu = \frac{\Sigma \ln x}{n}, \quad \sigma^2 = \frac{\Sigma(\ln x - \ln \bar{x})^2}{n - 1},$$

$$GM = \exp \mu, \quad GSD = \exp \sigma,$$

$$\text{Arithmetic mean} = \frac{\Sigma x}{n},$$

where x is the concentration of the substance in a sample, n the number of samples, Σ the sum, ln the natural logaritham, μ the average of log transformed measurements, and σ^2 is the variance of log transformed measurements. The arithmetic mean (AM) provides the average of the exposure measurement. Besides the AM, GM, and GSD, the range, minimum, maximum or 95 per cent confidence intervals are also often reported.

The GM and GSD change with monitoring time, in contrast to the AM, which should be fixed, and approaches have been described to make them comparable for different monitoring times (Spear *et al.* 1986; Kumagai and Matsunaga 1994). The AM is commonly used to calculate an index of cumulative exposure (exposure intensity × exposure duration), although sometimes the GM is also used. The choice may depend on the shape of the exposure–response relationship as Seixas *et al.* (1988) reported. They suggested that when adopting a linear exposure model, the AM is the appropriate measure. In other models, such as the linear-log (outcome proportional to logarithm of exposure) the GM would be more appropriate. The maximum likelihood estimator (MLE) may be preferred instead of the AM because of minimum variance (Selvin and Rappaport 1989; Attfield and Hewett 1992).

Where exposure concentrations are low the amount of agent collected by the air monitor may be insufficient, not allowing detection by the laboratory analysis method; in other words, the exposure may be below the limit of detection (LOD) and are termed as 'censored' data. However, statistical analyses require that a number be assigned to these censored values. For accurate estimation of the mean and standard deviation, Hornung and Reed (1990) suggest using LOD/$\sqrt{2}$ when data are not highly skewed, and LOD/2 when data are highly skewed (GSD approximately >3). Perkins *et al.* (1990) describe a technique that uses the mean and standard deviation of the quantitated values and the number of censored values, in conjunction with a table to obtain the overall mean and standard deviation. It can be used when a large number of data is available. Measurements below the detection limit can also be modelled by assigning a distribution to measurements between 0 and the detection limit and randomly assign a value of this distribution to a value under the detection limit.

Exposure generally varies from day to day for any given subject and from subject to subject, often referred to as the within and between subject exposure variability, respectively. The within and between subject variability can be estimated when repeated exposure measurements have been obtained using analysis of variance models (see Chapter 6). Besides variability caused by subjects there may be other determinants of exposure such as source strength or ventilation and these need to be identified to get a better understanding of what is causing the variability in exposure. This will be discussed further in Chapters 6 and 12.

1.6 Ecological vs. individual exposure estimates

To obtain exposure estimate(s) for a population in an epidemiological study, two main approaches are available: (a) individual and (b) exposure grouping. In the first, exposure estimates are obtained at the individual level, for example, every member of the population is monitored either once or repeatedly. In the second approach, the population is first split into smaller subpopulations, or more often referred to as exposure groups, based on specific determinants of exposure, and group or ecological exposure estimates are obtained for each exposure group. In environmental epidemiological studies, exposure groups may be defined, for example, on the basis of presence or absence of an exposure source (e.g. gas cooker or smoker in the house), distance from an exposure source (e.g. roads or factories), or activity (e.g. playing sport or not). In occupational epidemiological studies, exposure groups have been defined on the basis of (a) work similarity, that is, having the same job title and/or carrying out similar work, (b) similarity with respect to particular substances, and (c) similarity of environmental conditions, for example, process equipment and ventilation. These exposure groups have been referred to as homogenous exposure groups or exposure zones (Corn and Esmen 1979). The underlying assumption is that subjects within each exposure group experience similar exposure characteristics, including exposure levels and variation. A representative sample of members from each exposure group can be personally monitored, either once or repeatedly. If the aim is to estimate mean exposure, the average of the exposure measurements is then assigned to all the members in that particular exposure group. Alternatively, other exposure estimates can be assigned to the groups, for example, data from ambient air pollution monitors in the area where the subjects live. Ecological and individual estimates can be combined, for example, in the case of chlorination by-products where routinely collected trihalomethane measurements providing ecological estimates are combined with individual estimates on actual ingestion, showering, and bathing (see Chapter 15).

Intuitively, it is expected that the individual estimates provide the best exposure estimates for an epidemiological study. This is not often true, however, because of the variability in exposure and the limited number of samples. In general, in epidemiological studies, individual estimates lead to attenuated, though more precise, health risk estimates than ecological estimates. The ecological estimates, in contrast, result in less attenuation of the risk estimates, albeit less precise (Heederik *et al.* 1996; Kromhout *et al.* 1996; Seixas and Sheppard 1996; Nieuwenhuijsen 1997). These differences can be explained by the classical and the Berkson type error models (see Chapter 12). The between-group, between-subject, and within-subject variance can be estimated using analysis of variance models (see Chapter 6) and this information can be used to optimize the exposure–response relationship, for example, by changing the distribution of exposure groups (Kromhout and Heederik 1995; Nieuwenhuijsen 1997;

van Tongeren *et al.* 1997). In this case, the aim is to increase the contrast in exposure between exposure groups, expressed as the ratio between the between-group variance and the sum of the between- and within-group variance, while maintaining reasonably precise exposure estimates of the groups (see Chapter 6).

1.7   Exposure classification, measurement, or modelling

Exposure can be classified, measured, or modelled and different tools are available for this, such as questionnaires, air pollution monitors, and statistical techniques, respectively. The methods are often classified as direct and indirect (Fig. 1.5).

The main aim of an exposure assessment is to obtain accurate, precise, and biologically relevant exposure estimates in the most efficient and cost-effective way. The cost of the exposure assessment increases with an increase in the accuracy and precision, and therefore the assessment is often a balancing act with cost on one side and accuracy and precision on the other (Armstrong 1996). The choice of a particular method depends on the aim of the study and, more often, on the financial resources available. Misclassification of the exposure can lead to attenuation in health risk estimates or loss of power in the epidemiological study, depending on the type of measurement error model (classical or Berkson), and should therefore be minimized (see Chapter 12).

Subjects in an epidemiological study can be classified based on a particular substance and on an ordinal scale, for example, as exposed:

- yes/no
- no, low, medium, high.

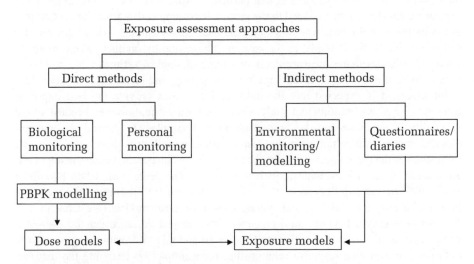

Fig. 1.5 Different approaches to human exposure assessment.

This can be, for example, achieved by

(1) Expert assessment, for example, a member of the research team decides, based on prior knowledge, whether the subject in the study is exposed or unexposed, for example, lives in an area with highly contaminated soil or not.

(2) Self-assessment by questionnaire, that is, the subject in the study is asked to fill out a questionnaire in which he or she is asked about a particular substance, for example, pesticides. Questionnaires are often used to ask a subject if she or he is exposed to a particular substance and also to estimate the duration of exposure.

Questionnaires can be used not only to ask the subject to estimate the duration of their exposure but also to obtain information related to the exposure, such as where people spent their time (time micro-environment diaries), work history including the jobs and tasks they carried out, what they eat and drink, and where they live (see Chapter 2). These variables could be used as exposure indices in the epidemiological studies or translated into a new exposure index, for example, by multiplying the amount of tap water people drink and the contaminant level in the tap water to obtain the total ingested amount of the substance. When used on their own they are often referred to as exposure surrogates.

Expert and self-assessment methods are generally the easiest and cheapest, but can suffer due to the lack of objectivity and knowledge and may therefore bias exposure assessment (see Chapter 8). Both experts and subjects may not know exactly what the subjects are exposed to or at what level and therefore may misclassify the exposure, while diseased subjects may recall certain substances better than subjects without disease (recall bias) and cause differential misclassification leading to biased health risk estimates (see Chapter 12).

A more objective way to assess exposure, particularly concentration, is through measurement. Some examples:

(1) Levels of outdoor air pollution can be measured by stationary ambient air monitors (i.e. ambient or environmental air monitoring). These monitors are placed in an area and they measure the particular substance of interest in this area. Subjects living within this area are considered to be exposed to the concentrations measured by the monitoring station. This may or may not be true depending on, for example, where the subject in the study lives, works, or travels. The advantage of this method is that it could provide a range of exposure estimates for a large population (see Chapters 3, 4, and 14).

(2) Levels of air pollution can be measured by personal exposure monitors (i.e. personal exposure monitoring). These monitors are lightweight devices that are worn by the subject in the study. They are often used in occupational studies and are being used with increasing frequency in environmental studies too. The advantage of this method is that it is likely to estimate the subject's exposure better than, for example, ambient air monitoring. The disadvantage is that it is often labour intensive and expensive (see Chapter 5).

(3) Levels of water pollutants and soil contaminants can be estimated by taking water and soil samples respectively, and analysing these for substance of interest in the laboratory. Often these need to be combined with behavioural factors such as water intake, contaminated food intake or hand-to-mouth contact to obtain a level of exposure.

(4) Uptake levels of the substance into the body can be estimated by biomonitoring. Biomonitoring consists of taking biological samples such as urine, exhaled breath, hair, adipose tissue, or nails, for example, the measurement of lead in serum. The samples are

subsequently analysed for the substance of interest itself or for a metabolite in a laboratory. Biomonitoring is expected to estimate the actual uptake (dose) of the substance of interest rather than the exposure (see Chapter 11).

The measurement of exposure is generally expansive, particularly for large populations. Modelling of exposure can be carried out preferably in conjunction with exposure measurements either to help build a model and/or to validate a model. It is particularly important that the model estimates be validated.

Modelling can be divided into:

(1) *Deterministic modelling* (i.e. physical) in which the models describe the relationship between variables mathematically on the basis of knowledge of the physical, chemical, and/or biological mechanisms governing these relationships (Brunekreef 1999). A deterministic model would be one where indoor air particle concentrations are explained by including in the modelling, for example, the sources, volume of rooms, air exchange rate, and settling velocity of the particles (see Chapter 3).

(2) *Stochastic modelling* (i.e. statistical) in which the statistical relationships are modelled between variables. These models do not necessarily require fundamental knowledge of the underlying physical, chemical, and/or biological relationships between the variables. An example is the relation between personal exposure to nitrogen dioxide and determinants such as traffic exhaust, cigarette smoke, and gas cooking, which are modelled using statistical regression techniques and an existing dataset (see Chapter 6).

All these different approaches are not exclusive and often are combined to obtain the best exposure index. This involves some form of modelling. At times it may be difficult or impossible to measure the exposure to the actual substance of interest and therefore exposure to an 'exposure surrogate' is estimated. This is often the case in environmental epidemiology, where sample sizes may be large. In occupational epidemiology 'job title' is also frequently used as a surrogate. It is important that the surrogate marker is as closely correlated as possible to the actual substance of interest. For example, the presence of gas cooker or electric cooker could be a surrogate for the exposure to nitrogen dioxide (yes/no exposure). Living distance from a factory could be a surrogate for the emission of pollutants from the factory. However, there is some uncertainty in these cases regarding actual exposure, for example, the gas cooker may not actually be used often or the subject is out of the house while cooking takes place and therefore there should be some validation. The National Research Committee (NRC) in the US came up with a ranking of exposure data and surrogate measures around point sources such as landfill sites (Table 1.2).

The data at the top of this hierarchy will provide some fairly good information on the exposure of the subjects, while at the bottom the exposure estimates are the worst and they may not be helpful in the interpretation of an epidemiological study. Of course there are still other issues that are important in the ranking, for example, many quantified area measurements may be better than a few quantified personal exposure measurements.

Other surrogate exposure measures can actually be measured and quantified. In bakeries, workers are exposed to inhalable (flour) dust, flour aeroallergen, and α-amylase (enzymatic bread improver), the latter two are potent sensitizers and can cause occupational asthma. They are also more difficult to measure than inhalable dust and therefore

Table 1.2 Hierarchy of exposure data and surrogates for fixed-source contaminants

Type of data	Approximation to actual exposure
(1) Quantified personal measurement	Best
(2) Quantified area measurements in the vicinity of the residence or sites of activity	
(3) Quantified surrogates of exposure (e.g. estimates of drinking water use)	
(4) Distance from the site and duration of exposure	
(5) Distance or duration of residence	
(6) Residence or employment in the geographical area in reasonable proximity to the site where exposure can be assumed	
(7) Residence or employment in a defined geographical geographical area (e.g. a county) of the site	Worst

Source: Adapted from NRC (1991).

it would be convenient if inhalable dust could act as an exposure surrogate. Inhalable dust comprises flour aeroallergen, α-amylase, and also other substances, further the composition may differ between different production areas. A recent study found that overall there was a good correlation between inhalable dust and flour aeroallergen ($r = 0.65$), but only a weak correlation between inhalable dust and α-amylase levels ($r = 0.42$) (Nieuwenhuijsen *et al.* 1999). Therefore inhalable dust could act as a reasonable surrogate for flour aeroallergen but may not be useful for α-amylase in an epidemiological study. However, it is important to remember that the use of this surrogate may lead to attenuation in risk estimates or loss of power in the study depending on the error models that apply (classical and Berkson error), but the magnitude of this can be quantified when the correlation between the true exposure and surrogate is known (see Chapter 12).

A related issue is that people are often exposed to a number of pollutants simultaneously (a mixture), for example, to pesticides, solvents, air pollution, and disinfection by-products, although the levels may differ. Since not all the substances can be measured, a surrogate measure or exposure marker is chosen, for example, in the case of chlorination by-products in drinking water where trihalomethanes were as used as a surrogate for other by-products (see Chapter 15). Mixtures of exposure may cause problems in the epidemiological analysis, for example, when the effects of different pollutants need to be disentangled. A possible way around this is to choose study sites where the exposure levels of the individual pollutants in the exposure mixture differ substantially and where there is a gradient of exposure.

1.8 Validation studies

In epidemiological studies, it is often not possible to obtain detailed exposure information on each subject in the study. For example, in large cohort study it is not feasible to take measurements from each subject and administer a detailed exposure questionnaire. In this case, it is desirable to carry out a small validation study on a representative subset of the larger population. Ideally this will be carried out before the main study begins and can utilize information from the literature. Questions in the questionnaire could be validated with measurements (see Chapter 2) and some exposure models could be constructed (see Chapter 6). The exposure assessment in the whole population could focus on key questions that have a major influence on the exposure estimates and thereby reduce the length of the questionnaire. Information on key determinants will also provide a better understanding of the exposure and how it may affect exposure–response relationships in epidemiological studies. Besides the validity, the reproducibility or reliability of various tools also can be evaluated in a subsample.

1.9   Retrospective exposure assessment

In epidemiological studies, when studying diseases with a long latency time, for example, cancer, it is not the current exposure that is of most interest for the study, but that in the past. A reconstruction of historical exposure often referred to as retrospective exposure assessment is therefore needed (see Chapter 7). In occupational epidemiology, retrospective exposure assessment has gained an important role. Retrospective exposure assessment is often difficult since there are usually many changes over time, for example, in production processes, job titles, and the tasks that are carried out within a job title. Factories may have closed over time and there is little information on which to base a retrospective exposure assessment. Often exposure surrogates need to be used such as exposure duration, process, and job title. Sometimes, exposure levels can be modelled with information on tasks, processes, exposure, and other determinants of exposure or using historical exposure measurements. Job-exposure matrices (JEM) have also been used with variable success to assign exposure to the subjects in the study (see Chapter 8).

1.10   Quality control issues

A well-designed and well-planned strategy carried out by well-trained personnel is essential for a successful exposure assessment. Issues such as cost, feasibility, accuracy, precision, validity, sample size, power, sensitivity, specificity, robustness, and reproducibility always need to be addressed (e.g. during sampling, storage, and analysis) (Table 1.3), while feasibility and pilot studies need to take place before the actual study. Any form of bias (e.g. bias in sampling, selection, participation, monitoring, information, and measurement error and exposure misclassification) should be avoided where possible, or if it cannot be avoided should be well described.

Clear protocols for sampling, storage, and analysis, including quality control should be written and be available at any time and researchers in the study should be properly trained. Potential sources of bias should be addressed at every stage.

Table 1.3   Terminology used in measurement issues

Accuracy: The degree to which a measurement or an estimate represents the true value of what is being measured.

Bias: Deviation of results or inferences from the truth, or processes leading to such deviation; any trend in the design, collection, analysis, interpretation, publication, or review of data that can lead to conclusions that are systematically different from the truth.

Limit of detection (LOD): The minimum concentration of an analyte, in a given matrix and with a specific method, that statistically is significantly greater than zero, that is, the lowest concentration that can be measured with a certain degree of confidence.

Precision: The degree of variability in a measurement or estimate, estimated, for example, by the standard error of measurements or the standard deviation in a series of replicate measurements

Power: The ability of a study to demonstrate statistically significant effects, which is determined by a number of factors including study design, magnitude of effect, and sample size.

Reliability: The degree of stability exhibited when a measurement is repeated under identical conditions, that is, the degree to which the results obtained by measurement procedure can be replicated.

Reproducibility/repeatability: A test or measurement is repeatable if the results are identical or closely similar each time it is conducted.

Robustness: A procedure is said to be robust if it is not very sensitive to departures from assumptions or variations in the conditions or practices under which it was set up.

Sensitivity: Is an index of the performance of a diagnostic tool, for example, for questionnaires: the proportion of truly exposed people in the population who are identified as exposed by the questionnaire. For measurement or analysis of exposure it refers to the response of the detector to a unit of analyte; the more sensitive the more response and hence a better detection limit.

Specificity: Is an index of the performance of a diagnostic tool, for example, for questionnaires: the proportion of truly non-exposed people in the population who are identified as non-exposed by the questionnaire. For measurement or analysis of exposure it refers to the response of the detector to a particular analyte, that is, whether only the substance of interest is measured or also other substances.

Validity: An expression of the degree to which a measurement measures what it purports to measure.

Source: Adapted from Last (1995).

Control measurements, for example, filters that are not exposed but are otherwise treated as exposed filters should be included (5–10% of total samples), particularly where measurements are close to the detection limit.

Samplers can measure with differing accuracy, for example, over or under sampling the true level and this should be addressed when different samplers are used in order to reduce or avoid bias. This can be done easily by comparative sampling with adjustments for any difference observed.

Monitors and laboratory techniques measure with differing precision. Precision can be represented by the coefficient of variation (CV) and contributes towards the total variability observed in the measured exposure levels. However this contribution is small compared to the environmental variability, caused by factors such as differences in working practices and environmental conditions. An analysis by Nicas *et al.* (1991) suggests that the CV is in general 15 per cent and that the GSD of the lognormal day-to-day environmental variability is in general 1.5 in which case the analytical variability contributes not more than 13 per cent to the total variability observed in measuring a worker's shift-average exposure level. The greater the environmental variability, the less the collection and analytical variability contributes towards the total variability. Even CVs of around 25 per cent contribute less than 20 per cent to total variability as long as the GSD of environmental variability is larger than approximately 1.8.

1.11   Conclusion

This chapter provided a brief overview of the basic issues in the exposure assessment of occupational and environmental epidemiological studies. In the following chapters many will be discussed in much greater detail. The focus is initially on some of the main methods and tools of exposure assessment, followed by newer tools such as PBPK modelling, which has rarely been used in this field but may provide a further refinement. The consequences of exposure misclassification and measurement error for epidemiological is discussed in great detail to show the importance of good exposure assessment and approaches to optimise it and the interpretation of epidemiological studies. The last five chapters discuss the more recent developments and research questions in exposure assessment of allergens, particulate matter, chlorination by-products, pesticides and radiofrequencies, including the consequences for and results of some epidemiological studies. These chapters show the great diversity and different levels of exposure assessment, but also the many commonalities. The following chapters attempt to describe the current status of the field, but are not meant to be exhaustive. They will encourage the reader to think of how to improve exposure assessments. Exposure assessment is a relatively new field and further developments and refinements are still needed.

References

Armstrong, B. K., White, E., and Saracci, R. (1992). *Principles of exposure measurement in epidemiology*. Oxford Medical Publications, Oxford.

Armstrong, B. (1996). Optimizing power in allocating resources to exposure assessment in an epidemiologic study. *American Journal of Epidemiology*, **144**, 192–7.

Attfield, M. and Hewett, P. (1992). Exact expressions for bias and variance of estimators of the mean of a lognormal distribution. *American Industrial Hygiene Association Journal*, **53**, 432–435.

Brunekreef, B. (1999). Exposure assessment. In *Environmental epidemiology: a text book on study methods and public health applications* (preliminary edn). WHO, Geneva.

Corn, M. and Esmen, N. A. (1979). Workplace exposure zones for classification of employee exposures to physical and chemical agents. *American Industrial Hygiene Association Journal*, **40**, 47–57.

Esmen, N. and Hammad, Y. (1977). Lognormality of environmental sampling data. *Environmental Science and Health*, **A12**, 29–41.

Heederik, D., Kromhout, H., and Braun, W. (1996). The influence of random exposure estimation error on the exposure–response relationship when grouping into homegeneous exposure categories. *Occupational Hygiene*, **3**, 229–41.

Hornung, R. W. and Reed, L. D. (1990). Estimation of average concentration in the presence of non detectable values. *Applied Occupational and Environmental Hygiene* **5**, 46–51.

Hughes, J. M., Weill, H., Randos, R. J., Shi, R., McDonald, A. D., and McDonald, J. C. (2001). Cohort mortality study of North American Industrial Sand Workers. II Case-referent analysis of lung cancer and silicosis deaths. *Annals of Occupational Hygiene*, **45**, 201–7.

Kromhout, H. and Heederik, D. (1995). Occupational epidemiology in the rubber industry; implications of exposure variability. *American Journal of Industrial Medicine*, **27**, 171–85.

Kromhout, H., Tielemans, E., Preller, L., and Heedrik, D. (1996). Estimates of individual dose from current measurements of exposure. *Occupational Hygiene*, **3**, 23–29.

Kumagai, S. and Matsunaga, I. (1994). Approaches for estimating the distribution of short-term exposure concentrations for different averaging times. *Annals of Occupational Hygiene*, **38**, 815–25.

Last, J. (ed.). (1995). *A dictionary of epidemiology*. Oxford University Press, Oxford.

National Research Committee (NRC). (1991). *Environmental epidemiology. I. Public health and hazardous waste*. National Academy Press, Washington DC.

Nicas, M., Simmons, B. P., and Spear, R. C. (1991). Environmental versus analytical variability in exposure measurements. *American Industrial Hygiene Association Journal*, **52**, 553–7.

Nieuwenhuijsen, M. J. (1997). Exposure assessment in occupational epidemiology: measuring present exposures with an example of occupational asthma. *International Archives of Occupational and Environmental Health*, **70**, 295–308.

Nieuwenhuijsen, M. J., Heederik, D., Doekes, G., Venables, K. M., and Newman Taylor, A. J. (1999). Exposure–response relationships of α-amylase sensitisation in British bakeries and flour mills. *Occupational and Environmental Medicine*, **56**, 197–201.

Perkins, J. L., Cutter, G. N., and Cleveland, M. S. (1990). Estimating the mean, variance and confidence limits from censored (<limit of detection), lognormally distributed exposure data. *American Industrial Hygiene Association Journal*, **51**, 416–19.

Seixas, N. S. and Sheppard, L. (1996). Maximazing accuracy and precision using individual and grouped exposure assessments. *Scandinavian Journal of Environment, Work and Health*, **22**, 94–101.

Seixas, N. S., Robins, T. G., and Moulton, L. H. (1988). The use of geometric and arithmetic mean exposures in occupational epidemiology. *American Journal of Industrial Medicine*, **14**, 465–77.

Selvin, S. and Rappaport, S. M. (1989). A note on the estimation of the mean from a lognormal distribution. *American Industrial Hygiene Association Journal*, **50**, 627–630.

Spear, R. C., Selvin, S., and Francis, M. (1986). The influence of averaging time on the distribution of exposures. *American Industrial Hygiene Association Journal*, **47**, 365–8.

van Tongeren, M., Gardiner, K., Calvert, I., Kromhout, H., and Harrington, J. M. (1997). Efficiency of different grouping schemes for dust exposure in the European carbon black respiratory morbidity study. *Occupational and Environmental Medicine*, **54**, 714–19.

Vineis, P. (ed.) (1999). *Metabolic polymorphisms and susceptibility*. IARC pub 148, IARC, France.

2. Questionnaires

Mark J. Nieuwenhuijsen

2.1 Introduction to questionnaires

Questionnaires are frequently used in the exposure assessment of occupational and environmental epidemiological studies. Questionnaires may be the method of choice for assessing exposure because no other sources of information are available, or because they provide the most efficient study design, allowing a larger study size and greater statistical power than would be possible with other more accurate measurement techniques. They may be used in combination with other methods too. Information on presence of exposure (yes/no), duration, frequency, and pattern of exposure is often obtained by questionnaire or, to a much lesser extent, observation. Very few if any standardized questionnaires that have been validated are available in this area. The design of new questionnaires often depend on the experience acquired with previous questionnaires.

Questionnaires are used and administered in a number of ways to obtain information (see later). At times it may not be possible to obtain information from the subject in the study because of death or disease, for example, Alzheimer's and it may therefore be necessary to obtain the information from a so-called proxy respondent such as relative, friend, or colleague. This may require some modification of the questionnaire, but has been carried out quite successfully (Hansen 1996; Debanne *et al.* 2001). All the different forms of questionnaires require careful consideration of design and administration issues, including, for example, the length, detail of the required information, logistics, participation and completion rate, and costs involved (Armstrong *et al.* 1992). Questionnaires often tend to be too long and not all the information from the questionnaire is analysed and/or used in the epidemiological study. One of the main questions the researchers should always ask themselves is 'do we really require this answer of this question for our study aims?'. If there is no justification for it, the question should be left out. An important issue is that the exposures of interest may have been in the past and subjects may not be able to recall these, this may lead to underreporting (Infante-Rivard and Jacques 2000). Furthermore lack of understanding of the questions or knowledge of the exposure may bias the reporting. Recall bias, where those with disease are more likely to report certain exposures compared to those without disease even though there is no true difference, needs to be avoided and this requires careful consideration of the questions that are asked (Rothman and Greenland 1998).

2.1.1   Self-administered questionnaire

The self-administered questionnaire can be used to obtain information on present and past exposure. It is the easiest, cheapest, and requires the least involvement from both subject and researcher and can be handed out, sent to the subjects, or be computer administered. When sent out to the subjects it requires a valid address since otherwise the subject may not receive it leading to a lower response rate. The response and completion rates in this method tend to be somewhat lower compared to other methods (Brogger *et al.* 2002). Monetary incentives can increase the response rate considerably (Edwards *et al.* 2002). The response rate can be improved by handing out the questionnaire, for example, for children at schools. Personal contact tends to increase response rates (Edwards *et al.* 2002). Recorded delivery may improve the response rate considerably and particularly if the subject actually lives at the address (Edwards *et al.* 2002). Mailed out questionnaires can be easily binned or forgotten and often require re-mailing to obtain a good response rate. The questionnaires cannot be too long since this is likely to lower the response and completion rates (Edwards *et al.* 2002). The subjects should be able to complete the questionnaire within about 30–60 min, preferably less. The questions need to be straightforward and easy to answer, otherwise lack of understanding by the subject may result in low completion rate or inappropriate answers. The advantage of a questionnaire is that it gives subjects the time to think about the questions, and if necessary obtain further information from elsewhere.

2.1.2   Self-administered diary

The self-administered diary can be used (repeatedly) to obtain information on present exposures. They have been used frequently to obtain information on food and drink intake (Willett 1998) (Table 2.1), and to a lesser extent in situations where people spend their time in the form of micro-environment activity diaries, which are used to obtain information on, for example, exposure to air pollution (Künzli *et al.* 1997; Jantunen *et al.* 1998) (Table 2.2). The collected information has at times been used to represent a much longer period than the actual observation period, and as validation for questionnaires. However, this requires careful interpretation of the data since there may be considerable differences in people's exposure over short periods, for example, differences between weekdays and weekends and seasonal differences. Further, the issue of the short observation period being representative of a longer period necessitates careful consideration of exposure determinants. The diary data can be used to estimate day-to-day variability within subjects and variability between subjects, and hence attenuation in risk estimates (see Chapters 6 and 12) (Shimukora *et al.* 1998). The diaries need to be short and easy to fill out. The advantage of the diary is that it needs little, if any, recall, particularly if they are filled out as a routine process. Diary data can be combined with measurements to obtain improved exposure estimates. For example, Preller *et al.* (1995) administered a 14-day diary to pig farmers, in which they recorded their activities and factors related to endotoxin exposure, and measured the endotoxin exposure on two of the days. They used regression analysis to relate the measurements and diary data and build a model, which they then applied to the days without measurements to predict the endotoxin levels for a longer time period. The predicted estimates showed the least attenuated risk estimates when they modelled the relationship between endotoxin exposure and lung function decline (see Chapter 6 for more detail).

2.1.3 Face-to-face interview

Questionnaires used in face-to-face interviews have the advantage that an interviewer is present who can explain any question if necessary. Information can be obtained on present and past exposures. The interviewer can explain questions and explore the answers in more detail, if necessary. Particularly for a complex exposure situation this may be an advantage. It requires a well-trained interviewer, particularly to avoid any interviewer bias and obtain the most relevant information. This method may result in more socially acceptable answers since an interviewer is present, and this needs careful attention. The questionnaire/interview can be of a longer duration than some of the other methods (1–2 h). The logistics aspect is generally more difficult. Arranging face-to-face interviews at convenient times for both subject and interviewer can be difficult, particularly if they live far apart. Face-to-face interviewing can be very expensive and therefore is not used often in this field.

Table 2.1 A section (introduction and one day) of a seven-day water diary to determine fluid intake, showering, bathing, and swimming among pregnant women

Seven-Day Water Diary

Please complete one page of the diary for each consecutive day of the week, including the weekend. Include ALL drinks and other liquids consumed. Give the required information on activities carried out EACH day. Please try to be as accurate as possible.

If you did not carry out a particular activity or did not consume a particular liquid please put a zero for duration or amount.

Remember to quote liquid consumption using the following guide (or a more precise measure if possible):

A 'glass' like the one pictured below is 200 cc (so five glasses equals 1 litre), a mug equals one glass and a bowl equals two glasses.

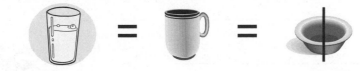

Table 2.1   *Continued*

Date ————————

(A) *Cooking and washing up*

	Duration (min)
Cooking involving boiling water	
Washing up by hand (excl. drying)	
Dishwasher running	

(B) *Washing yourself*

	Number	Duration (min)	Time spent in bathroom after bath/shower (min)
Shower			
Bath			

(C) *Food and drink*

	At home	At work/college	Elsewhere
Tap water (*glasses*)			
Bottled water (*glasses*)			
Tea (*mugs*)			
Coffee (*mugs*)			
Hot chocolate (*mugs*)			
Plain milk (*glasses*)			
Squash* (*glasses*)			

*including drinks made with powders

	At home	At work/college	Elsewhere
Soft drinks** (*glasses*)			
Beer (*glasses*)			
Wine (*glasses*)			
Spirits (*glasses*)			

**including fruit juices and fizzy drinks

	At home	At work/college	Elsewhere
Soups (*bowls/mugs*)			

(D) *Swimming*

	Length of session (min)
Swimming in a pool	

Table 2.2 Time micro-environment activity diary used by the EXPOLIS study

Date: _____

		Location													Activities		
		I am travelling by...					I am currently at...								I am...		Someone is smoking in the same room
							home		work		other						
Time	Briefly describe your activities	foot/ bike	motor-cycle	car/ taxi	bus	train	inside	outside	inside	outside	inside	outside	cooking	smoking	
6	0	○	○	○	○	○	○	○	○	○	○	○	○	○	○
	15	○	○	○	○	○	○	○	○	○	○	○	○	○	○
	30	○	○	○	○	○	○	○	○	○	○	○	○	○	○
	45	○	○	○	○	○	○	○	○	○	○	○	○	○	○
7	0	○	○	○	○	○	○	○	○	○	○	○	○	○	○
	15	○	○	○	○	○	○	○	○	○	○	○	○	○	○
	30	○	○	○	○	○	○	○	○	○	○	○	○	○	○
	45	○	○	○	○	○	○	○	○	○	○	○	○	○	○

2.1.4   Telephone interview

Questionnaires used in telephone interviews have the advantage that subjects can ask the interviewer to explain any question, if necessary. Information can be obtained on present and past exposures. The interviewer can explain questions and explore the answers in more detail, if necessary, although perhaps to a lesser extent than the face-to-face interview. As for the face-to-face interviews, it requires a well-trained interviewer, particularly to avoid interviewer bias and obtain the most relevant information. The advantage compared to face-to-face interviews is that they are easier to organize and carry out as no visits are required; further nowadays most people have a phone, so the costs involved are much lower. Subjects also may provide less socially accepted answers compared to the face-to-face interview. The interview duration needs to be much shorter, around 30–45 min. Telephone interviews facilitate direct entry into an electronic database, which reduces the time spent on data entry, although it is important to avoid mistakes by incorporating quality control checks. Interviews may need to be taped for quality control purposes. Examples of questions for self-administered, face-to-face, and telephone interviews are given in Tables 2.3 and 2.4.

2.1.5   Observation

Researchers may want to observe subjects to obtain information on exposure-related behaviour, for example, the extent of hand-to-mouth contact among children, which may result in uptake of a particular substance (Freeman *et al*. 2001). The observation needs a questionnaire in the form of a checklist to be used by the researcher. Using a hand-held computer, the information can be linked to other information that is collected simultaneously such as measurement data. Observation is used to obtain information on present exposures. The observation period is thought to be representative of a much longer period when there is no observation, but the validity of this depends under what conditions the observation was carried out, that is, was it carried out under conditions representative of other periods and did the subject behave in the same way. This method may be more accurate and objective than some other methods, but it is also more time consuming and costly. At times it may be the only method to obtain exposure information since the subjects of interest, for example, young children, cannot provide the information by filling out questionnaires. The observation can take place in 'real time' or video recordings can be made and analysed later. The advantage of the method is that it requires little involvement from the subject and there is little problem with recall. However, it cannot be used for all subjects in an epidemiological study, only a subpopulation to obtain information for an exposure model or to validate a model.

2.1.6   Obtaining information from records

Researchers may want to obtain information from existing records, for example, job titles and names of substances from company records. A questionnaire is needed to obtain the information in a systematic way and to note any problems with the information. The approach can be used to obtain information on past and present exposures. Although the information obtained from records may be at times more objective, it also

Table 2.3   Example of questions on painting the house in a reproductive study

1   **Were any home improvements such as decoration or painting made to your house just before or during the first 3 months of your pregnancy with *Childname?***

Yes	1
No	2 Go to next section
Don't know	3

Did this involve any of the following?

2   **Paint stripping?**

Yes	1
No	2 Go to Q5
Don't Know	3

3   **Did you yourself do any paint stripping?**

Yes	1
No	2 Go to Q5
Can't remember	3

4   **Approximately how many hours did you spend paint stripping altogether?**

5   **Did the decoration involve painting?**

Yes	1
No	2 Go to next section
Can't remember	3

6   **What kind of paint was used?**

Gloss	1
Emulsion	2
Don't know	3

7   **Did you personally do any painting?**

Yes	1
No	2 Go to next section
Can't remember	3

8   **How many hours did you spend painting altogether?**

Table 2.4   Example of questions on work in a reproductive study

The next section is about work and hobbies.

1   **Were you employed during the first 3
        months of your pregnancy with
        Childname?**

        Yes | 1 |
        No | 2 | Go to next
                                                                    section

*The following question will ask you details about your place of work. Please feel free not to
answer if you do not wish to identify your place of work.*

2   **What was the name and address of the company
        or organisation in which you worked?**

3   **In which department did you work?**

4   **What was your job title?**

5   **How many <u>hours per week</u> did you
        work in this job?**

6   **Until which week of your pregnancy
        with *Childname* did you continue to
        work?**

7   **Please state <u>your main tasks</u> at work
        and how many hours you spent at
        each task.**

Task	Number of hours per week

has its limitations. The terminology used may differ over years and between companies
(or other archives) and the organization of the information may not meet the needs of
the study, for example, for payment purposes. In factories, most of the workers may be
classified as production workers for payment purposes, and this may not be specific
enough for epidemiological studies, where more information is needed on the type of
work that was actually done and the substances they worked with. Information may
have been kept in books that have not been archived properly and may be difficult to
read, therefore careful interpretation is needed. Questionnaires in this case can guide the
researcher and enable the recording of the quality of the data, which can be analysed at
a later stage.

2.2 The design of questionnaires

The aims of exposure questionnaire design are:

(1) to obtain indices of exposure essential to the objectives of the study;
(2) to minimize errors in these indices;
(3) to create an instrument that is easy for the interviewer and subject to use, and for the researcher to process and analyse (Armstrong *et al.* 1992).

To keep the process on track, questionnaire design needs clear aims and objectives, a selection of items that need to be translated into questions, and a logical order. For example, when designing a questionnaire to study the exposure to chloroform, a by-product of the chlorination of drinking water taken up through ingestion, skin absorption, and inhalation during drinking, showering, bathing, and swimming, the aims and objectives can be defined as follows:

Aims

To assess the duration of exposure to the primary chloroform-related water activities

Objectives

At the end of the interview, we will have information on
    The amount of ingested tap water
    The duration of showering
    The duration of bathing
    The duration of swimming

Each of the objectives can then be translated into questions, for example, for tap water ingestion:
    How many glasses of tap water do you drink per day? ———glasses/day
    How many cups of tea do you drink per day? ———cups/day
    How many cups of coffee do you drink per day? ———cups/day

This information could subsequently be combined with information on the concentration of chloroform in tap water and some other factors to give an estimate for the actual intake of chloroform (see Chapter 15). It is important to note that a number of uncertainties are introduced, for example, it is unclear how large a cup or glass is as people use different sizes. Assumptions would need to be made. Also there may be temporal variability in the number of glasses and cups. On the other hand people cannot be asked how many (milli)litres of tap water they drink per day. It is difficult to provide a good estimate of variability over a long-time period, particularly when going back far into the past. It will be very difficult for people to remember how many glasses of tap water they drank 20 years ago. Similarly, people tend to know reasonably well how often they shower, but they are not very good at giving an accurate estimate of the duration of a shower (in minutes) and it may not be useful to include the latter in a questionnaire.

2.3 Issues in questionnaire design

Asking a question is one thing, getting a good answer another. It is extremely important to get a relevant answer of high quality to a question since otherwise time and effort are wasted. There are a number of issues that need to be considered when designing a questionnaire (Armstrong *et al.* 1992). There is often a tendency to design a questionnaire that is too long and provides so much information that not all the answers to the questions can be used in the epidemiological analysis. The length of the questionnaire is dependent on the administration method (see earlier). A long questionnaire may reduce the response and completion rates considerably and therefore it is important to consider if each question contributes to the overall aims and objectives of the questionnaire. If it does not make a significant contribution then it should not be used. Also, it needs to be clear at this stage how the answer is going to be analysed and how the answer relates to other answers in the study. Is useful new information obtained or does it repeat a previous question? High response and completion rates are essential for the success of a study (Rothman and Greenland 1998).

Avoid questions that go into too much detail and ask for information that the subjects cannot provide, or will provide, but is not of good quality, particularly in the case of past exposures. The subject may remember that they used a pesticide a number of years ago and the broad category, but they are unlikely to remember the name of the pesticide or the active ingredient (Engel *et al.* 2001). In certain situations it may be helpful to use more than one questionnaire, for example, a basic questionnaire and additional questionnaires, for example, specific job questionnaire. The latter can be used for more in-depth questions on particular topics after the subject indicates in the former that these take place. This kind of approach has been used for occupational questions in community-based studies.

The longer the recall time, the less likely it is that the subject will give an answer of sufficient quality to be included in the analysis. The longer the recall period the less detail can be expected from the subject. Complex exposure scenarios may occur, for example, where the subject is exposed to various substances over different time periods. This makes it difficult to design a simple and straightforward questionnaire and the complexity may overwhelm the subject and reduce the quality of the answers. In this case it is important to focus on key events. Rare events are likely to be remembered by the subjects only if they made a significant impact on their life or are somehow connected to other events.

There are still few, if any, standardized questionnaires for exposure assessment that have been validated. Many researchers therefore start from scratch, or base their design on previous experiences with questionnaire data. A critical evaluation of questionnaires that have been used in previous studies in the particular area, including how the answers were used in the analyses will be very helpful in the design of a new questionnaire. At times it is advisable to use the same questionnaire as in the previous study, even though it could be improved, so that an exact comparison can be made with results of the previous study. Designing the questionnaire is often a very long process and many changes will be made along the way.

2.4   Open-ended or closed-ended questions

Open-ended questions are questions without restrictions on the answers of the subjects, while closed-ended questions have restrictions in the form of a limited number of possible answers, for example, categories that subjects have to pick (Tables 2.3 and 2.4). Open-ended questions are used to record simple factual information such as name, weight, age, and occupational title. They are often used in occupational and environmental epidemiology, while closed-ended questions are often used in nutritional epidemiology, for example, in food frequency diaries (Willett 1998). The answer can be considerably different depending on whether the question is a closed- or open-ended question (Teschke *et al.* 1994). For closed-ended questions the answer may differ depending on the number of categories that are provided as a possible answer. However, most of the evidence comes from outside the field of occupational and environmental epidemiology and little research has been done specifically within this field. Open-ended questions need to be coded by a trained researcher before they can be analysed, for example, their occupation or tasks, and this may take a lot of time and careful interpretation of some of the answers and may itself introduce bias.

2.5 Wording

The words used in the questionnaire should be understood by the subjects and they should neither be too difficult nor too simple (Armstrong *et al.* 1992). The questions should be clear, unambiguous, short, and to the point and the subject should not have to figure out what is actually being asked. There should be no unexplained or vague terms, jargon, or abbreviations. Only one question at a time should be asked and the questions should be unbiased. Questions cannot be too precise and the subject needs to be familiar with it. In case of closed-ended questions the answers need to be mutually exclusive. The answers should allow linkage to the aims and objectives of the questionnaire.

Here are some examples of questions that have problems:

'Do you drink tap water regularly?' This appears to be a straightforward question but it is unclear what is meant by 'regularly'. In this case it would be better to define what is meant by 'regularly', for example, at least once a day or once a week

'Do you take a shower and/or bath, and how often?' Here we have a number of questions in one question and these should be separated. For example,

1a Do you take showers?
    Yes (go to question 1b)
    No (go to question to 2a)

1b How many showers do you take per week? ——

2a Do you take baths?
    Yes (go to question 2b)
    No (go to question 3)

2b How many baths do you take per week? ——

It is also tempting to ask how long the person showers or bathes, but this is difficult for a person to know without timing their shower or bath. On the other hand, without timing the answer will be 5 or 10 min for a shower and it is questionable if this is the true duration, and it may not be very useful in any analyses since it is more or less the same for everyone. On the other hand it is unlikely to be far off the actual duration. In this case, the frequency of showers is likely to be the more important factor when estimating the total duration of showering per week, and adding a question on the duration of showering, which results in an inaccurate answer, may be a waste of space.

'Where does your highest exposure to NO_2 take place?' Many subjects will not know what NO_2 is and even writing it down as 'nitrogen dioxide' will not help. Furthermore, in general people will have little knowledge where nitrogen dioxide is present let alone where their highest exposure takes places. In this case surrogate questions should be used, for example, questions on the use of gas cookers and time spent near (busy) roads or in smoky places, which are all associated with nitrogen dioxide exposure.

'How many minutes per week are you exposed to traffic fumes?' This question may be too precise and the subjects will probably have to estimate first their duration each day and then add them up to get a total for each week, which may be too complicated in many cases. Also subjects are unlikely to know exactly what they should count as traffic fumes. Are they exposed to traffic fumes when walking along a road, when they sit inside a car, when they live near a busy road, or in all three cases?

'Have you used any pesticides?' First, the time period is unclear in this question. Second, many subjects will not know what exactly is a pesticide and as such what they should count. Besides home and garden pesticides do they include herbicides, shampoos against lice, pet collars against fleas, fly spray, mothballs or bleach? Do they need to include both organic and non-organic pesticides? This apparently simple question is unlikely to provide a satisfactory and easily interpretable answer and should therefore be explained in more detail and broken up into a number of questions.

'Did you use any pesticides in 1973?' Besides the problems discussed previously, the additional problem in this case is the very precise time period, which is a long time ago. People are unlikely to remember this kind of detail. Introduction questions to aid their memory may help at times, for example, if interested in garden pesticides the researcher could ask if they had a garden in that particular year, followed by questions on particular pests they may have had.

2.6   Format of the questionnaire

The format of the questionnaire is as important as the actual questions. Remember that it is easy for people to bin the questionnaire. In the case of paper questionnaires long and complex looking ones do not encourage the subject to start filling them out. Make sure that the questionnaire looks nice, tidy, and appealing, but do not go over the top, and use a large enough letter type and easy to read font (Armstrong *et al.* 1992). Using different colours for different questionnaires can be helpful at times. Make sure to provide clear instructions on how to answer the questions, but do not make it too long since this will put off the subject. Use a logical order for your questions and start with some simple questions to get the subject going. Use the order in such a way that the subjects stay interested and that there is a natural flow. The former may be difficult when asking many exposure-related questions, particularly when a subject does not know how this relates to a particular disease or, in a case–control study, when asking controls. The response rate among controls often tends to be lower compared to the response rate among cases. Subjects are often not interested or do not know about, for example, chemicals, but they know about particular events (e.g. job, moving house, births) in their life and this could be used in the questionnaire to obtain relevant information. Not only may these events be related to particular exposures, but they may also keep the subject interested and increase response rates (Edwards *et al.* 2002). Thank the subjects at the end and remind them what to do with the questionnaire.

Branching off, that is, going into more detail for particular questions is not easy with paper questionnaires since it will take up a lot of space on a page and a subject may get confused about what to answer. However, it is possible to use this with computer aids and in particular with telephone interviews inputting data straight into the computer. This could be very useful and provide more specific information, for example, on occupational exposures (Stewart *et al.* 1998).

When asking for a job history the use of matrices can be very helpful at times, for example, with rows for each job and columns for job title, industry, tasks, and start and finishing date. A job title and the type of industry can provide substantial information about potential exposures, but the job titles used may vary in different companies. If possible, further information may need to be obtained about particular tasks that the subject carried out, particularly those that may be related to the exposure of interest (Stewart *et al.* 1998). Job history matrices can be coded and expressed as a job exposure matrix (see Chapter 8), where the researcher codes the job information and relates it to certain exposures. For a good coding of occupation, it is generally necessary to have a few open-ended questions on company, job, and activities.

2.7 Aids to recall

As mentioned earlier, subjects may find it difficult to remember particular facts and need some help to answer questions. Multiple-choice questions or cards with alternative answers given by the researcher may be very helpful, particularly when there are a limited number of possible answers. A tiered approach can be very helpful, for example, when trying to estimate the exposure to a particular chemical at work, the questionnaire may ask first of all:

- the employer the subject worked for,
- followed by the type of industry,
- the job title,
- the particular task that s/he carried out,
- the type of chemicals that s/he worked with,
- the name of chemicals that s/he worked with.

This approach has a further advantage that even if the subject does not know the answer to the last question, answers from the previous questions could be used for some analyses in an epidemiological study, for example, disease in relation to the type of industry or the type of industry and job title. The information on the industry and job title can subsequently be coded by an expert (see Chapter 8).

A calendar may also be used as an effective aid to recall. When studying risk factors of birth outcomes, a calendar could be helpful to determine where subjects lived or where they worked before conception and during different stages of various pregnancies. Pregnancies and everything around it are usually events that are clearly remembered.

In case of the use of household pesticides, rather than asking the subjects directly if they used any flea sprays, which they may not directly recall, it may be useful to ask first if the subjects had

- any pets, followed by
- if they had any problems with fleas,
- if they did do something about it,
- if so, if they used a spray, collar or other method,
- if so, what the name was of the product.

However, at times the subjects may not admit that they have had fleas in which case, the questions that follow will not be asked and the information is lost if they answered incorrectly.

Introducing these aids takes up more space in the questionnaire and there will always be a balancing act between space and the quality of the answers. In many circumstances, rather than asking for particular exposure to chemicals or other risk factors, surrogates are asked for. For example, in the case of nitrogen dioxide exposure, the use of gas cookers.

2.8   Coding

Information from the questionnaire needs to be coded for analysis. In the case of closed-ended questions, this is straight forward, but it is more difficult for open-ended questions. It is important to formulate a coding scheme early on in the study, which helps to focus the analyses. Humans make mistakes and therefore a good quality-control scheme needs to be carried out. Information may also need to be further translated, for example, in the case of a job history for which a job exposure matrix may be needed. Trained experts are required in this case to set up a job exposure matrix and carry out the coding, which may be a laborious task and provide mixed results (see Chapter 8).

2.9   Pilot testing

Pilot testing is an extremely important part of questionnaire design, and sufficient time should be allocated for it (Sudman and Bradburn 1983). Before pilot testing the questionnaire on people who are representative of the target population, it should be evaluated by a number of other researchers, particularly those who have used similar questionnaires and used the answers in an epidemiological study. This may be followed by a sample of convenience, for example, relatives, friends, or colleagues. After this, the questionnaire should be tested on a sample of people representative of the target population. At this stage it may become clear if the intentions of the researchers are sufficiently understood by the subjects. In some cases it may take a number of pilot tests to get the questionnaire right and at this stage the researcher should be critical of their work and open to suggestions. The better the pilot testing the less regrets there will be at the end of the study. Throughout the process written comments should be obtained that can be evaluated by a number of researchers.

During pilot testing the words and interpretations of questions are evaluated. At times this may be difficult to establish and it may need more in-depth discussion with the pilot subjects to determine how they interpreted the question and what they thought when giving an answer. Also, the researcher needs to evaluate how the answers can be interpreted and if they can be analysed and used for the epidemiological study. This is extremely important at this stage, particularly since questions still can be changed. More simple facts such as if all the questions were answered are easier to establish (Armstrong *et al.* 1992).

2.10   Translation

More and more, international multi-centre studies are carried out, for example, in Europe, and this may require translation of questionnaires into different languages. Furthermore, the (large) influx of immigrants also requires translation of the questionnaire since they may not be sufficiently familiar with their new language to be able to answer any questions satisfactorily. In these cases, the questionnaire should be translated and back translated, preferably by a number of experts familiar with the language and the topic. The researchers should be aware of cultural differences and take these into account in the questionnaire. After the translation has been carried out the questionnaire should be pilot tested again to make sure that no information has been lost in the process and the questions are interpreted in the same way as the original questionnaire.

2.11   Validity

A questionnaire may look good and the response to the questions may be good, but does the questionnaire actual measure what it needs to measure, that is, what is the validity of the questionnaire? Are those reporting longer exposure to environmental tobacco smoke (ETS) actually exposed to more ETS, are the subjects working with solvents actually exposed to higher solvent levels, do people who report drinking five glasses of tap water per day actually do so? Ideally all questions and answers should be validated, that is, compared to a gold standard. This could be done in a subset of the study population. However, often this is not possible, for example, because the questions relate to exposure in the past, there is no method to measure the substance of interest, or it is unclear what the gold standard is. Relatively few questionnaires have been validated.

Up to a certain extent, diaries can be used to validate a water ingestion questionnaire (Shimokura *et al.* 1998; Barbone *et al.* 2002), ETS exposure with personal exposure monitoring of nicotine (Coghlin *et al.* 1989; Eisner *et al.* 2001), or biomonitoring solvent metabolites (hippuric acid or methylhippuric acid) in urine in case of aromatic solvent exposure (Tielemans *et al.* 1999). The validation may only need to be carried out on a proportion of the population, and may provide invaluable information for the interpretation of the epidemiological study. The sensitivity, specificity, and predictive value of the various questions or the correlation between different questions from different methods can be determined and therefore the extent of exposure misclassification, if any, and the effect on risk estimates (Chapter 12).

Table 2.5   Sensitivity, specificity, and predictive values

		Biomonitoring 'truth'		
		Yes	No	
	Yes	a (100)	b (70)	$a + b$ (170)
Questionnaire				
	No	c (30)	d (800)	$c + d$ (830)
		$a + c$ (130)	$b + d$ (870)	

$$\text{Sensitivity} = \frac{a}{a + c} = \frac{100}{100 + 30} = 77\%$$

$$\text{Specificity} = \frac{d}{b + d} = \frac{800}{70 + 800} = 92\%$$

$$\text{Positive predictive value} = \frac{a}{a + b} = \frac{100}{100 + 70} = 59\%$$

$$\text{Negative predictive value} = \frac{d}{c + d} = \frac{800}{30 + 800} = 96\%$$

Sensitivity is the probability of a positive answer when the exposure is truly present while specificity is the probability of a negative answer when the exposure is truly absent (Table 2.5). Positive predictive value is the probability that a person is actually exposed given that he or she gave a positive answer, and the negative predictive value is the probability that a person has truly has no exposure given a negative answer.

Using a hypothetical example of a question validated with biomonitoring, it can be seen that in this case specificity is higher than sensitivity (Table 2.5). In epidemiological studies, specificity has a stronger effect on the risk estimates compared to sensitivity and it is therefore important to keep the specificity as high as possible, even if this may reduce the sensitivity slightly (see Chapter 12).

Tielemans *et al.* (1999) used biomonitoring to assess the validity of their various questionnaire methods and found sensitivity and specificity coefficients of around 0.30–0.55 and 0.77–0.92 respectively when using a generic questionnaire for solvent exposure, while this increased to 0.40–0.70 and 0.75–0.93 respectively when using a detailed job specific questionnaire, which elicited details on occupational tasks, products, and frequency of activity. A population-specific job exposure matrix showed higher sensitivity (0.58) but lower specificity (0.73). The highest positive predictive value was found for the job specific questionnaire (0.52). Shimokura *et al.* (1998) compared questionnaire data and diary data for water-related activities and found that there was a good correlation between drinking water intake ($r = 0.78$) and for the time spent showering ($r = 0.68$), but found that the actual amount of reported drinking water intake was considerably higher when using the questionnaire compared to the diary (0.75 vs. 0.40 l/day^{-1}). The difference for showering was less (10.5 vs. 9.8 min day^{-1}). Eisner *et al.* (2001) found a moderate correlation ($r = 0.47$) between questionnaire reporting of

ETS and personal measurements of nicotine, while Coghlin *et al.* (1989) found a much higher correlation ($r = 0.91$). A possible explanation of the difference may be the higher nicotine levels in the former study compared to the latter, which shows the importance of taking into account population characteristics. Teschke *et al.* (1994) found differences in the performance in questionnaires depending on whether they were closed- or open-ended questions (Teschke *et al.* 1994). The former generally showed higher sensitivity, although slightly lower specificity.

Besides the validity, there is the repeatability of the questionnaire, that is, are the answers reproducible, do we always get the same answer when we administer the questionnaire repeatedly (at times the term reliability is used here too). This can be assessed by administering the questionnaire twice to a proportion of subjects in the target population, and estimate, for example, the correlation between the answers (van der Gulden 1993; Westerdahl 1996; Farrow *et al.* 1996; Künzli *et al.* 1997; Barbone *et al.* 2002). The question raised often is whether the reproducibility of the questionnaire is measured or the variability in exposure. The interval between the two occasions should be long enough to provide independent observations, but not too long to avoid true variation in exposure. Some researchers tried to assess the reproducibility of a questionnaire, but used different methods of administration, for example, mailing and telephone or self-administered questionnaire and a face-to-face interview. This may introduce additional variation into the process and should be avoided. Künzli *et al.* (1997) used a number of different questionnaires to assess long-term ambient ozone exposure and found some differences in the reproducibility showing the importance of assessing different questionnaire methods. Barbone *et al.* (2002) found a good reproducibility for their questionnaire to assess tap water-related activities ($r = 0.6$–0.9).

References

Armstrong, B. K., White, E., and Saracci, R. (1992). *Principles of exposure measurement in epidemiology.* Oxford University Press, Oxford.

Barbone, F., Valent, F., Brussi, V., Tomasella, L., Triassi, M., Di Lieto, A., Scognamiglio, G., Righi, E., Fantuzzi, G., Casolari, L., and Aggazzotti, G. (2002). Assessing the exposure of pregnant women to drinking water disinfection byproducts. *Epidemiology*, **13**, 540–4.

Brogger, J., Bakke, P., Eide, G. E., and Gulsvik, A. (2002). Comparison of telephone and postal survey modes on respiratory symptoms and risk factors. *American Journal of Epidemiology*, **155**, 572–6.

Coghlin, J., Hammond, S. K., Gann, P. H. (1989). Development of epidemiologic tools for measuring environmental tobacco smoke in pregnant women. *American Journal of Epidemiology*, **130**, 696–704.

Debanne, S. M., Petot, G. J., Li, J., Koss, E., Lerner, A. J., Riedel, T. M., Rowland, D. Y., Smyth, K. A., and Friedland, R. P. (2001). *Journal of the American Geriatrics Society*, **49**, 980–4.

Edwards, P., Roberts, I., Clarke, M., DiGuiseppi, C., Pratap, S., Wentz, R., and Kwan, I. (2002). Increasing response rates to postal questionnaires: systematic review. *British Medical Journal*, **324**, 1183–92.

Eisner, M. D., Katz, P. P., Yelin, E. H., Hammond, K., and Blanc, P. (2001). Measurement of environmental tobacco smoke among adults with asthma. *Environmental Health Perspectives*, **109**, 809–13.

Engel, L. S., Seixas, N. S., Keifer, M. C., Longstreth, W. T. Jr., and Checkoway, H. (2001). Validity study of self-reported pesticide exposure among orchardists. *Journal of Exposure Analysis and Environmental Epidemiology*, **11**, 359–68.

Farrow, A., Farrow, S. C., Little, R., and Golding, J. (1996). The repeatability of self-reported exposure after miscarriage. ALPAC study team. Avonmouth study of pregnancy and childhood. *International Journal of Epidemiology*, **25**, 797–806.

Freeman, N. C., Jimenez, M., Reed, K. J., Gurunathan, S., Edwards, R. D., Roy, A., Adgate, J. L., Pellizzari, E. D., Quackenboss, J., Sexton, K., and Lioy, P. J. (2001). Quantitative analysis of children's microactivity patterns: The Minnesota Children's Pesticide Exposure Study. *Journal of Exposure Analysis and Environmental Epidemiology*, **11**, 501–9.

Hansen, K. S. (1996). Validity of occupational exposure and smoking data obtained from surviving spouses and colleagues. *American Journal of Industrial Medicine*, **30**, 392–7.

Infante-Rivard, C. and Jacques, L. (2000). Empirical study of parental recall bias. *American Journal of Epidemiology*, **152**, 480–6.

Jantunen, M. J., Hänninen, O., Katsouyanni, K., Knöppel, H., Kuenzli, N., Lebret, E., Maroni, M., Saarela, K., Sram, R., and Zmirou, D. (1998). Air pollution exposure in European cities: The "Expolis"-study. *Journal of Exposure Analysis and Environmental Epidemiology*, **8**, 495–518.

Künzli, N., Kelly, T., Balmes, J., and Tager, I. B. (1997). Reproducibility of retrospective assessment of outdoor time activity patterns as an individual determinant of long-term ambient ozone exposure. *International Journal of Epidemiology*, **26**, 1258–71.

Preller, L., Kromhout, H., Heederik, D., and Tielen, M. J. (1995). Modeling long-term average exposure in occupational exposure–response analysis. *Scandinavian Journal of Work Environment and Health*, **21**, 504–12.

Rothman, K. J. and Greenland, S. (1998). *Modern epidemiology* (2nd edn). Lippincott-Raven Publishers, Philadelphia.

Shimokura, G. H., Savitz, D., and Symanski, E. (1998). Assessment of water use for estimating exposure to tap water contaminants. *Environmental Health Perspectives*, **106**, 55–59.

Stewart, P. A., Stewart, W. F., Siemiatycki, J., Heineman, E. F., and Dosemeci, M. (1998). Questionnaires for collecting detailed occupational information for community-based case-control studies. *American Industrial Hygiene Association Journal*, **59**, 39–44.

Sudman, S. and Bradburn, N. M. (1983). *Response effects in surveys. A review and synthesis*. National Opinion Research Center Monographs in Social Research, Aldine, Chicago.

Teschke, K., Kennedy, S. M., and Olshan, A. F. (1994). Effect of different questionnaire formats on reporting of occupational exposures. *American Journal of Industrial Medicine*, **26**, 327–37.

Tielemans, E., Heederik, D., Burdorf, A., Vermeulen, R., Veulemans, H., Kromhout, H., and Hartog, K. (1999). Assessment of occupational exposures in a general population: comparison of different methods. *Occupational and Environmental Medicine*, **56**, 145–51.

Van de Gulden, J. W., Jansen, I. W., Verbeek, A. L., and Kolk, J. J. (1993). Repeatability of self-reported data on occupational exposure to particular compounds. *International Journal of Epidemiology*, **22**, 284–7.

Willett, W. (1998). *Nutritional epidemiology* (2nd edn). Oxford University Press, New York.

Westerdahl, J., Anderson, H., Olsson, H., and Ingvar, C. (1996). Reproducibility of a self-administered questionnaire for assessment of melanoma risk. *International Journal of Epidemiology*, **25**, 245–51.

3. Environmental measurement and modelling: introduction and source dispersion modelling

Roy Colvile, David Briggs, and Mark J. Nieuwenhuijsen

3.1 Introduction

Exposure assessment in environmental epidemiology often relies on environmental measurement and modelling, as opposed to personal exposure measurement and modelling, in contrast to occupational epidemiology where the opposite occurs. This is partly due to the differences in the size of study populations, which can be very large for environmental epidemiological studies and makes only environmental modelling and monitoring feasible, and the differences in nature and the temporal and spatial distribution of the exposure. Examples of environmental pollutants and their main exposure pathways and routes are

A) everyday indoor and outdoor pollutants such as particulate matter, NO_2, CO, and volatile organic compounds (VOCs), from sources such as traffic, gas cooking, (passive) smoking, with uptake through inhalation;

B) water contaminants such as arsenic, nitrate and nitrite, pesticides and chlorination by-products from geological sources, agriculture and water treatment respectively with uptake mainly through ingestion, and sometimes skin absorption and inhalation (e.g. trihalomethanes);

C) soil contaminants such as pesticides, metals, dioxins and VOCs from agriculture, industry and landfills with uptake through ingestion (including hand-to-mouth contact), and inhalation; and

D) food contaminants from deposition of air pollutants, uptake from soil, with uptake through ingestion.

Environmental measurements and models may not take into account differences in ingestion, inhalation, and skin absorption rates and differences in pathways of subjects and may therefore under or overestimate personal exposure or uptake, but there may still be a good correlation between environmental and personal exposure estimates, which is essential for epidemiological studies (see Chapter 12). Validation studies should be carried out to examine these issues.

Exposure assessment in environmental epidemiological studies often makes use of temporal and spatial variability in environmental levels of exposure. Some studies have used distance from a source such as a factory, radio and TV transmitters, roads, or landfill (Dolk *et al.* 1997, 1999; Elliott *et al.* 2001; Hoek *et al.* 2002). Epidemiological study designs for outdoor air pollution such as the time-series studies have related temporal (day-to-day) variation in air pollution to day-to-day variability in morbidity and mortality (Katsouyanni *et al.* 1995; Dockery and Pope 1997). Other studies such as the 'Six Cities Study' have used the spatial differences in air pollution to define the exposure index (Dockery *et al.* 1993; Dockery and Pope 1997). The environmental measurements for most of these studies were obtained from stationary ambient monitoring stations that routinely measure the air pollution levels at one or more points in the area where the subjects lived. Specific monitoring campaigns can be conducted to measure environmental exposure levels, but only for current exposure and these are often thought to be too expensive. An important issue is how well do these environmental measurements represent the subjects' actual exposure, this is discussed in Chapter 14.

Epidemiological studies of water contaminants such as chlorination disinfection by-products have used water treatment practices or routinely collected trihalomethane levels in a water zone or distribution network as their exposure index. Occasionally these environmental measurements have been combined with personal data on ingestion, showering, or swimming obtained by questionnaire to obtain more specific exposure indices (see Chapter 15).

Where routine measurements are used it is important to ensure that a quality control programme is in place to evaluate the quality of the measurements to avoid any bias as a result of differences in the measurement methodology and interpretation of results.

Certain areas within environmental epidemiology rely less on routinely collected data. For example, epidemiological studies of the effects of environmental tobacco smoke have often used questionnaires (e.g. whether spouse is smoking or not) or biomonitoring (e.g. cotinine) to obtain exposure estimates. The latter only indicates recent exposure, but can be used to validate questionnaire data (Etzel 1997; Wu 1997). Biomonitoring (e.g. blood lead) has also been used frequently in studies on the effect of lead exposure (Bellinger and Schwartz 1997). Studies on radon and electromagnetic fields have relied on a mixture of questionnaire data, expert knowledge, environmental measurements, and modelling of determinants (Brownson and Alavanja 1997; Savitz 1997). Studies examining house dust for metals, house dust mite allergen, or pesticide residues have their own specific methods; adapted vacuum cleaners hoover a specified area (e.g. 1 m^2) for a specific time period (e.g. 2 min) (Keegan *et al.* 2002). Similarly, soil sampling involves the collection of multiple samples (e.g. $n = 20$) of top soil (e.g. 0–5 cm) at specific locations in the study area (Keegan *et al.* 2002). The information can be combined with information on hand-to-mouth contact or consumption of vegetables grown in the soil (and uptake of contaminant into vegetables) to obtain more specific exposure indices.

Issues involved in the measurement of environmental exposure such as what and where to measure, for how long and how many measurements to take, and how to assess the variance components and exposure determinants are discussed in the chapters on personal monitoring (Chapter 5) and modelling (Chapter 6) respectively. Many of the issues involved are fairly similar, however there are some differences. For example, stationary ambient monitors can be larger than personal monitors and can collect more material for further analysis and measure lower levels because of the larger volume of air sampled. In this chapter and the next the main focus is on source dispersion modelling and geographical approaches to exposure assessment. The focus throughout the chapter is air pollution, but similar approaches can also be applied to soil and water.

3.2 Geography and exposure

3.2.1 Basic principles

The fact that a geographical approach to exposure assessment can be taken is based on a simple assumption: that environmental exposures show geographic variation. In fact, usually more is needed than this in order to estimate exposures with any degree of confidence. There is also a need for this geographical variation to be reasonably systematic (rather than random) and at a sufficiently coarse scale to enable the detection of these variations with the tools that are available. Systematic variation is important, because it enables the prediction of variations in exposure. This means that exposures do not have to be measured everywhere, but can be estimated on the basis of other factors. The scale of variation is important both because the methods of exposure assessment are inevitably only approximate, and because people are not static but move around in the environment. If levels of pollution vary dramatically over very short distances, we may therefore end up with serious errors in the exposure estimates. This may not matter much if, in the study design, population groups or areas with large differences in average exposure still can be identified—in those circumstances any association with health will be diluted but should not be removed. It matters much more where we are seeking effects of quite subtle variations in exposure, for in those cases we may not be able to reliably distinguish different levels of exposure within our population.

Fortunately, in many cases, these requirements can be satisfied. Many forms of pollution do show considerable systematic spatial variation. This occurs because most pollution derives from specific sources (often associated with some form of human activity), from which it disperses into the environment. During dispersion, it inevitably tends to spread out and concentrations become progressively diluted. The simple fact that the emission sources are geographically distributed (and often clustered) in some way nevertheless means that levels of pollution vary. The pathways of dispersion in the environment are also strongly constrained, so that dispersion is limited. As a result— unfortunately for those who live in more polluted environments but luckily for epidemiologists (who usually don't)—levels of exposure vary geographically. Indeed, like many other phenomena, pollution tends to conform to what has been dubbed Tobler's 'first law of geography': that all things are related to everything else, but near things are more related than those far apart (Tobler 1970).

3.2.2 Geographic approaches and methods

Based on Tobler's law, many different geographical approaches and techniques can be used to assess levels of exposure to environmental pollution. Classifying these different methods in any rigid way is difficult, for they tend to overlap and increasingly they are often used in combination. One important factor that distinguishes between them, however, is whether they are based on monitored pollution (or exposure) data, or whether they derive estimates from data on source activities. Another factor is their level of sophistication—essentially the extent to which they take account of local variation in exposures and in human activity.

Whatever method of assessment might be used, it is important to remember that we need to deal with exposures, not only pollution. It is not enough, therefore, simply to estimate patterns of pollution in the environment. These also need to be related to the population of interest. At some stage, therefore, geographic approaches to exposure assessment have to combine information on the environment and population. With new tools, such as geographic information systems (see Chapter 4), this is becoming relatively easy. One of the main factors that limits the reliability of many exposure measures, however, is this link. People are not distributed evenly across the world. Even within an urban area, major variations in population density occur. Further, the socio-economic characteristics of the population also vary geographically. Since these socio-economic factors may themselves affect health, they also need to be taken into account in epidemiological studies, and often we need to control for their potential confounding effects. Therefore just as much attention needs to be paid to the population that is studied as to the environmental patterns of pollution.

These different approaches to exposure assessment can also be applied within different epidemiological study designs. The most obvious application is in what are often called 'ecological' designs, in which comparisons are made between whole groups of people, usually based on where they live. In these cases, data are not available on individual exposures (or other relevant characteristics), but everyone in each area is treated as if they were the same. Exposures are therefore averaged across an entire area, such as a city or administrative district. Equally, aggregate estimates of this type are often used in time-series studies. In these, the focus of attention is on changes in exposure and their associations with health outcome, over time (e.g. from day-to-day). Spatial variations (e.g. differences in exposure between one area and another on any one day) are ignored. But geographic techniques may equally be applied to estimate exposures at the individual level, for example, by predicting the pollutant concentration at the place of residence of each participant. This allows them to be used in other study designs, such as case–control, cohort, or panel studies. Indeed, with some of the newer techniques that are now being developed, we can even model exposures as people move through the environment, as we will see later in Chapter 4.

3.2.3   Data needs and availability

One reason to use geographic methods of exposure assessment is, as we have already seen, the limited availability of direct measurements of exposure. Frustratingly in many cases, one of the most serious challenges that these methods face is also lack of data. Three types of data are generally required: monitored concentrations (or exposures) for the pollutants of interest; data on the distribution and characteristics of the sources from which they are derived; and information on the target population. With some methods (e.g. dispersion modelling), a wide range of other data may also be required, for example, on meteorological conditions. Because geographic methods generally need to be used over large study areas, and often retrospectively, these data can rarely be collected using purposively designed monitoring or sampling campaigns. Instead, for the most part, they have to be acquired from existing, often routine sources. Because these have usually been set up for other reasons other than exposure assessment or epidemiological research, they tend to be far from optimal.

Some indication of the problems that can be faced may be given by considering the sorts of data sets that might be needed for a study on air pollution in Great Britain. The number of monitoring stations for most of the pollutants of interest is small: there are only about 80 automatic monitoring sites for NO_2 or PM_{10}, to represent an area of some 250,000 km^2, and a population of almost 60 million people. The number of monitoring sites for other pollutants, such as VOCs and ozone is considerably fewer. Emission data are available for several pollutants, including PM_{10}, NO_x, SO_2, and VOCs, on a 1-km grid across the country, categorized by source. But these provide estimates only of average annual emissions and give no indication of short-term variations, which in many cases are substantial. Data on crucial meteorological factors, such as wind speed and wind direction, are available for only about 100 monitoring stations, and many of these tend to be clustered in coastal or relatively rural areas. Detailed population data are provided on a routine basis by the decennial census. Until 2001, these were reported for enumeration districts, which covered about 250 households (from 2001 they will be reported by census 'output area'). In urban areas enumeration districts are small; in the countryside, however, they may be anything up to 10 km^2 or more in extent. Inter-censual estimates are provided only for local authority districts, which cover areas of several hundred square kilometres. Using any of these data for exposure assessment thus poses serious challenges; and in many cases even the best data become limited by the worst when they have to be linked and combined. All this pertains to probably the best-served area in terms of pollution, namely air pollution. With other issues, such as drinking water quality, soil pollution, or noise the available data are even more restricted. Great Britain, of course, is extremely rich in data compared to many other countries, especially in the developing world. It is not surprising that exposure assessment is often seen as an attempt to squeeze as much information as possible out of inadequate and imperfect data sets!

Where there is little measured data, modelling becomes important and there are a number of different approaches. In the following sections (3.3 and 3.4) source dispersion modelling is discussed, including some of the basic concepts in dispersion modelling, and a number of examples are provided. Chapter 4 discusses the use of GIS in geographical approaches to exposure assessment, including in section 4.3.2 how source dispersion modelling can be integrated into GIS.

3.3   Source dispersion modelling

3.3.1   Mass balance model for a well-mixed box

The first type of model we will describe is not widely used directly in exposure assessment, but provides an understanding of the physical and chemical processes that control the spatial and temporal variability of a pollutant concentration in the environment. It is important that these should be understood before designing any modelling or even measurement-based exposure assessment study. If the wrong spatial resolution or averaging time is used, gross exposure misclassification can occur. Many studies produce information that is a lot less useful than it should be, because of failure to take into account the basic science that controls the spatial and temporal variability of the pollutants of interest, and this problem becomes most acute when trying to compare the results of studies of different pollutants, where it is vital to know how and why two pollutants might have different spatial and temporal variability.

To gain a quick understanding of such matters, we therefore consider the simplest possible case of a box containing a certain volume of the environment, within which the pollutant of interest can be considered to be well-mixed with constant concentration everywhere in the box. The rate of increase of the amount of pollutant in the box is given by the sum of the sources minus the sum of the sinks of that pollutant.

The typical sources are as follows (units are given, to allow calculation of rate of change of pollutant concentration in $kg\ m^{-3}\ s^{-1}$):

- emissions (e.g. kilogram per second from a chimney inside that grid cell, divided by the volume of the box);
- advection (concentration at the upwind edge ($kg\ m^{-3}$) multiplied by the speed of the wind or current flowing into the upwind side of the box ($m\ s^{-1}$), multiplied by the area of that side of the box (m^2), divided by the volume of the box (m^3));
- chemical reaction (concentration of each reagent ($kg\ m^{-3}$) multiplied by reaction rate constant ($m^3\ kg^{-1}\ s^{-1}$ for a reaction with two reagents)).

The main sinks, similarly, are as follows:

- deposition (concentration in the cell ($kg\ m^{-3}$) multiplied by deposition velocity ($m\ s^{-1}$), multiplied by area of base of box (m^2), divided by volume of box (m^3);
- advection (concentration inside the box ($kg\ m^{-3}$) multiplied by speed of the wind or current flowing into the upwind side of the box ($m\ s^{-1}$), multiplied by the area of that side of the box (m^2), divided by the volume of the box (m^3))—(*this is zero in a Lagrangian model*);
- chemical reaction (concentration ($kg\ m^{-3}$) multiplied by concentration of any other reagents ($kg\ m^{-3}$), multiplied by reaction rate constant ($m^3\ kg^{-1}\ s^{-1}$ for a reaction with two reagents)).

For a concentration that is not changing in time, the sum of the sources is equal to the sum of the sinks. In most advanced models, the equations are used to calculate the rate of change in concentrations. For our purposes, though, it will often be most instructive to consider a steady state averaged over a short period of time (e.g. an hour, during which weather conditions and emissions are assumed to be constant in an air pollution model). Note that the sinks are all proportional to the concentration in the box. When the sources and sinks are equated, straightforward algebraic rearrangement of the resulting equation gives the steady-state concentration in the box.

The spatial variability of a pollutant concentration can now be understood by examining the extent to which the forementioned six terms vary from one place to another, and which are the largest contributions to the balance of mass of pollutant in the box. We can think of the environment as being a three-dimensional grid of such boxes in rows and columns and stacked on top of each other (this is called a *Eulerian* model).

For oxides of nitrogen (NO_x) in the atmosphere, the most significant source term in an urban area is emissions, and the most significant sink is advection. If we take boxes of size 1 km $\times$ 1 km in the horizontal, in a typical region of interest containing a mixture of urban, suburban, and rural areas, emissions per square kilometre can vary by several orders of magnitude in rural and urban grid squares. Within an urban area, emissions can vary by a factor of 2–10 in adjacent grid squares. The advection sink is similar across the whole region, as wind speed at any given time only changes by a factor of two or less over quite large distances. We can therefore expect spatial variability of at least a factor of 10 in the NO_x concentration over a region of tens of kilometres, at a resolution of 1 km. The emissions usually vary less in time (maybe a factor of five between day and night, at most), while the wind speed controlling the advection sink varies by one or two orders of magnitude. This immediately tells us why air pollution time-series tend to have an apparently lognormal distribution, with frequent occurrence of wind speeds between 1 and 10 ms^{-1} giving a factor of 10 variability in pollutant concentration, and rarer events of wind speeds below 1 ms^{-1} giving rise to pollution episodes with concentrations a factor of a hundred or so higher than the annual average. If we go down to shorter length-scales, we find that within an urban 1-km grid square typically half the emissions come from one or more major roads only a few metres in width, and half come from domestic and commercial combustion of natural gas that are more evenly distributed throughout the square. If the roads are lined with buildings on both sides, the advection sink term in the box model is much smaller due to the way the buildings shelter the road from the wind, and so the concentrations there can be significantly higher.

Usually, nitrogen dioxide (NO_2) is of more interest for exposure assessment than oxides of nitrogen (NO_x, where $NO_x = NO_2$ plus NO, a mixture of oxides of nitrogen). Most NO_x is emitted as nitric oxide (NO), and this is then converted to NO_2 by chemical reactions in the atmosphere. The most important source of urban NO_2 is production by chemical reaction of nitric oxide with ozone (O_3). At a spatial scale of 1 km, the reaction occurs much more quickly than the time taken for pollution to blow (advect) from one box to the next. At this scale, NO_2 is therefore formed in the box from emissions of NO and advected out, resulting in spatial and temporal variability very similar to that of NO_x. At shorter distances, however, close to a single major road, the time taken for NO to be oxidized to NO_2 is about the same as the time taken for the plume of NO_x to move about 10 m, so the spatial variability in NO and NO_x is greater than that of NO_2.

The final air pollutant examined on this basis is fine particles (PM_{10}), which provides a good contrast to NO_x. Like NO_2, a large fraction of PM_{10} is a secondary pollutant produced by chemical reactions instead of being emitted directly from sources. Unlike NO_2, the chemical reactions producing PM_{10} from the precursor gases (mostly emissions of NO_x and sulphur dioxide SO_2) are slow. In a Eulerian model with fixed boxes of air on a fixed grid, the dominant terms are advection, with only a fraction of the precursor gases being converted to PM_{10} in the time taken for air to advect from one box to the next, even at grid resolutions of tens of kilometres. If we abandon the Eulerian framework and instead allow our box of air to move downwind carrying the pollution with it, the advection terms become zero and we obtain what is called a Lagrangian framework. We now see that the rate of chemical reaction is linked directly to the spatial variability in the pollutant concentration. Reaction taking hours to days in a parcel of air moving at a few kilometers per hour results in concentrations of PM_{10} building up over hundreds to thousands of kilometres. The deposition and chemical reaction sinks for these secondary particles are also amongst the smallest for any pollutant (exceptions are CO_2, N_2O, and CFCs, which are even longer lived and that are generally of no interest for exposure assessment). For PM_{10}, the dominant source term at length scales up to 100 km is usually advection, and the dominant sink term is the same. In a Eulerian model for PM_{10}, the particles that have been produced upwind simply blow into the box at one side, pass through and out the other. The result is a pollution field that spatially varies very little over rather long distances. Only very close to the strongest sources, such as within tens of metres of a road with heavy diesel-engined traffic, are primary sources of PM_{10} sufficiently influential to give significant spatial variability. The implications of this for exposure assessment and environmental epidemiology are potentially profound.

Last, we should see briefly how the box model approach can be used in other media. The example of trihalomethane in drinking and bathing water referred to earlier (and later) implicitly relied upon an assumption that everyone in a water zone has water containing similar levels of this substance. The same Lagrangian modelling approach can be used to check if this is a valid assumption, by tracking a small quantity of water flowing through the distribution network, and checking if the sources and sinks of trihalomethane are sufficiently large for any significant change in concentration to occur during the time taken for water to travel from the initial supply to the furthest customer.

3.3.2   Plume modelling

The consideration of air pollution in the previous section has omitted one of the most important processes that occurs at short range in the atmosphere, and which also occurs when pollution migrates through soil or water. That is the spreading of pollution horizontally and vertically, perpendicular to its direction of average movement. In the atmosphere, the spreading is caused by turbulence. If we are sure that chemical sources and sinks, and sinks due to deposition, are small over the distances of interest (in the atmosphere, typically up to about 50 km), a plume model provides a lot more information about the distribution of pollutant concentrations in the environment downstream or downwind of the source, more easily than any Eulerian or Lagrangian box modelling approach. Consequently, it is plume models that have most often been used in emission-based exposure modelling, alongside the more empirical methods that rely on environmental measurements.

The simplest case for movement of pollution through the environment is emissions from a single point in a homogeneous body of air, water, or soil. On average, the random nature of the spreading causes the concentration to assume a Gaussian distribution, just as any other random process (such as measurement error) causes a Gaussian distribution around an average value. The maximum concentration is found directly downwind of the source, with steadily decreasing levels of the pollutant being found as one moves perpendicular to the direction of the average wind away from the line of maximum concentration.

The Gaussian plume model will be briefly described here.

The Gaussian plume model is appropriate when modelling in the near field (0–100 km). In this model, the plume has a Normal (Gaussian) distribution of concentration in the vertical (z) and lateral directions (y). The concentration χ at any point is given by

$$\chi = \frac{Q}{2\pi \bar{u}\sigma_y\sigma_z}\exp\left(-\frac{y^2}{2\sigma_y^2}\right) \times \left[\exp\left(-\frac{(z-H)^2}{2\sigma_z^2}\right) + \exp\left(-\frac{(z+H)^2}{2\sigma_z^2}\right)\right],$$

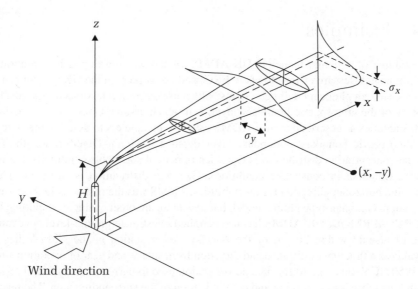

Fig. 3.1 Gaussian plume distribution.

where Q is the pollutant mass emissions rate ($\mu g\,s^{-1}$), $\bar{u}$ is the wind speed (in $m\,s^{-1}$), x, y, and z are the along wind, crosswind, and vertical distances (in m) respectively, H is the effective stack height (the height of the stack + the plume rise (in m)). The parameters σ_y and σ_z measure the extent of plume growth, and are the standard deviations of the horizontal and vertical concentrations in the plume (in m) (Fig. 3.1).

At plume centreline, $y = 0$, and ground level, $z = 0$, the equation reduces to give ground level concentration below the plume centreline

$$\chi = \frac{Q}{\pi \bar{u} \sigma_y \sigma_z} \exp\left(-\frac{H^2}{2\sigma_z^2}\right)$$

such that

(1) concentrations are directly proportional to emission rate Q, as in the box model;
(2) unless the source is at ground level, the maximum concentration will occur at a point some distance downwind from the stack;
(3) the distance to the maximum concentration increases with increasing effective stack height;
(4) the maximum concentration will decrease with increasing effective stack height.

The effective stack height is determined by plume buoyancy (if it is warmer than the surrounding air), or momentum (if it is released at a high velocity). To model a point source, data is needed on stack height and diameter, exit velocity or volume flow rate, temperature, and emission rate of each pollutant in grams per second; suitable topographical and meteorological data is also necessary.

3.4   Examples

An example of a plume model is UK-ADMS, which was developed by Cambridge
Environmental Research Consultants (CERC) and co-workers in the UK. In contrast to
earlier Gaussian plume modelling systems, which use discrete categories to describe the
stability of the atmospheric boundary layer, and which assume Gaussian distributions
in all stabilities as described earlier, ADMS uses two parameters to describe the state of
the atmospheric boundary—boundary layer depth and Monin–Obukhov length. The
vertical concentration distribution is Gaussian in neutral and stable conditions, but is a
skewed Gaussian in convective conditions. Gaussian distribution is assumed in the
crosswind horizontal direction for all stabilities. ADMS was the first so-called 'second-
generation' Gaussian-type plume model, but now there are other examples including the
USEPA's AERMOD. UK-ADMS has been applied to estimate ground-level concentrations of arsenic within 20 km of the Nováky Power station in the Nitra Valley in
Slovakia as a function of distance and direction from source and year of operation since
the 1950s (Colvile *et al.* 2001). The power station used to burn arsenic rich coal resulting in high emissions of arsenic and contamination of the surrounding area. The results
of modelling were used in an epidemiological study of arsenic and skin cancer around
the power station (Pesch *et al.* 2002). The epidemiological study needed historical estimates of arsenic, but very few measurements were available. Only arsenic emission levels were available since the opening of the power station, plus details of how emissions
were shared between a number of chimneys of varying height: from 100 m during the
early years of operation to 300 m today. The emissions reached their peak in the 1970s
after which they declined (Fig. 3.2). Air dispersion modelling was used to estimate the

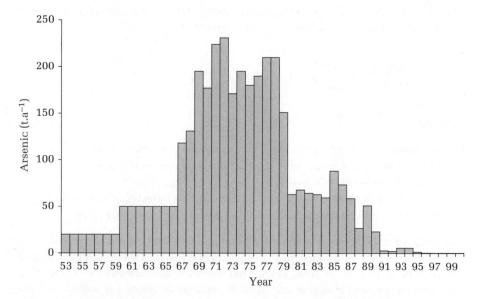

Fig. 3.2   Arsenic emission levels of a power station in the Nitra Valley.

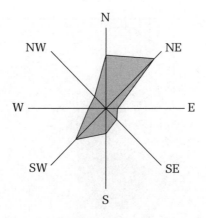

Fig. 3.3 Wind direction climatology (1990–3 inclusive) at Prievidza, showing channelling of local wind by the valley.

arsenic profiles around the power station and over time, using the arsenic emission levels and a number of assumptions.

To construct a model input that describes the local climatology, four years (1990–93) of observations were used, obtained from a weather station near the plant. The relevant data for each year were in the form of monthly average temperature and wind speed at 7 a.m., 2 p.m., and 9 p.m., monthly average cloud, and monthly frequency of occurrence of each wind direction by 45° sector. Figure 3.3 shows that it is relatively rare for the wind direction to be from the west or east. This was clearly because of the valley, which runs from north to south, channelling the wind.

Apart from the wind direction, the other notable feature of the Nitra Valley climatology was the high incidence of calms, which account for 13 per cent of the observations and as much as 32 per cent of the calmest month September 1990. UK-ADMS, like any Gaussian-type dispersion model, ceases to represent atmospheric physics realistically at wind speeds less than about 1 m s^{-1}. It is an unavoidable problem when using such a model that it becomes invalid at just the time when pollution concentrations can be highest. A simple box model was used to estimate the possible contribution of calms as follows. Emissions were assumed to become homogeneously mixed throughout a volume of air equal to that of the valley in the immediate vicinity of the Nováky Power station. An average calm was assumed to last 8 h (i.e. overnight), during which time no significant removal of arsenic from the volume of air is assumed to occur. At the end of the calm, the contents of the volume of air were assumed to be removed instantly by advection. These assumptions were clearly approximate, but were designed to be sufficient to carry out an order-of-magnitude estimate of the contribution of calms to the annual average atmospheric arsenic concentration.

Figure 3.4 shows the annual average ground-level concentration of arsenic modelled for the era of operation when emissions were highest, averaged over all times when wind speed was greater than 1 m s^{-1}. The three main features of the concentration

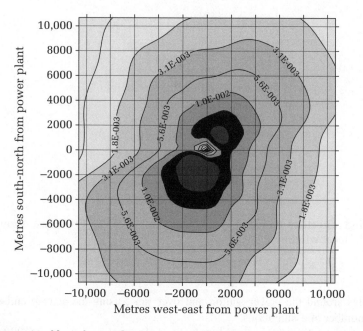

Fig. 3.4 Profiles of annual average ground level concentrations of arsenic ($\mu g\,m^{-3}$), modeled using ADMS for the era of operation 1973–5 around a power station in the Nitra Valley.

map are

(1) the concentration bands are not circular, as has been assumed for much previous epidemiological exposure estimation work, but are stretched along the valley because of the rarity of winds blowing across;

(2) the maximum of concentration is not immediately adjacent to the plant, but is displaced about 2 km to the north-east and south-west, because the pollution does not disperse vertically downwards from the elevated source;

(3) the concentration falls off rapidly with distance from the source, decreasing by a factor of 30 from 2 km away to 10 km away.

The modelled estimates were compared with some measurements that were available for the study period and they showed that there was a reasonable agreement between the estimates and measurements over the years and geographically, as long as the rough calculation of the contribution of concentrations accumulating during calm weather was included (Colvile *et al.* 2001). Soil sampling showed that the exposure profiles for the arsenic air modelling and arsenic in soil were fairly similar, with the highest levels measured near the power station and falling to background levels approximately 10 km from the power station (Keegan *et al.* 2002). The epidemiological study found an association between skin cancer and cumulative arsenic estimates based on the long-term air dispersion modelling estimates, taking into account changes over time, but not when simple distance measures were used, based on where subjects were living at the time of the study (Pesch *et al.* 2002).

The example used here is for point sources, but this approach can also be used for mobile sources or a combination of the two. For example, ADMS-Urban (CERC 1999) is a tool for investigating air pollution problems in cities and towns. It can be used to examine emissions from thousands of sources simultaneously, including road traffic, industrial, and background grid emissions. De Hoogh (1999) used this model, the Design Manual for Roads and Bridges (DMRB) model (Department of Transport 1994), and the Gaussian plume dispersion model CALINE-3 (Benson 1992) to estimate exposure to NO_2 for a sample of 1800 children in Sheffield, UK for whom data on respiratory symptoms were available (Strachan and Carey 1995). Model results were validated by comparing predicted concentrations with measurements at 28 sites, using passive samplers, deployed for five two-week periods over a year. The results showed that all three dispersion models gave good, relative predictions of monitoring NO_2 levels at the sample sites, with Spearman correlation coefficients of 0.83 (CALINE) to 0.93 (DMRB). However, both CALINE-3 and ADMS-Urban, in the way they were applied for this work, showed non-linear relationships between modelled and monitored concentrations, and ADMS-Urban substantially underestimated concentrations at monitoring sites. Logistic regression was used to explore the relation between modelled concentrations at the place of residence and school (both separately and respiratory symptoms, with and without confounders, but no significant associations were found).

This kind of modelling approach can also be used at a smaller scale for micro-environments. One example of this type of model is INDAIR, which estimates exposures to NO_2 in indoor environments (Dimitroulopoulou *et al.* 2001). INDAIR comprises two model components: a physical model, used to calculate hourly indoor air pollution concentrations for different micro-environments, as a function of outdoor concentrations, building characteristics, and indoor sources; and an exposure model used to calculate personal exposure to NO_2 for typical individuals through a series of micro-environments, depending on how much time they spend in each micro-environment. Both the physical and exposure models were developed in EXCEL using Visual Basic. The physical model is a simple, dynamic-compartment model that calculates the concentration C_i in the indoor micro-environment i over time t, by considering the air exchange rate between indoors and outdoors (λ_r), the exchange rate between indoor micro-environments (λ_t), the volume (V_i) and surface area (A_i) of each micro-environment, building fabric (f), the deposition velocity of the pollutant (V_d), and the emission rate of the pollutant in each micro-environment i. C_O is the outdoor concentration at the urban background-monitoring site. It is thus identical to the box model described previously, but the concept of a box is a much more natural one when considering air enclosed within a room. The model solves the following differential equation to consider each of the physical processes as C_i changes over time t:

$$dC_i/dt = [-V_d(A_i/V_i)C_i] + [\lambda_r fC_O - \lambda_r C_1] + [\lambda_t(C_j - C_i)] + [Q_i/V_1].$$

The first term of the equation is the pollutant mass deposited on the internal surfaces in the room. The second term determines the net pollutant mass entering the micro-environment compartment from outdoors, with the third term explaining the pollutant mass leaving the same micro-environment compartment. The fourth term explains the mass of pollutant moving between micro-environment compartments (e.g. kitchen to living room). The physical model considers several different types of micro-environment compartment: kitchen and living room at home, office, classroom, and outdoors. In terms of time spent in different micro-environments, the other important compartment is bedroom. The bedroom is not included in the physical model, but is assumed to be 2 ppb lower than the concentration in the living room, based on UK field data.

In addition, similar modelling methods are also used to estimate exposures from water, for example, for chlorination by-products. In Colorado each water district is required to monitor THM levels at least once per quarter in four different locations in their distribution systems. Gallagher *et al.* (1998) estimated total THM levels by summation of concentrations of four constituent species (Chloroform, BDCM, CDBM and bromoform) and used the hydraulic characteristics of each drinking water system to determine the geographic extent to which trihalomethane samples represented 'exposure level' in the drinking water distribution system in census block groups contiguous to each trihalomethane monitoring point. The hydraulic characterization was achieved using a computer simulation model, EPANET, which was developed by the US Environmental Protection Agency. The model analyses flow in water distribution systems using a network of pipes (links) intersecting at pipe junctions (nodes). The user must specify the length, diameter, and roughness of each link and the elevation and demand (water consumption) at each node until they are accurately determined throughout the system. This information can then be used to determine hydraulically unique 'zones' for any point in the system. Using this approach they determined that concentrations at the sampling points were reliable surrogates for THM concentrations in 28 of 86 census block groups.

References

Bellinger, D. and Schwartz, J. Effects of lead in children and adults. In *Topics in environmental epidemiology* (ed. K. Steenland and D. Savitz), pp. 314–49. Oxford University Press, New York.

Benson, P. E. (1992). A review of the development and application of the CALINE3 and CALINE4 models. *Atmospheric Environment*, **26B**, 379–90.

Brownson, R. C. and Alavanja, M. C. R. (1997). Radiation I. Radon. In *Topics in environmental epidemiology* (ed. K. Steenland and D. Savitz), pp. 314–49. Oxford University Press, New York.

Colvile, R. N., Stevens, E. S., Keegan, T., and Nieuwenhuijsen, M. J. (2001). Atmospheric dispersion modelling for assessment of exposure to arsenic in the Nitra Valley, Slovakia. *Journal of Geophysical Research—Atmospheres*, **106**, 17421–32

De Hoogh, C. (1999). *Estimating exposure to traffic related pollution within a GIS environment.* PhD thesis. University College Northampton and University of Leicester.

Department of Transport. (1994). *Design manual for roads and bridges*, Vol. 11: Environmental assessment, Section 3, Part 1: Air quality. HMSO, London.

Dockery, D. W., Pope III, A., Xu, X., Spengler, J. D., Ware, J. H., Fay, M. E., Ferris, B. G., and Speizer, F. E. (1993). An association between air pollution and mortality in six US cities. *The New England Journal of Medicine*, **329**, 1753–9.

Dockery, D. W. and Pope, C. A. (1997). Outdoor air I: particulates. In *Topics in environmental epidemiology* (ed. K. Steenland and D. Savitz), pp. 119–66. Oxford University Press, New York.

Dimitroulopoulou, C., Ashmore, M. R., Byrne, M. A., and Kinnersley, R. P. (2001). Modelling of indoor exposure to nitrogen dioxide in the UK. *Atmospheric Environment*, **35**, 269–71.

Dolk, H., Elliott, P., Shaddick, G., Walls, P., and Grundy, C. (1997). Cancer incidence near high power radio and TV transmitters in Great Britain: II. All transmitter sites. *American Journal of Epidemiology*, **145**, 10–17.

Dolk, H., Thakrar, B., Walls, P., Landon, M., Grundy, C., Suez Lloret, I., Wilkinson, P., and Elliott, P. (1999). Mortality among residents near cokeworks in Great Britain. *Occupational and Environmental Medicine*, **56**, 34–40.

Elliott, P., Briggs, D., Morris, S., de Hoogh, C., Hurt, C., Kold Jensen, T., Maitland, I., Richardson, S., Wakefield, J., and Jarup, L. (2001). Risk of adverse birth outcomes in populations living near landfill sites. *British Medical Journal*, **323**, 363–8.

Etzel, R. A. (1997). Environmental tobacco smoke. I: Childhood diseases. In *Topics in environmental epidemiology* (ed. K. Steenland and D. Savitz), pp. 200–26. Oxford University Press, New York.

Gallagher, M. D., Nuckols, J. R., Stallones, L., and Savitz, D. A. (1998). Exposure to trihalomethanes and adverse pregnancy outcomes. *Epidemiology*, **9**, 484–9.

Hoek, G., Brunekreef, B., Goldbohm, S., Fischer, P., and van den Brandt, P. A. (2002). Association between mortality and indicators of traffic related air pollution in the Netherlands: a cohort. *Lancet*, **360**, 1203–9.

Katsouyanni, K., Zmirou, D., Spix, C., Sunyer, J., Schouten, J. P., Ponka, A., Anderson, H. R., LeMoullec, Y., Wojtyniak, B., Vigotti, M. A., and Bacharova, L. (1995). Short-term effects of air-pollution on health—a European approach using epidemiologic time-series data—the Aphea Project—background, objectives, design. *European Respiratory Journal*, **8**, 1030–8.

Keegan, T., Bing Hong, Thornton, I., Farago, M., Jakubis, P., Jakubis, M., Pesch, B., Ranft, U., and Nieuwenhuijsen, M. (2002). Assessment of environmental arsenic levels in Prievidza District. *Journal of Exposure Analysis Environmental Epidemiology*, **12**, 179–85.

Savitz, D. A. (1997). Radiation II: Electromagnetic fields. In *Topics in environmental epidemiology* (ed. K. Steenland and D. Savitz), pp. 295–313. Oxford University Press, New York.

Strachan, D. P. and Carey, I. M. (1995). Home environment and sever asthma in adolescence: a population based case–control study. *British Medical Journal*, **311**, 1053–6.

Tobler, W. R. (1970). A computer movie simulating urban growth in the Detroit region. *Economic Geographer*, **46**, 234–40.

Pesch, B., Ranft, U., Jakubis, P., Nieuwenhuijsen, M. J., Hergemöller, A., Unfried, K., Jakubis, M., Miskovic, P., Keegan, T., and the EXPASCAN Study Group. (2002). Environmental arsenic exposure from a coal-burning power plant as potential risk factor for non-melanoma skin carcinoma: results from a case-control study in the District of Prievidza, Slovakia. *American Journal of Epidemiology*, **155**, 798–809.

Wu, A. H. (1997). Environmental tobacco smoke II: Lung cancer. In *Topics in environmental epidemiology* (ed. K. Steenland and D. Savitz), pp. 200–26. Oxford University Press, New York.

4. Environmental measurement and modelling: geographical information systems

David Briggs

4.1 GIS as a tool for exposure assessment

4.1.1 What are GIS?

This chapter builds on what is discussed in Chapter 3. Geographical approaches to exposure assessment are not new. They are often (though perhaps with some generous reinterpretation of history) traced back to the classic study of cholera in London, by John Snow in the mid-nineteenth century (Snow 1855). For many years, however, the right tools have been needed. Traditional cartographic techniques could be used in a relatively simple way to describe and display patterns of pollution and show simple associations with population distribution or with health, but the instruments required to analyse these data in any rigorous way were lacking. In the last decade or so, these have become available in the form of geographical information systems (GIS).

In simple terms, GIS are computerized mapping systems. As such, they comprise a computer, software, data, and whatever other devices are needed to capture and display the data (e.g. scanner, plotter, printer). GIS, however, can do more than simply map data. They also provide the capability to integrate the data into a common spatial form, and to analyse the data geographically. It is these capabilities that give GIS their special power in relation to exposure assessment. The ability to integrate the data implies that they can be used to bring together data on the environment, on population, and on health—all of which may have been collected in very different spatial formats (e.g. as points, lines, or areas, at different spatial scales)—and convert them into a common geography. This allows them to be linked, combined, and compared. The analytical functions available in GIS enable these data then to be queried and manipulated in many different ways. They can be used, for example, to examine the spatial associations between different features (e.g. people, sources of pollution, and pollution monitoring sites) and to determine how closely these are connected in space. They can be used to explore spatial patterns in the same features, and fit models that summarize the patterns that are found. We can then use these models to interpolate between our sample points, and hence to estimate conditions at locations for which we do not have data.

In addition, we can use GIS in combination with other models (e.g. dispersion models) to simulate the ways in which pollutants propagate in the environment, and the exposures that occur thereby.

Although many of these methods are now being used in environmental epidemiology, in truth most studies still use relatively simple techniques. This is largely perhaps because of unfamiliarity with GIS and what they can do. Sometimes there is also rightful suspicion about technologies such as GIS: they may be powerful, and GIS are certainly persuasive, but that does not always mean that the answers they provide are right. Some degree of scepticism is certainly merited with any method of exposure assessment, and in most cases we would be wise to validate our estimates against independent data. For this reason, geographical methods do not stand apart from other techniques, such as personal monitoring, but are complementary. Few of the techniques we will consider in the following sections also depend entirely on GIS. Many can be applied in other ways. But the use of GIS undoubtedly makes them more practicable and above all provides the capability to extend them to larger areas or populations with relative ease.

4.1.2   Geographic data and GIS

As mentioned in Chapter 3, there are some problems in acquiring the data needed to carry out geographic methods of exposure assessment. In using these techniques another issue comes to the fore: all the data that are used must be *georeferenced*. This means that it must be possible to relate every data point or observation to a geographic location, defined in terms of its two-dimensional (or, where height is also important, three-dimensional) geographic coordinates. Georeferencing can be done in several different ways. Sometimes it is direct: for example, pollution monitoring sites or places of residence may be referenced by their latitude and longitude or x,y coordinates (e.g. in metres from a specified origin). In other cases, georeferencing is more indirect. Populations might only be available for census districts, or whole cities or regions, so their spatial connection is only to an area. It is this area that is then formally georeferenced, usually by digitally encoding its boundaries (e.g. by digitizing them onto a base map within the GIS).

Georeferencing of the data serves several vital functions. First, it enables every feature to be fixed in space and thus to be mapped. Second, it allows the features to be linked geographically, and in this way matched to a common geography. Third, it provides information on the *topology* of these features. We can tell, for example, which administrative areas are adjacent to each other, where two roadlines intersect, or where a power line passes through a housing estate. This enables us to make stronger inferences about the relationships between the features we have mapped, and the possible pathways and processes of exposure that might exist. It is important to realize, however, that the way in which we conceptualize space is highly fluid. The entities and objects that we recognize in the world, and which we may then try to map, are not always so clear-cut, but to a large extent are constructs of our minds. A roadway, for example, can be seen as a continuous feature in its own right, or just as a rather irregular gap between houses. In particular, the way in which we conceive of any feature depends upon the scale of analysis we use. A feature such as a landfill site might be seen as an area at one scale, but effectively represented as a point at another. How we conceive of, and georeference, features in a GIS, therefore, depends on circumstances and need. We do, however, have to be aware of the implications of representing space in these different ways, for when we change the form of spatial representation, we may also change the implied topology. When represented as part of a continuous network, for example, stream water monitoring sites are connected in a very specific way. If represented as unconnected points, the topological connections are lost. If we used these two different constructs to model, say, the distribution of the pollution within the river network, we might obtain very different results.

4.2   Interpolation methods

Tobler's (1970) first law of geography implies that in things geographical distance is the key (see Chapter 3). In so far as this is true, it means that two people who live close to each other are likely to have more similar exposures than two people who live further apart. Where data on pollution levels are available from a number of sampled locations, therefore, spatial interpolation techniques can be used to model the pollution surface, and thereby estimate conditions at unsampled locations, simply on the basis of their relative proximity to the sampling points. By intersecting the resulting map with the population distribution, an assessment of exposures can then be made. Explicitly or implicitly, these principles are commonly used as a basis for exposure assessment in many different fields.

4.2.1   Point in polygon techniques

Interpolation is something we carry out intuitively—so much so, in fact, that we often do not realize that we are doing it. It is simply the art of estimation on the basis of the evidence that surrounds us. It is a technique that is used almost universally in epidemiological studies, for rarely if ever do we have complete data on pollution levels or exposures, either over time or space. We therefore have to fill in the gaps by interpolation.

Geographically, probably the simplest way in which this is done is by point-in-polygon techniques. Essentially, this involves taking data from a single sample point and extending it to its surrounding area. This methodology is so simple that it does not need sophisticated mapping tools. It is done routinely in many time-series studies of air pollution, merely by assigning populations to the monitoring stations within their city. Daily concentrations from the monitoring stations are then computed (e.g. by averaging data from all the available sites within a city) and assigned to everyone living within that city. Associations may then be sought between this averaged pollution concentration and health outcome (e.g. mortality or numbers of hospital admissions) from day to day. The same technique can also be used for studies of long-term exposures and chronic health effects. It was used, for example, in the seminal 'Six Cities Study' in the US (Dockery *et al.* 1993). This study compared rates of respiratory illness, including mortality, across six cities with contrasting levels of pollution, each city being classified by averaging long-term data from the available monitoring stations. A strong gradient was found for several health outcomes, especially with particulate (PM_{10}) and

SO_2, and results from this study have become the foundations of many of the air quality guidelines adopted across the world.

This approach to exposure assessment is evidently very naïve, in that it takes no account of spatial variations in exposure: everyone within each area is assumed to get the same exposure. Slightly more sophistication can be introduced, however, by allocating different areas to different monitoring or measurement stations. This raises the question of which stations get assigned to which areas. One way of doing this is by simple proximity: each area is considered to be represented by its closest monitoring station. A GIS technique known as Thiessen tessellation is useful for this purpose: this can be used to create polygons around each monitoring station so that every location in the city is associated with its nearest station (Fig. 4.1). Populations can thus be assigned to, and represented by, their nearest monitoring site.

4.2.2   Inverse distance weighting

The simple methods described above are clearly a very crude approximation of reality. If we look at the pollution surfaces that they produced, we would find that they consisted of flat areas, within which the pollution levels are assumed to be the same, separated by abrupt changes. In the real world, of course, pollution surfaces tend to be much smoother. In order to model these more realistically, therefore, methods need to be used that treat the pollution field as a continuously varying surface, not as a set of discrete blocks.

Many different methods are now available to do this, and classifying them is not easy. Some methods, however, are essentially deterministic, and model the surface as

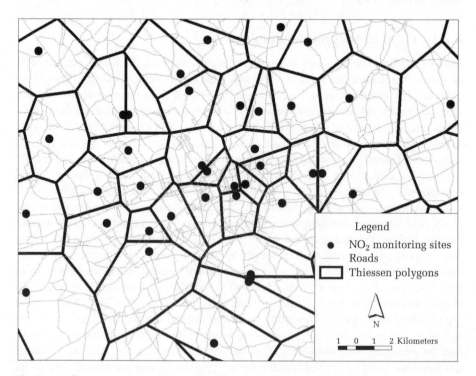

Fig. 4.1   Thiessen polygons around NO_2 monitoring sites in London.

a function of the inverse distance between the monitoring sites. The user determines what type of function to apply, and the software then calculates the estimated pollution level at each location based on the distance from, and measured pollution levels at, each of the surrounding monitoring sites. This approach thus rigorously applies Tobler's law in assuming that nearer monitoring sites are likely to provide better estimates of pollution levels at any location than those further away. In some cases a simple linear function of distance is used ($1/d$), but more commonly some form of inverse power function is used, on the principle that the 'influence' of more distant sites declines more than proportionally to distance. Probably the most common is an inverse square ($1/d^2$).

Inverse distance models can be applied in several different ways. One of the most common approaches is to use what are known as triangulated irregular networks (TINs). These involve taking each group of three sampling points to form a triangle. This triangle can thus be seen to describe a plane, the shape of which is determined by the distance function used, and anchored in place by the monitored pollution values at each corner. By joining these triangular surfaces, a complete pollution map is obtained, from which the concentration at any point can be read. If appropriate, the surface can be smoothed (e.g. by using the moving window techniques described later), to remove the artificial jaggedness that otherwise occurs.

Moving window techniques are relatively simple and essentially deterministic. The 'window' is typically a square or circular area that is moved across the map, centring on each location in turn. The pollution concentration at that location is then determined by taking the inverse distance-weighted average of all the monitoring sites that fall within the window. The size (and shape) of the window is selected by the user, and should be chosen to ensure that it contains enough monitoring sites to provide a reliable estimate for each location, but not so many that it ends up over-smoothing the surface.

Both TINs and moving window approaches have the advantage that they are relatively easy to apply, require no data other than the monitored pollution concentrations and locations of each monitoring site, and are available as standard functions in almost any GIS. They nevertheless have some disadvantages. First, the results they produce depend upon decisions made by the user (e.g. the choice of inverse distance function and—in the case of the moving window methods—the window size). They also work effectively only where there is a reasonably dense network of monitoring or sample sites; otherwise, areas tend to occur within which the estimates may be highly generalized and unreliable.

In practice, they have also had surprisingly little use in environmental epidemiology. This is partly, perhaps, because the data available usually do not meet the requirements of the techniques: monitoring stations are often too sparse or too clustered. More generally, however, it may be because epidemiologists are not always aware of the existence of these techniques. Certainly they should not be ignored, for by providing area-weighted estimates of pollutant concentrations, rather than simple averages, they can undoubtedly improve exposure assessment and allow some of the local spatial variation in exposures to be taken into account.

4.2.3 Geostatistical techniques

As already mentioned, one of the problems with deterministic techniques such as TINs and moving windows is their dependence on decisions of the user—decisions that in many cases are inevitably not always well informed. In general, it would therefore seem more justifiable to use stochastic methods of surface modelling, which allow the data to decide. One such approach, which is increasingly being used, is geostatistics. Geostatistical techniques include a wide range of different methods, amongst which kriging is the best known. Various forms of kriging are now available as a standard function in a number of GIS, including ArcGIS.

Kriging comprises a varied suite of techniques, all based on the same underlying assumptions, namely that spatial variation in the phenomena of interest can be sub-divided into three main components: systematic variation (or drift), random but spatially correlated variation, and random, spatially uncorrelated variation (or noise). Kriging models the components of variation by examining spatial patterns in the available data. Generically, kriging thus attempts to solve the following equation:

$$Z_i(x) = m(x) + j(x) + \varepsilon, \tag{4.1}$$

where $Z_i(x)$ is the value of the variable Z_i at location x; $m(x)$ is a measure of the systematic variation at x; $j(x)$ is a stochastic, locally varying component of variation at x, and ε is the residual variation or noise.

Under the simplest forms of kriging (ordinary kriging), $m(x)$ is assumed to be zero— that is, there is assumed to be no systematic variation or trend. The spatially correlated random component of variation then becomes the focus of attention, and this is mod-elled by analysing the association between the difference in the measured values at each pair of sample points and their distance apart (or lag). This is done by measuring the semivariance, which is defined as:

$$\gamma(h) = \tfrac{1}{2}(n) \cdot \Sigma [Z_{x_i+h} - Z_{x_i}]^2, \tag{4.2}$$

where h is the distance between the n pairs of sites, and $Z(x_i)$ is the value of variable Z_i at site x.

Different models may then be fitted to the data (e.g. spherical, exponential, Gaussian), and the optimum one chosen using cross-validation techniques or other methods. The resulting semivariogram typically shows two diagnostic features: a small 'nugget' effect, where the model intersects with the y-axis (reflecting the residual error or noise), and a relatively steep rising limb to a 'sill', where it then levels off. The distance to the sill is referred to as the 'range' and shows the distance from each point within which the spatially correlated variation is effective. In other words, it indicates the area around each location from which sample points may be drawn to make estimates.

Ordinary kriging, as described above, provides a relatively straightforward way of modelling pollution levels in areas where there is a reasonably dense network of sample points, and no strong trend or drift. If a regional trend is present, however, it can lead to biased estimations, especially where monitoring stations are relatively far apart. In these circumstances, universal kriging needs to be applied. This also models the regional trend in the data, to various polynomial orders (e.g. linear, quadratic, cubic). The trend component can also be modelled either globally (i.e. a single trend across the whole data set) or locally (by generating a local surface for the subset of surrounding points): in the latter case, the user has to determine how many local points (i.e. what percentage of data points) should be used.

Once computed, the model is then applied to all the unsampled locations within the study area. This is done by passing a filter (moving window) across the map, visiting each location in turn. The pollutant concentration at each location is then computed based on the model derived from the sample data. The size of the moving window is defined by the user, either by setting minimum and maximum numbers of sample points (monitoring stations) to be used for each computation, or by delimiting a search radius. The search radius is usually set to be at least equivalent to the 'range' defined by the semivariogram, in order to ensure that it captures all the relevant information from the surrounding monitoring sites.

Kriging techniques attracted attention in the earth sciences relatively early—they originated from geology and quickly spread into applications such as soil mapping (Burrough and McDonnell 1998). They are being used only recently for pollution mapping and exposure assessment, but under some circumstances they have proved to be highly effective. Liu and Rossini (1996), for example, used ordinary kriging to assess short-term ozone concentrations in Toronto, while Cressie (2000) illustrates its use to model daily PM_{10} concentrations in Pittsburgh. Järup (2000) also describes the application of ordinary kriging to model the distribution of cadmium in moss, in Mönsterås, Sweden, as a basis for assessing associations with urinary cadmium.

In all cases, one of the key strengths of kriging is that it not only provides an approximation of the pollution surface but also yields estimates of its standard error at each location. This enables the reliability of the modelled surface to be examined, and exposure estimates to be weighted accordingly. Nevertheless, kriging does have its limits. Like other methods of interpolation, it works best when the monitoring sites are evenly and densely spread. It is also less effective where the pollution surface shows complex structural variations (e.g. associated with local emission sources) that are not well represented by the monitoring stations. It is thus constrained by the available monitoring data, and as we have seen this is often severely limited.

4.3 Source-based modelling

The lack of monitored data on pollution concentrations or exposures means that, for many applications, we cannot rely on them for exposure assessment. Instead, we are often better served by trying to generate measures of exposure from information on the sources of pollution, and on its pathways through the environment. As Table 4.1 shows, this can be done in a range of different ways—from using relatively simple proxies, such as distance from source, to more sophisticated models that simulate the processes of dispersion and propagation of the pollutant through the environment.

4.3.1 Distance and proximity measures

In this context, as with spatial interpolation, Tobler's law might seem to apply. If things that are closer together tend to be more similar, equally, levels of pollution might be expected to decline with distance from source. Distance from, or proximity to, the sources of pollution thus appears to offer a useful and easily applicable measure of exposure. It is certainly an approach that has been used widely, especially in the context of air pollution.

Many studies of traffic-related air pollution, for example, have classified exposures in terms of the distance to the nearest main road, the road traffic volume on the nearest

Table 4.1 A classification of geographic exposure modelling techniques

	Activity-based	Interpolation
Simple spatial models	Distance and proximity measures	Point-in polygon techniques
Surface models	Dispersion modelling	Inverse distance weighting techniques (Moving-windows, TINs) Geostatistical techniques (Ordinary and universal kriging)
	Hybrid methods (Cokriging, regression modelling)	
Time–space models	Dynamic time–space exposure models	Micro-environmental exposure models

road, or the road density or total traffic intensity (vehicle kilometres) within the surrounding area. Proximity has equally been used to classify exposures from industrial pollution. In studying associations between urban air pollution and lung cancers, for instance, Barbone *et al.* (1995) defined five exposure zones, based on the land use zone in which people live (rural, residential, mixed, industrial, or city centre). Comparisons between these showed that people living in rural areas had somewhat reduced risks of cancer compared to those living in residential areas, while those in the industrial areas and city centre had slightly increased risks.

Another example of this approach is in the study of congenital malformations and low birthweight around landfill sites in Great Britain (Elliott *et al.* 2001). In this case, the rationale for using a simple distance measure to define exposed and unexposed groups was based on several considerations. One was the relatively poor quality of the data on landfill sites: exact boundaries of these were rarely known, and most were identified only by a point location (usually the gateway). More importantly, neither the exact pollutants being emitted from the landfill sites, nor the pathways of dispersion (e.g. by air or groundwater) were known. For both these reasons, the use of sophisticated models was not considered worthwhile. On the other hand, what little work had been done previously clearly suggested that exposures, by any route, were likely to be confined close to the sites, and certainly within a kilometre or two. At the same time, the large number of sites that had to be considered (some 19,000 in all), and their often close clustering, meant that many people lived within a few kilometres of a number of different landfill sites. Without real knowledge about the spatial variation in exposures, however, the cumulative risks from these multiple sites could not be reliably assessed. In consequence, it was decided to use a simple threshold distance (2 km) to distinguish between 'exposed' and 'unexposed' populations. Using buffering techniques in a GIS, therefore, circles 2 km in radius were drawn around each of the landfill sites, and these were then intersected with the postcodes of residence (Fig. 4.2). Based on this, the birth of every child between 1983 and 1998 could be allocated either to the 'exposed' group or 'unexposed' group, depending on how far away their parents lived from the landfill sites.

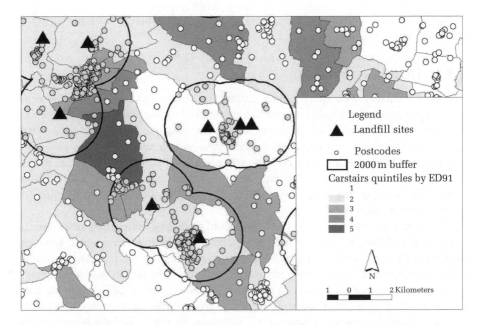

Fig. 4.2 Buffering around landfill sites and intersection with postcodes.

Using this exposure measure, the authors found that about 80 per cent of births were to mothers living within 2 km of landfill sites. They also reported slightly increased risks of a number of congenital malformations amongst the 'exposed' group, especially for abdominal wall defects and neural tube defects. Interestingly, however, some of these excesses existed even *before* the landfill sites were opened, suggesting that waste disposal might not be the cause of the observed health effects. This example thus carries a salutary lesson: we should be careful about interpreting results from simple geographic studies, particularly when we lack a clear, *a priori* hypothesis about the aetiological processes involved. Spatial correlation rarely if ever implies cause.

Other problems with these relatively simple source-based measures also need to be recognized. Implicit within them, for example, is that pollution spreads uniformly away from its source. This is clearly not always the case: wind direction determines the dispersion of air pollution; slope angle may constrain the spread of pollution in the soil; in networks, such as rivers or drinking water supply systems, pollutants will be channelled along specific and complex pathways; in other systems, such as the food supply chain, distance is likely to be an extremely poor proxy for dispersion. Because they are inherently non-specific (they do not relate to a particular pollutant nor exposure pathway), they can also be difficult to interpret. They might suggest that people living in certain areas suffer increased health risks, but they do not tell us why. It is perhaps partly for this reason that the health risks from both types of sources (road traffic and landfill sites) remain only poorly assessed and controversial. Almost certainly, we need more specific and more powerful measures of exposure if we are to detect and measure these risks reliably, against the large background of 'noise' with which we have to contend in epidemiological studies.

4.3.2   Dispersion models

The main difficulty with using simple distance or proximity to source as a measure of exposure is clearly that they are no more than crude proxies for the processes that determine the distribution of pollutants in the environment. Where we have better understanding of the environmental systems involved, however, we can use more sophisticated models to simulate both the processes and pathways of pollutant propagation in the environment, and thereby begin to obtain more realistic and dynamic estimations of exposures. One way of doing this is through the use of dispersion (or pollutant propagation) models.

The principles and procedures of dispersion modelling have been discussed in more detail in Chapter 3, so they need not concern us here. In general terms, however, dispersion models consist of mathematical representations of the processes that generate pollutants and control their movement, dilution, and fate in the environment. As Chapter 3 showed, dispersion modelling is far more firmly established in the field of air quality than in other areas. Most of the applications for exposure assessment have thus tended to focus on atmospheric pollution. Examples include the use of the Danish Operational Street Pollution Model (OPSM) to assess exposures to nitrogen dioxide (NO_2) in a study of traffic-related air pollution and cancer (Berkowicz *et al.* 1994), and the Dutch CAR model to estimate exposures to the same pollutant in a case–control study of respiratory illness in Haarlem (Oosterlee *et al.* 1996). Nyberg *et al.* (2000) used the AIRVIRO model to map concentrations of NO_2 and SO_2 between the 1960s and 1980s in Stockholm. Exposures were then estimated for *c.* 1000 cancer cases and 2000 controls by dropping the place of residence onto the pollution maps within a GIS. When adjusted for confounding by smoking, the results showed a small, but statistically significant, increased risk of lung cancer for exposures to NO_2, though not to SO_2. Since NO_2 is largely generated by road traffic, while SO_2 tends to come from stationary combustion sources such as domestic heating systems, the implication was that this risk is primarily a function of traffic-related air pollution.

So long as the processes are sufficiently well understood and can be simulated by the available data, propagation models can also be applied to other forms of pollution. One example is noise pollution. Concerns about the health effects of noise have grown considerably in recent years, and several studies have suggested associations with cognitive development in children and possible cardiovascular illness, as well as sleep loss and anxiety (Evans and Lepore 1993; Babisch 2000; Rosenlund *et al.* 2001). In the face of these concerns, stronger policies on noise are being implemented in many parts of the world, including Europe. Sophisticated noise models are being developed, both from road traffic and aircraft (e.g. Probst and Huber 2001). In the future, we may also expect to see similar approaches increasingly used in environmental epidemiology, often together with GIS, for other forms of environmental pollution, such as groundwater and soil pollution (e.g. Aral *et al.* 1994).

4.4 Hybrid methods

The ability to use dispersion modelling for exposure assessment—and, indeed, the reliability of these models—depends primarily on the availability of the necessary input data. As Chapter 3 showed, these data requirements are often demanding, and far beyond the capabilities of many epidemiological studies. In air pollution modelling, for example, as noted earlier, detailed data may be needed not only on the characteristics of the emission source (e.g. traffic volume, composition, speed, emission control technologies, percentage of cold starts), but also on meteorological conditions (wind speed, wind direction, mixing height, etc.), surface topography, and building characteristics. Approximation of these data inputs (e.g. by using proxy data or data from other areas) is sometimes feasible and, but for the occasionally overzealous concerns of modelling experts, might be done more frequently. Nevertheless, it also carries risks of reducing both the reliability and the acceptability of the results. As with interpolation techniques, therefore, data availability represents an important limitation.

One solution to this dilemma is to try to make use of all the data available, and to combine both source-based and monitoring information. A number of what might be called hybrid methods have been developed with this in mind. Typically these methods use information on covariates of pollution (that have been measured more extensively) together with monitored pollution data to improve the methods of interpolation.

Co-kriging, for example, is an extension to ordinary and universal kriging, which allows other variables to be included in the interpolation model. Obvious candidates include measures of source activity or intensity (e.g. traffic volume, emission rate) and factors affecting dispersion rates (e.g. altitude, soil type, slope angle). As yet, however, there are few examples of its use for pollution or exposure modelling. Where it has been tried, it does not always perform better than ordinary kriging or the types of regression mapping approach outlined below.

Regression mapping uses data from a 'training' set of monitoring stations to develop regression-based models of the associations between pollution levels and relevant environmental variables. These models are then applied to each location within the study area to develop an exposure estimate. The approach was used by Briggs *et al.* (1997), for example, to model NO_2 concentrations in Huddersfield, Amsterdam, and Prague, as part of a European study on traffic-related air pollution and health. In each case, passive samplers (Palmes tubes) were deployed at up to 80 sampling locations for periods of 2 weeks, on four occasions throughout the year. Using GIS techniques, a range of potential covariates were then extracted, including data on road traffic density (e.g. traffic volume, road length), land use (e.g. areas of industrial, urban, residential land), and altitude in the surrounding area. Slightly different models were developed in each city, because of differing availability of data. In Huddersfield, however, NO_2 concentrations were found to be effectively predicted by a model comprising three variables: a measure of road traffic volume (vehicle kilometres) in the surrounding 40 and 300 m buffer zones, a measure of the area of intensively built-up land in the surrounding 300 m buffer zone, and altitude. This was used to map NO_2 concentrations across the study area, at a resolution of 10 m. The map was also validated against independent data from additional monitoring sites. Subsequently, the model was further adapted and applied to model NO_2 concentrations in three other cities, as well as in Huddersfield for a later year (Briggs *et al.* 2000). Again, validation showed that it gave reliable estimates of air pollutant concentrations, with a standard error of estimate of only $5-10\,\mu g\,m^{-3}$ ($<20\%$ of the mean concentration).

4.5   Time–space models

Strictly, all the methods outlined above are essentially measures of pollutant concentrations, rather than exposure, in that they take no direct account of where people are. Exposures are assessed usually by dropping the place of residence of the individual participants onto the resulting pollution map, or by computing some form of population-weighted average across an area. Notably, in all these situations people are seen as static and tied to their home. As we all know, this is rarely the truth. Most of us spend a considerable part of the day outside the home, often in far-flung places. Indeed, there are several anomalies in doing exposure assessment in this way. We are likely to be at our home, for example, mainly at night. In many cases, however, the times of greatest environmental pollution are during the day, when road traffic and industry are most active. The geographies we use to estimate pollution and population distributions are therefore curiously mismatched. To make matters worse, when we are at home we tend to be indoors. Yet—in studies of air pollution especially—we tend to use estimates of *outdoor* pollution as the basis for our exposure measure. Sometimes it seems quite surprising that studies using these types of exposure estimation find anything at all! Yet it is also these associations between health and outdoor pollution levels that are then used as a basis for setting pollution standards and guidelines in many cases.

If we are to obtain more realistic estimates of exposure we clearly need to move away from this rather naïve view of the world. We need to recognize that people move, and that they do not spend all their time at home (but outdoors). This requires a far more sophisticated type of exposure model—one that takes account of human time–activity patterns and pollution levels in the sorts of micro-environment (e.g. bedroom, kitchen, living room, commuting to work, work, and pub) in which they spend their time. Thus:

$$E = \Sigma(t, C)_{ij}, \tag{4.3}$$

where E is the amount of exposure for periods $i = 1, \ldots, n$; t_{ij} is the amount of time during period i spent in environment j; C_{ij} is the pollutant concentration in micro-environment j during period i.

In applying this approach, we thus wish to model the exposures of individuals, or groups of individuals, as they move through a changing pollution field.

In recent years, a number of exposure models have been developed on this basis, though few have yet been used in any significant way as part of epidemiological studies. They can be broadly divided into what might be termed micro-environmental (or box) models and dynamic exposure models. The former do not try to simulate the trajectory or movement of individuals through the environment, but instead simply compute the time-weighted exposures within each micro-environment. The exposure can be either measured (Klepeis 1990) or modelled (Dimitroulopoulou *et al.* 2001) using, for example, outdoor and indoor sources in each micro-environment. One

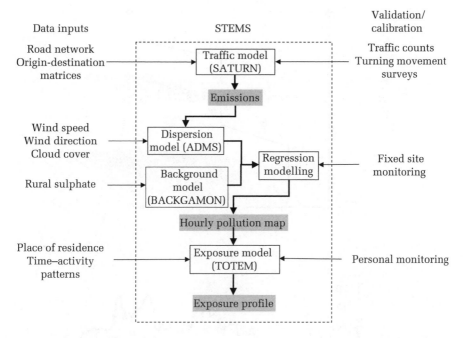

Fig. 4.3 The STEMS model.

example of this type of model is INTAIR, which estimates exposures to NO_2 in indoor environments and was discussed in Chapter 3 (Dimitroulopoulou *et al.* 2001).

Using GIS, more dynamic models can be developed. Jensen *et al.* (2001), for example, has created the AirGIS model in ArcView, which couples the OPSM dispersion model to a set of procedures for estimating exposures in different micro-environments based on aggregated time–activity data. Somewhat more sophisticated is the space-time exposure modelling system (STEMS), which is illustrated in Figs 4.3 and 4.4. This uses the functionality of GIS to loose-couple a number of different models, each calibrated and validated against field data, from which it derives a fine resolution air pollution map that is updated for each hour. It then uses time–activity data to simulate the movement of individuals across this changing pollution field, generating an exposure profile that passes across or lingers in each pixel on the map. Outputs from the system thus comprise exposure profiles either for individuals or for simulated groups of people.

4.6 Conclusions

Geographic methods of exposure assessment clearly have a great deal to offer in environmental epidemiology. Where monitored data are sparse, they provide a range of methods for estimating pollution levels at unsampled sites and constructing maps of pollution. They also provide the means to link these estimates of pollution to population

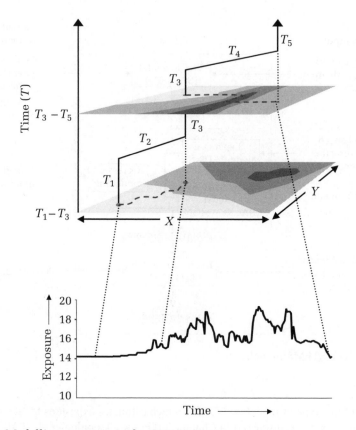

Fig. 4.4   Modelling exposure in the STEMS system.

distribution, and thereby assess exposures either for individuals or for population groups. To date, most applications of these methods have been relatively simple: many have used proximity or distance, and techniques such as point-in-polygon analysis or buffering, for exposure assessment. In most cases, little account has been taken of population dynamics; instead, exposures are usually in relation to the place of residence. These simplifications are often justifiable because of the general nature of the hypothesis being tested, uncertainties about the specific toxic agent involved, or the poor quality of the health data. But they do not need to be so. As Chapter 3 showed, powerful dispersion models are now available, and these are beginning to be used in epidemiology. With the help of GIS techniques it is now feasible to develop far more realistic models of exposure, including time–activity patterns of people.

Nor is the potential of these techniques confined only to the investigation of associations between environmental pollution and disease. Geographical exposure assessment equally offers a way of translating established dose–response functions into measures of health risk—that is for health impact assessment. By estimating the distribution of exposures across the population, they allow the attributable health risk, or the overall burden of disease, from a specified pollutant or source activity to be estimated. This is important for policy, for it is often on the basis of calculations such as this that issues are prioritized and the decision for action made. Just as important are the visualization capabilities of GIS. Maps are persuasive, and their ability to make maps of exposure or health risk more-or-less to need, and then to interrogate them interactively, means that GIS are especially powerful tools. Yet models and maps can also lie. So in using these techniques, we have to be careful. We need to remember that they are only approximations of reality. We need to recognize that few, if any, of the techniques we use are wholly neutral or objective: in various ways, sometimes explicitly, often implicitly, we make choices and decisions that influence the results we obtain. These results are also subject to uncertainty, so we should always try to check them by validation against independent data, such as personal monitoring. Above all, we should use and interpret them cautiously. Together with a little imagination and insight, these techniques can certainly help us to generate new and exciting hypotheses. But if we want to use them as part of a process of hypothesis testing, or as a basis for intervention and policy, we must at all times be guided by what is both environmentally and biologically plausible. Geography is thus just one of the sciences that we need to employ in pursuing questions about the effects of environmental pollution on health, or what we should do about them.

References

Aral, M. M., Maslia, M. L., Williams, R. C., Susten, R. A., and Heitgerd, J. L. (1995). Exposure assessment of populations using environmental modeling, demographic analysis, and GIS. *Water Resources Bulletin*, **30**, 1025–41.

Babisch, W. (2000). Traffic noise and cardiovascular disease: epidemiological review and synthesis. *Noise and Health*, **8**, 9–32.

Barbone, F., Boveni, M., Cavallieri, F., and Stanta, G. (1995). Air pollution and lung cancer in Trieste, Italy. *American Journal of Epidemiology*, **141**, 1161–9.

Berkowicz, R., Hertel, O, Sørensen, N. N., and Michelsen, J. A. (1994). Modelling air pollution from traffic in urban areas. *Proceedings of the IMA Conference on Flow and Dispersion Through Groups of Obstacles*. University of Cambridge, Cambridge.

Briggs, D. J., Collins, S., Elliott, P., Kingham, S., Fisher, P., Lebret, W., van Reeuwijk, H., van der Veen, A., Pryl, K., and Smallbone, K. (1997). Mapping urban air pollution using GIS: a regression-based approach. *International Journal of Geographical Information Science*, **11**, 699–718.

Briggs, D. J., de Hoogh, C., Gulliver, J., Wills, J., Elliott, P., Kingham, S., and Smallbone, K. (2000). A regression-based method for mapping traffic-related air pollution: application and testing in four contrasting urban environments. *Science of the Total Environment*, **253**, 151–67.

Burrough, P. A. and McDonnell, R. A. (1998) *Principles of geographical information systems.* Oxford University Press, Oxford.

Cressie, N. (2000). Geostatistical methods for mapping environmental exposures. In *Spatial epidemiology. Methods and applications* (ed. P. Elliott, J. C. Wakefield, N. G. Best, and D. J. Briggs), pp. 185–204. Oxford University Press, Oxford.

Dimitroulopoulou, C., Ashmore. M. R., Byrne, M. A., and Kinnersley, R. P. (2001). Modelling of indoor exposure to nitrogen dioxide in the UK. *Atmospheric Environment*, **35**, 269–71.

Dockery, D. W., Pope, C. A. III, Xu, X., Spengler, J. D., Ware, J. H., Fay, M. E., Ferris, B. G. Jr., and Speizer, F. E. (1993). An association between air pollution and mortality in six U.S. cities. *New England Journal of Medicine*, **329**, 1753–9.

Elliott, P., Briggs, D. J., Morris, S., de Hoogh, C., Hurt, C., Kold Jensen, T., Maitland, I., Richardson, S., Wakefield, J., and Jarup, L. (2001). Risk of adverse birth outcomes in populations living near landfill sites. *British Medical Journal*, **323**, 363–8.

Evans, G. W. and Lepore, S. J. (1993). Nonauditory effects of noise on children: a critical review. *Children's Environments*, **10**, 31–51.

Järup, L. (2000). The role of geographical studies in risk assessment. In *Spatial epidemiology. Methods and applications* (ed. P. Elliott, J. C. Wakefield, N. G. Best, and D. J. Briggs), pp. 415–33. Oxford University Press, Oxford.

Jensen, S. S., Berkowicz, R., Hansen, H. S., and Hertel, O. (2001). A Danish decision-support GIS tool for management of air quality and human exposures. *Transportation Research Part D*, **6**, 229–41.

Klepeis, N. E. (1990). An introduction to the indirect exposure assessment approach: modeling human exposure using microenvironmental measurements and the recent National Human Activity Pattern Survey. *Environmental Health Perspectives*, **107** (suppl 2), 365–74.

Liu, L. J. S. and Rossini, A. J. (1996). Use of kriging models to predict 12-hour mean ozone concentrations in Metropolitan Toronto—a pilot study. *Environment International*, **22**, 677–92.

Nyberg, F., Gustavsson, P., Järup, L., Bellander, T., Berglund, N., Jakobsson, R., and Pershagen, G. (2000). Urban air pollution and lung cancer in Stockholm. *Epidemiology*, **11**, 487–95.

Oosterlee, A., Drijver, M., Lebret, E., and Brunekreef, B. (1996). Chronic respiratory symptoms in children and adults living along streets with high traffic density. *Occupational and Environmental Medicine*, **53**, 241–7.

Probst, W. and Huber, B. (2001). Integration of GIS data into city-wide noise maps. *Proceedings of the Institute of Acoustics*, **23**, 29–36.

Rosenlund, M., Berglund, N., Pershagen, G., Järup, L., and Bluhm, G. (2001). Increased prevalence of hypertension in a population exposed to aircraft noise. *Occupational and Environmental Medicine*, **58**, 769–73.

Snow, J. M. (1855). *On the mode of communication of cholera* (2nd edn). Churchill Livingstone, London.

Tobler, W. R. (1970). A computer movie simulating urban growth in the Detroit region. *Economic Geographer*, **46**, 234–40.

5. Personal exposure monitoring

Mark J. Nieuwenhuijsen

5.1 Introduction

Personal exposure monitoring involves the monitoring of people's personal exposure rather than the environmental media around them, that is, environmental monitoring, for example, in the case of air pollution attaching an exposure monitor to the person rather than placing a sampler in the area where they live or work. Personal exposure monitoring is widely accepted and commonly used in occupational epidemiology (Nieuwenhuijsen 1997), and it is being carried out in environmental epidemiology with increasing frequency (Nieuwenhuijsen 2000). It is, increasingly, regarded as more informative and more representative than environmental monitoring in environmental epidemiological studies, although its use is often limited by practical issues. Smaller health risks and lower exposure levels require a more refined exposure assessment. Environmental exposure levels tend to be lower than occupational exposure levels and therefore require more sensitive methods of measurement. For example, exposure to particulate matter tends to be measured in milligram per cubic metre in the work place (Nieuwenhuijsen 1997), while levels in the general environment tend to be measured in microgram per cubic metre (Janssen 1998). Of course for many substances this distinction is not very clear and very sensitive methods are required in the workplace. Duration of occupational exposure (up to approximately 8 h a day) tends to be shorter than the duration of environmental exposure (up to 24 h a day) and this may require different sampling durations and strategies.

Exposure to any pollutant is characterized by its nature (e.g. its chemical form or particle size), the concentration, duration, and frequency of contact. Estimates of these characteristics can generally be obtained instrumentally (i.e. using a monitoring device), via questionnaires, through direct observation, or through the use of biomarkers. The emphasis in this chapter is on the measurement of personal exposure with instruments; these provide information mainly on the level of exposure. Information on duration, frequency, and pattern of exposure is generally obtained by questionnaire, observation, or from records and is discussed in Chapter 2. Biomonitoring is discussed in Chapter 11.

Personal monitoring is generally labour intensive, costly, and difficult to carry out. These factors restrict its use, even though the information obtained is generally more informative and relevant than other approaches, depending on the circumstances, and increase the scientific value of epidemiological studies. It is usually not possible to carry out personal monitoring on a large number of people. A more efficient use may be to use it to develop and/or validate (statistical) exposure models in a representative sample and/or time period of the population under study (Hornung *et al.* 1994; Preller *et al.* 1995; Burstyn *et al.* 2000). This is discussed in Chapter 6.

Personal exposure monitoring is perhaps most fully developed in relation to air pollution, particularly in the workplace. Many air pollutants, for example, particulate matter, Ozone, CO, NO_2 in the general environment and particulate matter, asbestos, crystalline silica, biological allergens, solvents, and isocyanates in the workplace have the ability to cause adverse human health effects given a sufficient level of exposure and therefore personal monitoring is necessary. In this chapter the focus will be on personal monitoring of air pollutants, although the same principles could also be applied for personal sampling of soil and water contaminants, however for the latter personal factors such as ingestion rate, obtained by questionnaire (see Chapter 2), are combined with environmental levels (see Chapters 3 and 4) to obtain exposure indices.

Once the decision has been made to use personal monitoring for an epidemiological study, a comprehensive sampling strategy needs to be designed, carried out, and the results interpreted. In the process, a number of choices need to be made that will fundamentally affect the way in which the study is carried out, and the value and inter-pretation of the results. These include whether to adopt a group or individual sampling approach, the number of measurements needed, the duration of monitoring and appro-priate averaging time, the type of monitor or method to be used, and how the data will be analysed, interpreted, and used for the epidemiological study. Crucial to these choices is the fact that, in most circumstances, marked variation occurs in exposure levels, both for the individual and between individuals for any given time. Thus, a single 'best estimate' of the average exposure level may not be sufficient; instead, data are needed on levels of variations in exposure. The challenge is to design a strategy that incorporates the variability to the advantage of the epidemiological study in the most efficient way whilst attempting to avoid potential bias.

Issues regarding the expression of results (e.g. geometric mean (GM) or arithmetic mean (AM)), treatment of data under the detection limit, and quality control are discussed in Chapter 1.

5.2   Group vs. individual approach

As discussed in Chapter 1, to obtain exposure estimate(s) for a population in an epidemiological study, two main approaches are available: (a) individual and (b) expo-sure grouping. In the individual approach, every member of the population is monitored either once or repeatedly, and data are obtained at the individual level. In the group approach, the population is first split into smaller subpopulations or exposure groups based on specific determinants of exposure. In environmental epidemiological studies, exposure groups might be defined, for example, on the basis of distance from an expo-sure source (e.g. roads or factories), while in occupational epidemiological studies, exposure groups may be defined *a priori* on the basis of (a) work similarity, that is, having the same job title and/or carrying out similar work, (b) similarity with respect to particular substances, and (c) similarity of environmental conditions, for example, process equipment and ventilation. The underlying assumption is that subjects within each exposure groups experience similar exposure characteristics, including exposure levels and variation. Subsequently, a representative sample of members from each exposure group is monitored, either once or repeatedly. If the aim is to estimate mean exposure, the average of the exposure measurements is then assigned to all the members in that particular exposure group (where a sufficient number of samples have been taken from a population, the population could be divided afterwards into exposure groups based on the statistical analysis of those samples).

Where possible repeated measurements on individuals should be taken. This enables the estimation of the within- and between-subject variance in the individual approach and within- and between-subject variance and between-group variance in the group approach. How to estimate these variance components will be discussed in Chapter 6, while the effect of the distribution of the variance will be discussed in Chapter 12.

5.3   Number of subjects and measurements

The number of subjects to be measured and the number of measurements to be taken on each subject depends on the chosen strategy and the distribution of variability in exposure across the population. In the case of the individual approach, every subject will be monitored. Repeated measurements are highly recommended so that the within- and between-subject variance can be estimated, and attenuation in health risk estimates reduced. The number of repeated measurements required can be estimated, and is dependent on the ratio of within- and between-subject variance and the level of attenuation (Liu *et al.* 1978, Chapter 12). In the group approach, the number of measurements depends on the ratio of between-group variance and between- and within-group variance, and the required precision of the estimated mean for each group (Kromhout and Heederik 1995; Kromhout *et al.* 1996). The number of measurements required for a certain precision can be calculated in various ways, for example,

$$n = ((t \times CV) / E)^2,$$

where n is the number of samples, t is the t-distribution value for the chosen confidence level and $n_0 - 1$ degrees of freedom (e.g. 1.96 for 95% confidence, infinite degrees of freedom), CV is the coefficient of variation (e.g. in geometric standard deviation/ln GM), and E is the chosen level of error (0.1 for 10% variation around the mean). It is important to note that repeated measurements on individuals contribute less to the overall precision of the subgroup mean.

Loomis *et al.* (1994) reported a more practical approach. They designed a study with a fixed target measurement size, based on considerations of precision and feasibility. They grouped jobs into three levels of presumed exposure. The number of measurements for each job was weighted such that the presumed medium- and high-exposure groups were respectively sampled with 3 and 5 times the frequency of the low-exposure group. Because the variance increases with an increase in exposure level, a greater number of measurements were needed in the more highly exposed groups to meet the desired precision criterion. The measurements were distributed within these levels in proportion to the relative size of the various companies involved. Workers were selected randomly and those in the medium- and high-exposure groups were monitored twice on randomly selected days. To enable the taking of so many measurements they send out the sampler through the mail.

The number of measurements can be increased by sending out (passive) samplers rather than handing them out or by self-monitoring (Loomis *et al.* 1994; Liljelind *et al.* 2001). In this way the number of measurements can be increased even though the method(s) may not be as reliable. The benefits of a larger number of samples however may outweigh the loss in reliability.

Whatever the approach, to avoid bias and to fulfil the assumptions of statistical programs, subjects and measurements should be selected randomly (see Chapter 6).

5.4   Duration of sampling

The duration of the sampling period (or averaging period) depends, amongst others, on the health outcome of interest in the epidemiological study, the detection limits of the measurement technique, and the level of the pollutant in the environment.

Chronic disease outcomes (e.g. the effects of potential carcinogens on cancer prevalence) generally require long sampling durations (many hours to days). Studies of acute disease outcomes (e.g. relationships between ammonia and irritant effects) require shorter sampling durations (minutes to less than an hour). Relatively long sampling times may also be necessary for less-sensitive measurement and analysis techniques, for example, use of passive samplers to measure exposure to nitrogen dioxide (NO_2), or where low-exposure concentrations are being investigated, such as particulate matter in the general environment compared with the workplace, to ensure that enough material is collected. In the latter case, the duration can be shortened if the flow rate of the sampler is increased, but this may also introduce other problems such as the increase in weight of the sampler. In general, the variance of the exposure measurements decreases with increasing monitoring time (LeClare *et al.* 1969; Coenen 1976).

At times it may not be known what the sampling duration should be so short- and long-term sampling may need to be carried out. Flour and its additives such as fungal α-amylase are well-known causes of bakers' asthma. Little is known about the duration, frequency, and levels of exposure required for the development of occupational asthma, that is, it is unknown whether short-term peak exposure levels or longer-term exposure levels (work shift) may be responsible for it. In a recent epidemiological study in bakeries and flour mills (Cullinan *et al.* 1994, 2001), group- and task-based approaches were used to characterize exposure. Personal exposure measurements of total dust were taken on a representative sample within each group for an entire work shift and during tasks that were expected to have high-dust exposure and analysed gravimetrically and for flour aeroallergen (FA) levels in the laboratory with an immunoassay (Nieuwenhuijsen *et al.* 1994).

Table 5.1 shows full shift and highest-exposed task levels of dust and FA in the main exposure groups in bakeries and flour mills. Short-term exposure levels during certain tasks were considerably higher than average full-shift levels. For example, flour millers experienced a 15-fold greater dust exposure level during spillage clean-up compared to their full-shift average exposure. Frequency and duration of peak levels differed, for example, some peaks occurred a few times during a day and others a few times a month (Table 5.2).

Table 5.1 Characteristics of the personal inhalable dust $(mg\,m^{-3})$ and FA exposure $(\mu g\,m^{-3})$ of the main exposure groups in the bakeries, flour mills, and packing stations (the GMs for the full-shift measurements and the highest-exposure tasks are given)

	Full shift			Task	
	Dust GM	FA GM	Highest-exposed task	Dust GM	FA GM
Bakeries					
Dispense/mixing	5.0	228.7	Floor cleaning	8.3	415.9
Bread production	0.9	176.6	Dusting flour	9.0	185.5
Bread wrapping	0.4	45.5	Floor cleaning	1.4	18.6
Roll production	2.4	215.3	Dusting flour	8.8	163.1
Roll wrapping	0.8	100.9	Floor cleaning	1.4	18.6
Conf/dough brake	6.4	208.5	Dusting flour	4.2	118.5
Conf/flour involved	1.6	252.0	Dusting flour	4.2	118.5
Conf/no flour inv.	0.7	80.2	–		
Despatch	0.5	64.5	–		
Hygiene inside	0.7	72.8	Cleaning bins	42.9	1138.5
Flour mills and packing stations					
Flour miller	2.4	248.3	Cleaning spills	39.3	3807.9
Mixing area	11.0	303.9	Cleaning floor	12.9	141.5
Packing area	5.7	227.6	Ripping/tipping	21.2	405.8

Source: Nieuwenhuijsen *et al.* (1994, 1995*b*).

Table 5.2 Frequency, duration, and level of exposure to inhalable dust and FA for various tasks of flour millers

	Frequency	duration	GM dust $(mg\,m^{-3})$	GM FA $(\mu g\,m^{-3})$
Flour millers				
Tipping additives *gluten, amylase, vitamix	1/day	20 min	8.8	63.6
Spillage/chokes cleaning	variable	variable	39.3	3807.9
Cleaning sifters	1/month	4 h	28.5	236.7
Cleaning floor	1/day	30 min	12.9	234.4
Cleaning dust collectors	1/month	4 h	34	1149.3

Source: Nieuwenhuijsen *et al.* (1995*b*).

In the bakeries and flour mills no correlation existed between duration of exposure and intensity indices of exposure (peak and average) for both dust and FA, suggesting that these can be used as independent exposure indices in the epidemiological analysis (Table 5.3) (Nieuwenhuijsen *et al.* 1995*a*). Moderate to good correlation existed between the various intensity measures of exposure for both dust and FA. Good correlations

Table 5.3   Spearman correlation coefficients (r_s) between various measures of flour exposure in a population with occupational exposure to flour in bakeries, flour mills, and flour packing stations

	Average dust level	Average allergen level	Cumulative dust exposure	Cumulative allergen exposure	Peak dust exposure	Peak allergen exposure
Exposure duration	0.05	0.07	0.59	0.64	−0.05	−0.07
Average dust level		0.86	0.73	0.60	0.73	0.73
Average allergen level			0.68	0.65	0.57	0.66
Cumulative dust exposure				0.93	0.46	0.49
Cumulative allergen exposure					0.39	0.47
Peak dust exposure						0.87

Source: Nieuwenhuijsen *et al.* (1995).

existed between measures of exposure to dust and measures of exposure to FA. Since the exposure variables were fairly well correlated, only full-shift dust measurements were used in the epidemiological analysis (Cullinan *et al.* 1994, 2001).

5.5   Active or passive sampling

To take personal airborne samples, equipment is needed that is light enough to be carried around without undue inconvenience to the subject and that will not significantly alter their usual behaviour patterns. The sampler should be placed such that it takes a sample of the inhaled air of the subject, often referred to as the breathing zone (within around 30 cm of the nose and mouth). Both active and passive samplers are available for this purpose.

For active sampling, air is drawn by a sampling pump through a collection unit, a sampling head with a filter inside for particulate matter or a Tenax tube for VOCs. The sampling flow rate is dependent on the requirements of the collection unit and may vary from less than 100 ml min^{-1} for VOC sampling to over 4 l min^{-1} or more for particulate matter sampling. The exposure concentration in air is determined by dividing the difference in the measured amount of the substance before and after the sampling period (e.g. for particulate matter, the weight on the filter before and after sampling is adjusted for blanks), by the volume of air (in m^3) drawn through the collection unit. The volume of air is the duration of air multiplied by the flow rate. Active sampling is generally used in workplace sampling, partly because of the relatively short sampling duration (up to 8 h per day).

Passive sampling is based on the principle of diffusion and does not require a sampling pump. It is widely used for gaseous substances, such as NO_2. Passive samplers for particulates are in the design stage (Brown *et al.* 1994). A problem in sampling environmental pollutants using passive samplers is that the concentration of pollutants present are often low, relative to the detection limits of the samplers. This implies the need for relatively long sampling durations and means that the samplers typically provide measures of long-term average concentrations only (e.g. over a week or longer period). There are also problems of accuracy and precision. On the other hand, passive sampling is generally less labour intensive and less costly than active sampling. This provides the possibility of taking more measurements for the same cost and of carrying out relatively intense spatial and temporal sampling (e.g. for use of estimating variance components). Recent advances in the design of passive samplers, the application of strict sampling protocols (including repeat measurements at each site), and the use of validation studies comparing passive samplers with more conventional methods, all offer scope to improve the performance of passive sampling.

Nitrogen dioxide is one of the substances where personal monitoring is used in exposure assessment for environmental epidemiological studies (Magnus *et al.* 1998; Krämer *et al.* 2000). This is partly due to its potential adverse health effects and its use as a marker for combustion-related, including traffic-related, pollutants. NO_2 is an air pollutant generated mainly by combustion. It occurs both in homes, primarily from gas stoves or heaters, and in outdoor environments, primarily as a result of emission from road vehicles. It is also relatively cheap and easy to monitor, using passive samplers such as the Palmes tube (Palmes *et al.* 1976) or the Willems badge (van Reeuwijk *et al.* 1998). NO_2 is absorbed on metal grids, coated with triethanolamine, and then extracted with sulponic acid and NEDA, which produces a coloured product that can be analysed in a photometer.

Krämer *et al.* (2000) measured outdoor ambient levels of NO_2 and personal exposure to NO_2 with Palmes tubes. They estimated personal exposure to NO_2 with a micro-environment model for an epidemiological study of children. Personal exposure levels to NO_2 (22–27 $\mu g\,m^{-3}$) were less than half the outdoor ambient levels of NO_2 (44–62 $\mu g\,m^{-3}$). There was only a weak correlation between personal and outdoor levels ($r = 0.37$), suggesting that outdoor levels were not a good indicator for personal exposure levels. Outdoor levels of NO_2 correlated stronger with the amount of traffic ($r = 0.7$) compared to personal exposure levels, suggesting that personal samples also included sources other than traffic. The correlation between personal exposure to NO_2 with Palmes tubes and estimated personal exposure to NO_2 with a micro-environment model was good ($r = 0.7$). Outdoor NO_2 levels were a stronger predictor of respiratory disease than personal NO_2 levels, perhaps because it was a better marker for traffic-related air pollution. Magnus *et al.* (1998) measured personal exposure to NO_2 with Palmes diffusion tubes and NO_2 levels in indoor (kitchen, sleeping room, and living room) and outdoor environments for a case–control study of bronchial obstruction in children. Outdoor levels (25.3 $\mu g\,m^{-3}$) were higher than personal (15.5 $\mu g\,m^{-3}$) or indoor levels (13.2–14.9 $\mu g\,m^{-3}$). There was weak correlation between personal and outdoor levels ($r = 0.36$), but stronger correlation between personal and indoor levels (e.g. living room $r = 0.52$, kitchen $r = 0.77$, sleeping room $r = 0.74$). The study found no association between exposure to NO_2 and the development of bronchial obstruction.

5.6   Continuous or average sampling

Depending on the collection unit used, exposure measurements can take the form either of continuous readings or an average over the sampling period. Continuous measurements are provided by direct reading instruments, such as the MINIRAM, TSI DustTrak ($PM_{2.5}$), TSI P-Trak (ultrafine), and GRIMM monitor for particulate sampling and the Langan CO Enhanced Measurer T15 monitor for CO (Fig. 5.1) (ACGIH 2001). They can be useful for the study of acute health effects. Wegman *et al.* (1992) used the MINIRAM to successfully examine the acute effects of dust in an occupational epidemiological study. Magari *et al.* (2002) measured continuous exposure to $PM_{2.5}$ with a TSI Inc. DustTrak to determine the relation between personal exposure to $PM_{2.5}$ and heart rate variability in 20 relatively young healthy male workers. The arithmetic mean $PM_{2.5}$ concentration over a 24-h period was 150 $\mu g\, m^{-3}$ (SD = 292 $\mu g\, m^{-3}$). As expected, smokers had a higher mean $PM_{2.5}$ than non-smokers with an arithmetic mean of 216 $\mu g\, m^{-3}$ (SD = 404 $\mu g\, m^{-3}$) compared to 96 $\mu g\, m^{-3}$ (SD = 158 $\mu g\, m^{-3}$) in non-smokers. The authors used 3-h $PM_{2.5}$ moving averages and found an association between $PM_{2.5}$ exposure and cardiac autonomic function.

Information from direct reading instruments can be stored in data loggers and downloaded to a computer, where they can be graphed and analysed. Although direct reading instruments can provide a very informative picture of the variation in exposure over the sampling period, their usage for epidemiological studies is relatively rare. The instruments

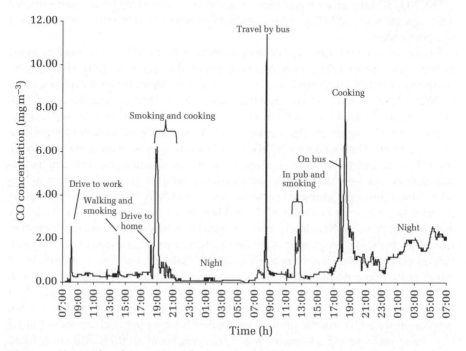

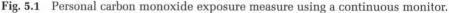

Fig. 5.1   Personal carbon monoxide exposure measure using a continuous monitor.

are often expensive, they are sometimes not very specific and accurate calibration is of considerable importance. Also, in case of chronic disease, short-term variations in exposure may not be considered important. More commonly monitoring is aimed at providing estimates of average concentrations over a measurement period, for example, a work shift (approximately 8 h), a day, or a few days. Only one concentration value is obtained per measurement period. As noted earlier, time-averaged data of this type are provided by both passive and active monitors.

5.7 Size-selective sampling

Over the years epidemiological studies have examined the health effects of airborne particulates. The health hazard from airborne particulates varies with its nature: physical, chemical, toxicological, and/or biological properties. An important property is the aerodynamic diameter, which determines how deeply the particle is likely to penetrate into the respiratory system. Particles have thus been categorized according to the region they are likely to reach in the respiratory system; to measure different size fractions, a personal sampler with different sampling heads is needed (ACGIH 2001). The inhalable particle fraction is the fraction that enters the nose and the mouth and has a 50 per cent cut point diameter of 100 μm. For example, an IOM sampler can be used to measure this at a flow rate of 2 1 min^{-1} (Mark and Vincent 1986). (Other samplers are discussed in Kenny *et al.* 1997.) This fraction is often measured in the workplace, but rarely in the general environment (ACGIH 2001). The thoracic fraction is the fraction that enters the thorax and has a 50 per cent cut point diameter of 10 μm; it is therefore referred to as PM$_{10}$. The PM$_{10}$ is often measured in the general environment, but rarely in the workplace. To measure this fraction, a special PM$_{10}$ sampling head is required, the most frequently used to date is the Harvard Impactor designed by Buckley *et al.* (1991), which runs at an airflow rate of 4 1 min^{-1}. The respirable fraction is the fraction that enters the lungs (the alveolar region). This has a 50 per cent cut point diameter of 4 μm and can be measured with special cyclones. PM$_{2.5}$, particles with a 50 per cent cut-off diameter of 2.5 μm, is the fraction that penetrates deep into the alveolar region. In environmental studies, cyclones are also used to measure this fraction, for example, the GK2.05 cyclone, which runs at 4 1 min^{-1}, is designed specifically for the EXPOLIS study (Jantunen *et al.* 1998). Among the new integrated methods to measure personal and micro-environmental air pollutant concentrations is the multi-pollutant sampler, which was developed to allow personal particulate and gaseous exposures to be measured simultaneously over 24-h periods (Chang *et al.* 1999). In its most complete form, the multi-pollutant sampler can be used to measure personal exposures and micro-environmental concentrations of PM$_{10}$, PM$_{2.5}$, the particle components elemental carbon (EC), organic carbon (OC), sulfate (SO$_4^{2-}$), nitrate (NO$_3^-$), and the elements, and also the gases ozone (O$_3$), sulphur dioxide (SO$_2$) and NO$_2$ simultaneously (see Chapter 14 for more details). A personal cascade impactor such as the eight-stage Sierra Marple 298 separates particulate matter by aerodynamic diameter and can be used to estimate the particle size distribution during the entire monitoring period, but tends to require higher particulate matter concentrations to collect enough matter on the different stages (Marple *et al.* 1987; Sandiford *et al.* 1994). This impactor was used in the study of occupational

Table 5.4   Particle size distribution by mass (%) in bakeries and flour mills taken with an eight-stage personal cascade impactor

50% Cut off diameter (μm)	Packing area		Dough brake	
	Dust	FA	Dust	FA
21.3	56.2	41.9	55.9	34.0
14.8	23.8	26.9	30.7	41.1
9.8	10.4	11.5	5.6	16.0
6.0	4.7	10.5	2.4	5.5
3.5	1.8	3.0	1.0	0.5
1.55	0.6	1.5	1.0	0.7
0.93	0.6	1.3	1.0	0.7
0.52	0.6	1.2	1.4	0.7
0.05	1.3	2.2	1.0	0.7

Source: Sandiford *et al.* (1994).

asthma mentioned earlier and most of the particles belonged to the extra thoracic fraction (Table 5.4).

5.8   Further laboratory analysis

Particulate mass and size are not the only important factors in the development of adverse health effects, the composition of particulates is also important. It is therefore useful to analyse particulate samples for their biological and elemental composition. A range of techniques are available for further analysis, including X-ray fluorescence (XRF), inductively coupled plasma-mass spectrometry (ICP-MS), gas chromatography-mass spectrometry (GC-MS), GC-FID, GFAAS, immuno-assays, electron scanning microscopy, or reflectance methods. Further information on these techniques can be found in, analytical chemistry books. Results for immuno-assays to measure FA are given in Tables 5.1–5.4.

5.9   Relationship between ambient and personal measurements

In environmental epidemiology, in contrast to occupational epidemiology, stationary ambient air pollution levels are often used as an exposure index rather than personal exposure measurements. How good a marker are ambient levels for personal exposure? Some of this can be illustrated by results from a study of personal exposure of children and adults in the Netherlands, conducted by Janssen (1998). She took repeated personal measurements of PM_{10} and fine particulates (FPs) (50% cut point approx. 3 μm) and compared these with measurements obtained by stationary ambient monitoring. As

Table 5.5 Average levels of personal and outdoor concentrations, and the correlation between personal and outdoor concentrations in Dutch children and adults (after Janssen 1998)

Population	Size fraction	n	Mean personal* ($\mu g\,m^{-3}$)	Mean ambient* ($\mu g\,m^{-3}$)	Median individual correlation	Cross-sectional correlation**
All subjects						
Adults	PM_{10}	37	62	42	0.5	0.34
Children	PM_{10}	45	105	39	0.63	0.28
Children	FP	13	28	17	0.86	0.41
Non-ETS exposed						
Adults	PM_{10}	23	51	41	0.71	0.50
Children	PM_{10}	25	89	40	0.73	0.49
Children	FP	9	23	18	0.92	0.84

* Mean of individual averages.
** Estimated cross-sectional R, by randomly selecting one measurement per subject.

expected, PM_{10} exposure levels were higher than FP levels (Table 5.5). Children had higher PM_{10} exposure levels than adults, mainly due to high concentrations in classrooms of coarse particles and/or suspension of soil material, caused by the activity of the children. Personal particulate exposure levels were higher than ambient exposure levels, as has often been observed, except perhaps in cases where the ambient exposure levels are very high (Wallace 1996). Higher personal PM_{10} exposure levels have commonly been attributed to the 'personal dust cloud', which is generally not observed with finer particulates (Wallace 1996). The results also showed that personal particulate exposure levels were considerably lower in adults and children not exposed to environmental tobacco smoke (ETS) than for the population as a whole; this confirms that ETS is one of the main sources of indoor air particulate exposure (Wallace 1996).

Janssen (1998) observed that the correlation was low between personal particulate exposure levels and outdoor fixed-point exposure measurements in the whole population when only one personal and one fixed-point outdoor exposure measurement was used for each subject. The correlation was considerably higher, however, for people not exposed to ETS, especially for FPs. Using repeated measurements of personal and fixed-point outdoor exposure measurements for each subject increased the correlation, in particular for subjects not exposed to ETS and for FPs. The median of the individual correlation coefficients was 0.9. This suggests that stationary ambient outdoor monitors might be a good indicator of personal exposure to FPs in epidemiological time-series studies that involve linking day-to-day variation in particulate exposure levels to day-to-day variation in health end points. The moderate to high correlation between repeated personal and stationary ambient outdoor measurements can be explained by the exclusion of 'fixed' indoor air particulate sources such as smoking and gas cookers, which are likely to change little from day-to-day compared to outdoor levels. Similar studies have been carried out for gasses such NO_2, and differences have been observed due to the physical and chemical nature of the substance (Magnus *et al.* 1998; Krämer *et al.* 2000) (see Section 5.5). In Chapter 14, there is a more detailed discussion of the various issues in personal exposure assessment of particulate matter in the general environment.

5.10   Conclusions

Personal monitoring is inevitably labour intensive and expensive. It is nevertheless a valuable technique, for it can dramatically improve exposure assessment in epidemiological studies, and thereby add to the scientific credibility of the studies. Intuitively, personal monitoring should provide more accurate exposure estimates than other methods. As has been shown, however, this is highly dependent on the quality and rigour of sampling, the putative agent, and the variability in exposure levels in the study population. Good exposure assessment thus requires careful design of personal monitoring campaigns. Estimates of average exposure levels also provide only one perspective on exposures; equally important are the sources and pathways of exposure and the distribution of variability in exposure levels (see Chapter 6). In many cases, an understanding of the major determinants of exposure can be as informative as measures of the exposure levels themselves.

More information on personal monitoring can be found elsewhere (National Research Council 1991; Keith 1996; Nieuwenhuijsen 1997, 2000; ACGIH 2001).

References

ACGIH (2001). *Air sampling instruments* (9th edn). ACGIH, Cincinnati, OH.

Brown, R. C., Wake, D., Thorpe, A., Hemingway, M. A., and Roff, M. W. (1994). Preliminary assessment of a device for passive sampling of airborne particulate. *Annals of Occupational Hygiene*, **38**, 303–18.

Buckley, T. J., Waldman, J. M., Freeman, N. C. G., Lioy, P. J., Marple, V. A., and Turner, W. A. (1991). Calibration, intersampler comparison and field application of a new PM-10 personal air sampling impactor. *Aerosol Science and Technology*, **14**, 380–7.

Burstyn, I., Kromhout, H., Kauppinen, T., Heikkilä, P., and Boffetta, P. (2000). Statistical modeling of the determinants of historical exposure to bitumen and polycyclic aromatic hydrocarbons among paving workers. *Annals of Occupational Hygiene*, **44**, 43–56.

Chang, L.-T., Sarnat, J., Wolfson, J. M., Rojas-Bracho, L., Suh, H. H., and Koutrakis, P. (1999). Development of a personal multi-pollutant exposure sampler for particulate matter and criteria Gases. *Pollution Atmosphérique*, **10**, 31–9.

Cullinan, P., Lowson, D., Nieuwenhuijsen, M. J., Sandiford, C., Tee, R. D., Venables, K. M., McDonald, J. C., and Newman Taylor, A. J. (1994). Work related symptoms, sensitisation and estimated exposure in workers not previously exposed to flour. *Occupational and Environmental Medicine*, **51**, 579–83.

Cullinan, P., Cook, A., Nieuwenhuijsen, M. J., Sandiford, C., Tee, R., Venables, K., McDonald, J. C., and Newman Taylor, A. J. (2001). Allergen and dust exposure as determinants of work-related symptoms in a cohort of flour-exposed workers; a case-control analysis. *Annals of Occupational Hygiene*, **45**, 97–103.

Coenen, W. (1976). Beschreibung des zeitlichen verhaltens von schadtstoffkonzentrationen durch einen stetigen Markow-process. *Staub-Reinhalt Luft*, **31**, 16–23.

Hornung, R. W., Greife, A. L., Stayner, L. T., Steenland, N. K., Herrick, R. F., Elliott, L. J., Ringenburg, V. L., and Morawetz, J. (1994). Statistical model for prediction to ethylene oxide in an occupational mortality study. *American Journal of Industrial Medicine*, **125**, 825–36.

Janssen, N. (1998). *Personal exposure to airborne particles. Validity of outdoor concentrations as a measure of exposure in time series studies.* PhD Thesis, Wageningen Agricultural University.

Jantunen, M. J., Hanninen, O., Katsounyanni, K., Knoppel, H., Kuenzli, N., Lebret, E., Maroni, M., Saarela, K., Sram, R., and Zmirou, D. (1998). Air pollution in European cities: the EXPO-LIS study. *Journal of Exposure Analysis and Environmental Epidemiology*, **8**, 495–518.

Keith, L. H. (1996). *Principles of environmental sampling* (2nd edn). American Chemical Society, Washington, DC.

Kenny, L. C., Aitken, R., Chalmers, C., Fabries, J. F., Gonzalez-Fernandez, E., Kromhout, H., Liden, G., Mark, D., Riediger, G., and Prodi, V. (1997). A collaborative European study of personal inhalable aerosol sampler performance. *Annals of Occupational Hygiene*, **41**, 135–53.

Kromhout, H. and Heederik, D. (1995). Occupational epidemiology in the rubber industry; implications of exposure variability. *American Journal of Industrial Medicine*, **27**, 171–85.

Kromhout, H., Tielemans, E., Preller, L., and Heedrik, D. (1996). Estimates of individual dose from current measurements of exposure. *Occupational Hygiene*, **3**, 23–9.

Krämer, U., Koch, T., Ranft, U., Ring, J., and Behrendt, H. (2000). Traffic-related air pollution is associated with atopy in children living in urban areas. *Epidemiology*, **11**, 64–70.

LeClare, P. C., Breslin, A. J., and Ong, L. D. Y. (1969). Factors affecting the accuracy of average dust concentration measurements. *American Industrial Hygiene Association Journal*, **30**, 386–93.

Liljelind, I. E., Rappaport, S. M., Levin, J. O., Stromback, A. E., Sunesson, A. L., and Jarvholm, B. G. (2001). Comparison of self-assessment and expert assessment of occupational exposure to chemicals. *Scandinavian Journal of Work, Environment and Health*, **27**, 311–17.

Liu, K., Stamler, J. A., Dyer, A., McKeever, J., and McKeever, P. (1978). Statistical methods to assess and minimize the role of intra individual variability in obscuring the relationship between dietary lipids and serum cholesterol. *Journal of Chronic Disease*, **31**, 399–418.

Loomis, D. P., Kromhout, H., Peipins, L. A., Kleckner, R. C., Iriye, R., and Savitz, D. A. (1994). Sampling design and field methods of a large randomized, multisite survey of occupational magnetic field study. *Applied Occupational and Environmental Hygiene*, **9**, 49–56.

Magari, S. R., Schwartz, J., Williams, P. L., Hauser, R., Smith, T. J., and Christiani, D. C. (2002). The association between personal measurements of environmental exposure to particulates and heart rate variability. *Epidemiology*, **13**, 305–10.

Magnus, P., Nafstad, P., Øie, L., Lødrup Carlsen, K. C., Becher, G., Kongerud, J., Carlsen, K.-H., Ove Samuelsen, S., Botten, G., and Bakketeig, L. S. (1998). Exposure to nitrogen dioxide and the occurrence of bronchial obstruction in children below 2 years. *International Journal of Epidemiology*, **27**, 995–9.

Mark, D. and Vincent, J. H. (1986). A new personal sampler for airborne total dust in workplaces. *Annals of Occupational Hygiene*, **30**, 89–102.

Marple, V. A., Rubow, K. L., Turner, W., and Sprengler, J. D. (1987). Low flow rate sharp cut impactors for indoor air sampling design and calibration. *Journal of the Air Pollution Control Association*, **37**, 1303–7.

National Research Council (1991). *Human exposure assessment for airborne pollutants. Advances and opportunities.* National Academy of Sciences, Washington, DC.

Nieuwenhuijsen, M. J. (1997). Exposure assessment in occupational epidemiology: measuring present exposures with an example of occupational asthma. *International Archives of Occupational and Environmental Health*, **70**, 295–308.

Nieuwenhuijsen, M. J. (2000). Personal exposure monitoring in environmental epidemiology. In *Disease and exposure mapping* (ed. P. Elliott, J. Wakefield, N. Best, and D. Briggs), pp. 360–74. Oxford University Press, Oxford.

Nieuwenhuijsen, M. J., Sandiford, C., Lowson, D., Tee, R. D., Venables, K. M., McDonald, J. C., and Newman Taylor, A. J. (1994). Dust and flour aeroallergen in flour mills and bakeries. *Occupational and Environmental Medicine*, **51**, 584–8.

Nieuwenhuijsen, M. J., Lowson, D., Venables, K. M., and Newman Taylor, A. J. (1995*a*). Correlation between different measures of exposure in a cohort of bakery workers and flour millers. *Annals of Occupational Hygiene*, **39**, 291–8.

Nieuwenhuijsen, M. J., Sandiford, C. P., Lowson, D., Tee, R. D., Venables, K. M., McDonald, J. C., and Newman Taylor, A. J. (1995*b*). Peak exposure levels for dust and flour aeroallergen in flour mills and bakeries. *Annals of Occupational Hygiene*, **39**, 193–201.

Palmes, E. D., Gunnison, A. F., Dimattio, J., and Tomczyk, C. (1976). Personal sampler for nitrogen dioxide. *American Industrial Hygiene Association Journal*, **37**, 570–7.

Preller, L., Kromhout, H., Heederik, D., and Tielen, M. J. (1995). Modeling long-term average exposure in occupational exposure-response analysis. *Scandinavian Journal of Work, Environment and Health*, **21**, 504–12.

Sandiford, C. P., Nieuwenhuijsen, M. J., Tee, R. D., and Newman Taylor, A. J. (1994). Determination of the size of airborne flour particles. *Allergy*, **12**, 891–3.

van Reeuwijk, H., Fischer, P. H., Harssema, H., Briggs, D. J., Smallbone, K., and Lebret, E. (1998). Field comparison of two NO_2 passive samplers to assess spatial variation. *Environmental Monitoring and Assessment*, **50**, 37–51.

Wallace, L. (1996). Indoor particles: a review. *Journal of the Air and Waste Management Association*, **46**, 98–126.

Wegman, D. H., Eisen, E. A., Woskie, S. R., and Hu, X. (1992). Measuring exposure for the epidemiologic study of acute effects. *American Journal of Industrial Medicine*, **21**.

6. Analysis and modelling of personal exposure

Alex Burdorf

6.1 Introduction

In the past decade personal exposure measurements have been increasingly used in epidemiological studies. Measuring exposures of individuals may render objective and quantitative results, but it is also expensive. These desirable features are generally thought to be superior to questionnaires and semi-quantitative approaches in every situation they are applied. However, there is growing evidence that the validity of measurement methods depends on circumstances particular to each epidemiological study.

In general, measurements of personal exposure are made for two main purposes: (1) assessment of current exposure levels in cross–sectional and cohort studies to be used in exposure–response relationships, and (2) estimation of past exposure levels in cross-sectional, retrospective cohort, and case-referent studies (Armstrong *et al.* 1992). For the first purpose, the best approach would be to obtain information for each subject on his exposure distribution over a sufficient period of time, for example, in an occupational setting, with measurements taken during a series of tasks in workplaces representative of his job. In most studies this approach can only be approximated by reducing the number of samples over time and over groups of persons. Thus, decisions have to be made about how to best allocate the available number of measurements on subjects and situations to be monitored. In Chapter 5, the basic considerations in designing a measurement strategy have been discussed.

For the second purpose, the strategy is complicated by the fact that exposure measurements have to be linked with information from the past, comprising, for example, time-dependent aspects (i.e. duration of exposure, time trends in exposure levels), environmental factors, and characteristics of workplaces and jobs in the past. This requires a linkage of practical tools, such as questionnaires, company records, or walk-through surveys, with quantitative exposure measurements. This approach requires knowledge about the important (historical) determinants of exposure and, subsequently, exposure models may be developed to predict (historical) personal exposure levels over time.

In both approaches exposure will always vary to some extent, due to differences in environmental factors, lifestyle, work conditions, and personal work techniques. This phenomenon of variability of exposure over time and among persons needs to be understood, since it affects the basic elements of any measurement strategy. Similarities in environmental conditions, work environments, job tasks, and identifiable exposures may not always be sufficiently large to assign subjects to exposure groups. This chapter will primarily focus on statistical methods that evaluate the impact of exposure variability on the exposure estimates to be used in epidemiological studies. The consequences of exposure variability on non-differential misclassification of subjects with respect to exposure and systematically incorrect estimation of exposure levels will be dealt with in detail in Chapter 12.

This chapter starts with a detailed description of statistical methods that are commonly used to evaluate assumptions on exposure variability and determinants. Examples are presented in which modelling of exposure was used to predict personal exposure in current and past situations. These examples are taken mainly from airborne agents in the occupational environment, but the principles are applicable to all sorts of physical, chemical, and biological contaminants in different compartments (air, soil, water) in the general and work environments, as well as in personal environment, and other various environmental levels.

6.2 Analysis of exposure variability

6.2.1 Estimation of variance components

Analysis of variance

In most measurement strategies, sampling of both subjects and exposure time is undertaken. A common approach is to predefine exposure strata (i.e. exposure groups) with assumed homogeneous exposure patterns. Stratification criteria may vary, for example, in occupational epidemiology these are often limited to job title and worksite. In environmental studies stratification criteria are used, such as random sampling that is performed within these strata with subjects chosen at random from all available subjects in each stratum, and sampling periods chosen at random from the total exposure duration of subjects to be monitored. This measurement strategy is generally affected by three principal sources of variability: between-group variance (do *a priori* defined groups really differ?), between-subject variance (are subjects *a priori* assigned to a homogeneous exposure group really similar?), and within-subject variance (do repeated samples on an individual show similar exposure levels?).

These variance components (Fig. 6.1) may be estimated by analysis of variance (ANOVA) techniques. ANOVA is useful for analysing the influence of classification variables, known as independent variables, on a continuous response variable, know as the dependent variable. In order to use an ANOVA, three basic assumptions have to be tested:

(1) *Variables are randomly selected*: Non-randomness of sample selection may result in dependency of exposure variables, heterogeneity of variances, or non-normal distributions (Sokal and Rohlf 1981).

(2) *Variables and error terms are normally distributed*: This is a basic assumption for many statistical techniques and evaluation of this assumption may reveal outliers or skewed distributions. Occupational and environmental exposure distributions are often lognormally distributed, hence, a logarithmic transformation may be required to obtain a normal distribution. In general, ANOVA is quite robust for non-normality of error terms and only very skewed distributions will have a marked effect (Sokal and Rohlf 1981).

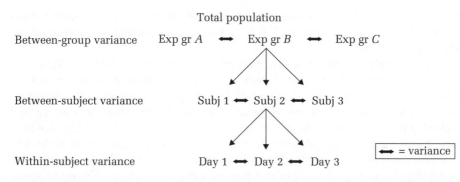

Fig. 6.1 Example of variance components in a study population. In the figure: Between-group variance, exposure variation due to differences in exposure levels between groups; Between-subject variance, exposure variation due to differences in exposure levels between subjects; Within-subject variance, exposure variation due to, for example, day-to-day variability in exposure within subjects; Exp gr, exposure group; and Subj, subject.

(3) *Variables have equal variances*: ANOVA can tolerate deviations from the equal variance assumption without introducing substantial flaws in the results, particularly when the data is balanced (i.e. equal numbers of observation for every combination of the classification variables). Differences in residual variances within groups up to a factor of 3–4 seem acceptable (Glantz and Slinker 1990). In occupational and environmental measurements heterogeneity may be introduced by large differences in duration of measurements in the groups monitored.

In ANOVA techniques, the variation in the response variable (e.g. exposure level) is separated into variations due to the classification variables (e.g. workers and factories) and variation due to random error. The random error includes the measurement error due to the coefficient of variation associated with the measurement technique. ANOVA models can be distinguished as random and fixed effect. Let us assume a survey on asbestos exposure in three factories with six measurements on fibre concentration in each factory. In a fixed-effect model the differences between the categories of the classification variable (e.g. three factories were specifically selected to reflect differences in technological development) are assumed to be fixed and repeatable. The purpose of the analysis is to estimate true differences between the average concentrations of fibres in the three selected factories. If there is a significant effect among the factories, then multiple comparison tests may be conducted to determine which factories differ from each other. In a random-effect model the factories are considered to be a random sample from all factories with asbestos exposure. The purpose of the analysis is to test whether the variance within each factory (the variance among the six samples) can (partly) explain the differences in average exposure among the three factories. In other words, the added variance due to the factories is estimated. The argument for selecting a fixed or a random model is not always obvious and sometimes a mixed-effect model may be preferred. This combines fixed and random effects into one model. Random-effect models are often applied to evaluate the impact of random exposure variability (interpreted as measurement error) on risk estimates in epidemiological studies. A mixed-effect model may be the best option when one is interested in predicting worker's exposure by production process, job title, or other exposure determinants (fixed effects), while accounting for the within-worker variability (random effect) (Burstyn *et al.* 1999).

A simple one-way ANOVA with random effects is presented in Table 6.1. Variable *A* has *k* classes and *n* is the number of observations per class; in the asbestos survey $k = 3$ and $n = 6$. To find the sum of squares (SS_e) among all 18 samples, the difference between each sample and the overall mean is calculated, these differences are squared and subsequently summed. The sum of squares (SS_a) among factories is calculated likewise by taking the mean difference between each factory and the overall mean. The *F*-statistics is used to test whether the variance of the means of factories is significantly larger than the average variance of observations within the factories. The mean square of error (MS_e) is an unbiased estimate of the residual variance (σ_e^2). The MS of variable *A* is an unbiased estimate of the variance due to the residual variance in each class (σ_e^2) and the added variance component due to differences among the classes of variable *A* ($n \times \sigma_a^2$). In the asbestos survey σ_e^2 is the within-factory variance and σ_a^2 is the between-factory variance.

A special case is the nested ANOVA. When measuring workers repeatedly in each factory it is obvious that differences may occur between- as well as within-workers. Differences within workers may result in observed differences among factories where in fact true differences among factories do not exist. The only way to separate the effects of variance between- and within-workers is to apply a nested model. In such a model the repeated measurements per worker are nested within each worker and the workers are nested within each factory. Nested effects can be looked upon as an interaction effect. The asbestos survey can be conducted by measuring in each factory ($k = 3$) three workers ($n = 3$) each twice ($q = 2$). The nested ANOVA with random effects is described in Table 6.2. Non-random selection of workers and monitoring periods can affect the

Table 6.1   An ANOVA random-effect model with balanced data

Source	Degrees of freedom	Mean square	*F*-value	E(MS)
Variable *A*	$k - 1$	$SS_a/(k-1)$	MS_a/MS_e	$\sigma_e^2 + n\,\sigma_a^2$
Error	$k(n-1)$	$SS_e/(k(n-1))$		σ_e^2
Total	$kn - 1$			

Table 6.2   A nested ANOVA random-effect model with balanced data

Source	Degrees of freedom	Mean square	*F*-value	E(MS)
Variable *A*	$k - 1$	$SS_a/(k-1)$	MS_a/MS_b	$\sigma_e^2 + q\sigma_b^2 + nq\,\sigma_a^2$
Variable *B* (in *A*)	$k(n-1)$	$SS_b/(k(n-1))$	MS_b/MS_e	$\sigma_e^2 + q\sigma_b^2$
Error	$kq(n-1)$	$SS_e/(kq(n-1))$		σ_e^2

variability of exposure and unequal variances across workers in the factory populations may violate the assumptions of the ANOVA model. Information on the magnitude of the variance components within-workers, between-workers, and between-factories can be used to optimize grouping of workers in epidemiological studies.

Exposure to inhalable flour dust

The application of the presented ANOVA models will be demonstrated with an example of characterization of exposure to inhalable flour dust in Swedish bakeries. In 12 bakeries, workers were monitored during their shift (Burdorf *et al.* 1994). The bakeries were randomly selected from all bakeries in Göteborg's environment. In all facilities workers were assigned *a priori* to an exposure group based on their principal task and, subsequently, measured during the execution of this task. All workers were assigned to one of the following *a priori* four exposure groups, distinguished according to the tasks:

(1) *Dough makers*: They tip flour and ingredients like solid fats, spices, yeast, bread improver, and salt in mixing machines, add water, and produce dough. These workers regularly handle flour, even when the production of dough is largely automated.

(2) *Bread formers*: They put pre-cut dough into baskets or on plates and handle machines for rolling out dough. Often some flour is scattered on work surfaces or in the baskets to prevent dough from sticking to it.

(3) *Oven workers*: The workers attending ovens and packing areas, and handling plates with ready-made products.

(4) *Packers*: These employees are involved in slicing, wrapping, and packing of the bakery products.

Concentrations of airborne inhalable flour dust in the breathing zones of workers were measured. In total, 111 personal measurements were conducted on 72 workers of which 77 samples were repeated measurements on 34 workers. Since all distributions differed significantly from the normal distribution, the data were log-transformed. The descriptive measures of exposure within the *a priori* exposure groups are presented in Table 6.3. There was a significant hierarchy in mean exposure of the groups; in descending order: dough makers, bread formers, oven workers, and packers. Within each group the measurements of worker's exposure to flour dust showed considerable

Table 6.3 Measurements of exposure to inhalable flour dust among bakery workers by task group (*n* is the number of measurements and *N* is the number of persons measured)

Task group	N	n	AM (mg m^{-3})	GM (mg m^{-3})	GSD	Range (mg m^{-3})
Dough makers	18	34	6.90	5.46	2.09	1.20–16.90
Bread formers	41	62	3.39	2.69	1.96	0.60–14.20
Oven workers	7	10	1.59	1.17	2.43	0.20–4.00
Packers	6	9	0.63	0.48	2.40	0.10–1.40

AM, arithmetic mean; GM, geometric mean; GSD, geometric standard deviation.

variation. The values of the GSDs within the task groups ranged from 1.96 to 2.43. These GSD values were smaller than the GSD in the total population (2.77), which indicates that the differences among workers within the groups were smaller than the differences among workers in the total population.

In order to investigate the homogeneity of each task group, one-way ANOVA with repeated measurements were conducted. If the between-worker variance is large compared with the within-worker variance, the workers are not uniformly exposed. The relative homogeneity of each task group can be expressed by the variance ratio λ, which is the ratio of the within-worker over the between-worker variance, estimated by $\sigma_{ww}^2/\sigma_{bw}^2$. Among the bread formers ($\lambda = 0.79$) and the packers ($\lambda = 1.09$) the within-worker variance almost equalled the between-worker variance, showing an important contribution of the within-worker variance to the total variability of exposure in these groups. Among the oven workers ($\lambda = 2.07$) the within-worker variance was markedly larger than the between-worker variance. The opposite pattern was found among the dough makers ($\lambda = 0.45$). The variance components may also be expressed by GSD values. The between-worker GSD_{bw} can be calculated by the equation $GSD_{bw} = \exp(\sigma_{bw})$. Since this parameter may be somewhat difficult to interpret, the use of the range ratio $R_{0.95}$ has been proposed. The range ratio is expressed by the ratio of the 97.5th percentile to the 2.5th percentile of the distribution of worker's mean exposure (Rappaport 1991). This ratio holds exactly the same information as the GSD_{bw} and is calculated by the equation $R_{0.95} = \exp(3.92 \times \sigma_{bw})$.

To investigate whether inhalable flour concentrations were determined by bakery characteristics and individual work techniques or by task groups, a nested analysis of variance was performed. While assuming only random effects, this technique allows the partitioning of the total variance among the measurements into its main components: between-group, between-worker, and within-worker variances. By varying the assignment of workers to specific exposure groups the optimum grouping strategy was evaluated. The optimum was defined as the classification into exposure groups that had the largest between-group variance. In Table 6.4 the total variability of exposure to

Table 6.4 Partitioning of the total variability in exposure to inhalable flour dust among bakery workers using different grouping strategies

	Grouping strategy					
	Strategy A		Strategy B		Strategy C	
Source of variance	σ^2	%	σ^2	%	σ^2	%
Between-group variance	0.69	61	0.71	61	2.25	69
Within-group variance	0.10	22	0.10	22	0.19	20
Within-worker variance	0.05	17	0.05	17	0.05	11

Grouping strategy A with four groups: dough makers, bread formers, oven workers, and packers. Grouping strategy B with three groups: dough makers, bread formers, oven workers + packers. Grouping strategy C with two groups: dough makers + bread formers vs. oven workers + packers. σ^2, estimated variance.

inhalable flour dust is partitioned into its different components using three alternative grouping strategies. The within-worker variance component was the same for all three grouping strategies, its contribution to the total variance varied from 11 to 17 per cent. The between-worker variance component was relatively constant over the three grouping strategies. Assignment of the oven workers and the packers to one or two exposure groups did not influence the exposure variability. For all grouping strategies the variance between task groups was the largest source of variance, ranging from 61 to 69 per cent (Burdorf *et al.* 1994). Thus, given the results of this exposure survey, a detailed questionnaire on occupational history, including tasks, may be sufficient for assessment of historical exposure patterns among all subjects under study.

6.2.2 Estimation of important determinants of exposure

Linear regression

In the previous section, ANOVA techniques have been described that focus on the analysis of factors determining the variability in exposure among individuals. An alternative approach is to use linear regression analysis to evaluate the influence of these factors on the actual measured personal exposure levels. A linear regression model enables the researcher to predict what exposure levels correspond to given values of determinants of exposure. Linear regression analysis with dichotomous variables can be considered as a specific type of ANOVA.

A mathematical expression of a linear regression model is described as:

$$\ln(C_{ij}) = \beta_0 + \beta_1 \text{var}_i + \beta_2 \text{var}_j,$$

whereby $\ln(C_{ij})$ is the natural logarithm of exposure concentration (Y), β_0 is the intercept, and β_1 and β_2 are regression coefficients of the independent variables (X). The intercept represents the exposure concentration when the independent variables equal zero. Hence, the intercept may be considered as the background exposure level. The regression coefficients represent the amount of change in the exposure level for each 1-unit change in the independent variables. For any given straight line, this rate of change is always constant. Independent variables may be expressed at a dichotomous level (e.g. presence or absence of local exhaust ventilation, indoor or outdoor activity) or interval level (e.g. hours spent on a specific task, time spent outdoors).

The mathematical expression becomes a statistical model, expressed in the form

$$\ln(C_{ij}) = \beta_0 + \beta_1 \text{var}_i + \beta_2 \text{var}_j + E,$$

whereby E denotes a random variable with mean 0, often called the error term. In this statistical model $\ln(C_{ij})$ is considered a random variable but in the mathematical expression $\ln(C_{ij})$ is fixed. The statistical model is used to analyse how well exposure determinants (known, fixed variables X) can predict the exposure level (Y) whereas the mathematical expression is used to assign exposure levels to subjects with unknown exposure levels, based on their time–activity, work and environmental and workplace characteristics. In the statistical model the independent variables are fixed, which is sometimes erroneously associated with the statement that these variables are measured without error. For making statistical inferences the practical implication of the statistical model is that error term E is the only random component on the right-hand side of the equation.

In order to use linear regression techniques there are five assumptions (Kleinbaum *et al.* 1988):

(1) For any value of the independent value X, Y is a random variable with a mean and variance: in other words, the mean and variance of the random variable Y depend on the value of X. Hence, changes in X are the cause of variations of Y.

(2) The Y-values are statistically independent of one other: this assumption may be violated when exposure levels are measured repeatedly on the same subject at different times. For example, if time–activity patterns of a particular subject partly determines his exposure it is to be expected that the exposure at one time would be related to the exposure at a later time.

(3) The mean value of Y is a linear function of X: this assumption specifies a straight-line function and non-linearity will contribute to the error term.

(4) The variance of Y is the same for any X: this assumption of equal variances is quite robust and some differences in variances seem acceptable.

(5) For any value of X, Y has a normal distribution: this is a basic assumption and for workplace and environmental measurements often a logarithmic transformation is required. If the normality assumption is not badly violated, the conclusions reached by a regression analysis will generally be reliable and accurate (Kleinbaum *et al.* 1988).

Procedures for selecting the best regression equation are based on goodness-of-fit tests, which closely resemble those used in ANOVA techniques. The differences between expected and observed values of Y contribute to the residual variance. The variance in Y, explained by X, is referred to as the explained variance, expressed by R^2 in percentage of the total variance. Standard techniques such as residual plots and outlier detection should be used to evaluate the models. For a more detailed review of regression techniques the reader is referred to statistical handbooks.

Exposure to endotoxins

The application of linear regression models will be illustrated by an example of the effect of farm characteristics on endotoxin concentrations among pig farmers (Preller *et al.* 1995). In the study among 198 Dutch pig farmers the effect of endotoxin exposure on lung function was evaluated. Exposure to inhalable dust containing endotoxins was determined by means of personal sampling. Measurements for 8 h were conducted for each participant during one shift in summer and one shift in winter. The farmers were requested to complete a diary on time spent in different activities during the day of measurement and the following 6 days. In addition, farm characteristics of all breeding compartments were registered during a walk-through survey. Information was recorded on number of animals, feeding methods, heating and ventilation, type of floor, bedding material, and degree of contamination. A linear regression model was fitted, based upon all factors that showed a significant influence on the endotoxin exposure.

Table 6.5 presents the overall results of the measurements, demonstrating a substantial variability in the concentration of endotoxins. The mean exposure in winter was significantly higher than in summer. In a linear regression model outdoor temperature, 12 farm characteristics, and 8 activities in pig farming explained about 37 per cent of the variation in log-transformed time-weighted average exposure to endotoxins. The intercept in the statistical model corresponded roughly to 80 $ng\,m^{-3}$ [exp(4.44)], indicating that the background endotoxin concentration in these pig farms was relatively

Table 6.5 Measurements of personal exposure to endotoxins among 198 pig farmers in the Netherlands (*n* is the number of measurements)

Season	*n*	AM (ng m^{-3})	GM (ng m^{-3})	GSD	Range (ng m^{-3})
Summer	182	111	78	2.4	5.6–825
Winter	168	150	109	2.3	10.6–1503
All	350	129	92	2.4	5.6–1503

AM, arithmetic mean; GM, geometric mean; GSD, geometric standard deviation.

high compared with the overall average concentration of 129 ng m^{-3}. The activities with the largest contribution to the predicted endotoxins exposure were teeth cutting ($\beta = 0.51$) and ear tagging ($\beta = 0.43$) and the most important farm characteristic was the presence of a convex floor ($\beta = -0.22$). Since a lognormal transformation was performed, the exposure level of teeth cutting is estimated to be 141.17 ng m^{-3} [exp(4.44 + 0.51)]. Since the regression model on log-transformed exposure data is multiplicative, the exposure among pig farmers involved in teeth cutting is a factor 1.67 [exp(0.51)] higher than those farmers not conducting this activity as part of their regular work.

6.2.3 Exposure variability and implications

Occurrence of exposure variability

It has been demonstrated that many occupational groups (i.e. job titles) are not uniformly exposed. In an evaluation of exposure patterns among 165 occupational groups, defined by job title and factory, it was illustrated that personal mean exposures within a group on average were within a 5-fold range. In fact, only 42 groups (25%) had 95 per cent of the individual mean exposures lying within a factor of 2, almost 30 per cent of the groups were over the 10-fold range, and 10 per cent of the groups showed a range of over 50-fold. In general, the within-worker variability exceeded the between-worker variability, suggesting larger differences in exposure among work shifts than among workers with the same job in the same factory. It was also shown that environmental and workplace factors had a clear impact on the within-worker variability, but less on the between-worker variability. The largest day-to-day variability was demonstrated among groups working outdoors, those working without local exhaust ventilation, groups with mobile workers, and groups working with intermittent processes (Kromhout *et al.* 1993). In the past 10 years the presence of exposure variability has been illustrated in many occupational groups described in various publications.

A classical illustration of exposure variability in environmental exposure is based on measurements of exposure to lead and nitrogen dioxide (NO_2). For lead on home floors (milligram lead in dust spot sample of 1 m^2) the within-room variance was substantially lower than the between-room variance ($\lambda = 0.39$). The measurements of personal exposure to NO_2 among mothers and children showed that the within-subject variance was also lower than the between-subject variance (λ of 0.33 and 0.44) (Brunekreef *et al.* 1987).

Exposure variability and exposure–response relationships

The consequences of exposure variability in epidemiological studies have primarily been explored in the context of their effects on the exposure–response relationship. In most research conditions a non-differential misclassification in exposure status (exposed vs. non-exposed) will result in an attenuation of the true association between exposure and response (see Chapter 12).

When exposure is characterized by a continuous variable, it has been demonstrated that in a study with measurements on all individuals the variance ratio λ (within-subject variance divided by between-subject variance) is directly linked to the attenuation in the observed risk estimate under the classical error model (Liu *et al.* 1978). Attenuation is expressed by the coefficient of reliability ρ_{xx} that can be approximated by the expression $1/(1 + \lambda)$. Hence, the accuracy of an exposure–response function depends on the degree to which the exposure assessment is successful in providing unbiased estimates of individual exposure levels. An illustration of the effect of exposure variability on attenuation of exposure–response relationships will be presented in Section 6.3.1.

An alternative approach, more common in epidemiologic surveys, is to monitor a random sample of subjects in each group under study. Subsequently, the average values of the parameters measured are used to characterize the exposure of the subjects within each group. An underlying assumption of this measurement strategy is that the mean exposure of the subjects sampled is supposed to be equal to the average of the whole group. In the analysis of an exposure–response relationship all subjects within the same group have been assigned the same exposure level. In general, in the grouping approach the attenuation is substantially less than in the individual approach, based on the Berkson error model (see Chapter 12), but confidence intervals are wider. Several authors have presented mathematical expressions for estimating group-based attenuation and have evaluated the effect of different grouping strategies on the observed association between exposure and health outcome (Van Tongeren *et al.* 1997; Werner and Attfield 2000). In the group approach the aim is to increase the contrast of exposure (ε) between exposure groups, expressed as the ratio between the between-group variance (σ_{bg}^2) and the sum of the between- and within-group (σ_{wg}^2) variance (i.e. $\varepsilon = (\sigma_{bg}^2)/(\sigma_{bg}^2 + (\sigma_{wg}^2)$, while maintaining reasonably precise exposure estimates of the exposure groups. The precision can be estimated as $1/\sqrt{(\sigma_{wg}^2/k + \sigma_{ws}^2/ kn)}$, where k is the number of subjects, kn the number of observations in each group, and σ_{ws}^2 the within-subject variance.

Choosing the best measure of exposure in epidemiological studies

Exposure variability may also have implications for the choice of the appropriate measure of exposure, since different measures may be associated with different patterns of exposure variability. A theoretically superior measure of exposure with expected high variability may be less attractive in an epidemiological study than a more proximal measure of exposure with less inherent variability. This point may be illustrated with the applicability of markers of exposure in biological monitoring. Although theoretical arguments may be in favour of biological monitoring, it has to be considered whether markers of exposure can be measured with higher accuracy than environmental agents. Few studies have been published on the utility of markers of exposure in relation to within- and between-subject variability in these markers. Hence, the choice between environmental exposure measurements and measurement of markers of exposure in human material partly depends on the variability in the parameter of interest.

The strengths and weaknesses of both measurement approaches were explored in a longitudinal study among boat workers exposed to styrene (Rappaport *et al.* 1995). The exposure assessment consisted of full-shift personal measurements of styrene exposure per worker carried out over 1 year on seven occasions. Sister chromatid exchanges (SCEs) were used as the marker of exposure, measured in lymphocytes from two venous blood samples per worker obtained during the measurement surveys. The correlation between styrene exposure and SCEs was low (11% explained variance). A variance ratio of 0.33 for styrene exposure was observed and of 2.21 for SCEs. If attenuation of the health risk estimates would be restricted to 10 per cent, 3 measurements per person would be required for airborne styrene exposure vs. 20 measurements per person for SCEs. The latter value would be impossible in epidemiological studies due to the invasive character of the technique and the associated costs. This study is but a mere illustration of the profound implications of variability in the measure of exposure for the design of an exposure assessment strategy in epidemiological studies.

6.2.4 Optimization of sampling strategies

In designing an efficient measurement strategy information is required on the expected variability in exposure among the subjects in the study population. General guidance has been presented in the literature on the potential effect of work process and workplace characteristics on the measurement strategy, based upon analysis of those factors that determine the variance components in occupational populations (see Section 6.2.3). As a rule of thumb, it is advised to increase the number of measurements with the following characteristics: working outdoors, intermittent process, no local exhaust ventilation, mobile worker, local sources, and manual tasks (Kromhout 2002). This information may not be specific enough, thus, a pilot study on exposure patterns and variance components may be required before deciding on the optimum sampling scheme for exposure measurements.

When enough information on exposure variability is available from other studies, mathematical equations can assist in the decisions on the most efficient measurement strategy. The appropriate number of measurements depends on the relative accuracy, study size, power, and significance level. Formulae have been presented to calculate the number of subjects in relation to the number of repeated measurements for each subject (Armstrong *et al.* 1992; White *et al.* 1994). These formulae combine the classical equations for determining the power of a study with the expressions for evaluating the influence of exposure variability on the precision of the average exposure. The efficiency of increasing the number of repeated measurements or, vice versa, increasing the number of subjects, is partly determined by the variance ratio (Phillips and Smith 1993). In addition, in most epidemiological studies cost considerations will become part of the discussion on the required efficiency of the sampling scheme (Lemasters *et al.* 1996).

For a more detailed discussion on sample size calculations and efficiency of measurement strategies the reader is referred to Chapter 12.

6.3   Predicting personal exposure

6.3.1   Modelling of determinants of exposure

Type of modelling

In all studies exposure data only cover a small proportion of the subjects and time periods to be assessed. It is sometimes feasible to apply modelling techniques in which unknown data are estimated by values derived from a prediction model fitted with the data from exposure surveys (on a subset of the population). Typically, such a model includes determinants of exposure, such as presence of ventilation, type of production process, residence characteristics, and time–activity patterns.

In a deterministic modelling approach exposure indices are calculated (conversion factors) based upon significant changes in exposure due to particular factors. In a mathematical expression these changes are regarded as fixed effects that raise or lower exposure levels among workers. Illustrations of the deterministic approach are presented in studies on historical exposure among painters (Fidler *et al.* 1987) and resin manufacture workers (Dosemeci *et al.* 1990). An interesting example is the reconstruction of historical exposure to man-made mineral fibres. Experiments were conducted to determine the effects on exposure of changes in product process (addition of oil), ventilation rate, and production rate. Conversion factors were derived for each of these modifications and applied to measured concentrations of fibres in recent periods. Subsequently, the history of engineering and process changes in the plant was used to assess historical trends in exposure among workers (Dodgson *et al.* 1987). The advantage of the deterministic approach is that it can be used when only few measurement data are available. It provides more consistent exposure estimates than other approaches and may be especially useful for describing historical trends in exposure (Kaupinnen 1994). However, this approach is most likely to be less accurate than more data-driven empirical modelling methods.

Empirical statistical modelling is perhaps the most comprehensive approach to exposure estimation but it requires a substantial amount of data (Seixas and Checkoway 1995). The common approach in statistical modelling is based on a simple linear regression model (see Section 6.2.2). These models can be refined to take into account dependence of repeated measurements of the same worker (Rappaport *et al.* 1999; Burstyn *et al.* 2000). One of the first applications of statistical modelling was in a mortality study among workers in an asbestos textile plant (Dement *et al.* 1983*a*). A detailed survey of plant processes and dust control methods over the period 1930–75 was conducted and linear statistical models were developed to reconstruct historic dust exposure levels, taking into account textile processes, dust control measures, and job assignments. Parameters of these statistical models were estimated using almost 6000 industrial hygiene sampling measurements covering the period 1930–75. The exposure estimates were combined with an assessment of mortality among workers at this plant to investigate exposure–response relationships (Dement *et al.* 1983*b*).

A clear drawback of these statistical models is the large amount of data required to develop a meaningful empirical model, especially when long-term trends over time are part of the modelling approach. In addition, models with limited predictive value for exposure have little use in the assessment of individual exposure. However, sometimes it may be worth the effort when various databases on measurements can be made available. Burstyn and colleagues were able to construct a large database on exposure among asphalt workers from 37 different sources in eight countries. This database enabled the researchers to present three models on the important determinants of exposure intensity of bitumen fume and vapour and polycyclic aromatic hydrocarbons (PAH) among paving workers. These statistical models explained 36–43 per cent of the total variability and revealed strong associations with various production factors, such as surface dressing, oil gravel paving, and asphalt temperature (Burstyn *et al.* 2000).

Another interesting statistical modelling approach was adopted in an analysis of factors that influence exposure to nitrogen oxides in the environment (Zipprich *et al.* 2002). Epidemiological studies that evaluate health effects associated with NO_x commonly rely upon outdoor concentrations of NO_x, NO_2 or residence characteristics as surrogates for personal exposure. In a study personal exposure over 48 h and corresponding indoor and outdoor concentrations of NO_x were measured for 48 subjects from 23 households. Demographic, time–activity patterns, and household data were collected by questionnaire and used to develop exposure prediction models. In a statistical model up to 70 per cent of the variation in personal NO_2 and NO_x exposure was explained by two variables (bedroom NO_2 and time spent in other indoor locations; bedroom NO_x and time spent in kitchen). These statistical models may reduce the measurement effort considerably in any epidemiological study, since the assessment strategy can largely rely on taking measurements of bedroom exposure to NO_2 and NO_x and on reporting of time–activity patterns in a diary or questionnaire (Zipprich *et al.* 2002).

Combining practical tools with exposure measurements

A prerequisite of the application of exposure modelling is that the information on potential determinants of exposure is readily available, for example, collected during a walk-through survey, from community or industry records, or by questionnaire. Particular fixed traits, such as residential characteristics, presence of ventilation, or job status, may be easily recorded without misclassification during field surveys with active monitoring programmes. In specific situations relevant information on frequency and duration of exposure may be retrieved from other records.

An example of the latter situation is an investigation on occupational cancer risks in pilots and flight attendants. Estimates of cumulative exposure were arrived at by combining company records on flight hours and transatlantic routes (altitude, latitude, travel route) of each individual worker with known levels of cosmic radiation at any latitude, altitude, and place at earth (Blettner *et al.* 1998).

In a study on residential exposure to pesticides and breast cancer GIS was used to estimate the relative intensity of past exposures at each study subject's addresses over the past 40 years, taking into account local meteorological data, distance, and direction from a residence to a pesticide use source area, size of the source area, application by ground-based or aerial methods, and persistent or non-persistent character of the pesticide applied. The resulting individual-level estimates of relative exposure intensity were used in conjunction with interview data to obtain more complete exposure assessment in the epidemiologic study (Brody *et al.* 2002).

Sometimes exposure models can be developed by linking practical tools to active monitoring of exposure. Studies on the association between exposures to airborne particulate matter (PM) and respiratory disease have shown that short-term peaks in PM exposures are critical to health effects. In a recent survey, magnitude and duration of peaks in PM exposures were measured by taking PM concentrations at 1-min time intervals for 1 week. A time-stamped voice recorder was used to document activity and location in real time. Although for each person patterns of PM exposure were remarkably consistent over the day, it was found that high PM levels occurred in relatively few of the minutes measured but comprised a substantial fraction of the total exposure. PM levels were significantly higher during subject-reported events including barbeque, yard work, being near pets or construction activities, cooking, and environmental tobacco smoke exposure, as compared to periods with no pollution events (Quintana *et al.* 2001). This analysis may be converted into an exposure prediction model to be applied to time–activity patterns determined by questionnaire.

In some studies individual assessments are arrived at by assessing the distribution of tasks among workers and exposure levels within separate tasks. Such an approach will be particularly fruitful in surveys with a limited number of tasks that dominate the exposure pattern. In one study on styrene exposure in fibreglass-reinforced polyester facilities, the long-term average exposure per worker was assessed by linking the average exposure during each work process with the frequency and duration of different work processes performed for several weeks as obtained from diaries filled out by each worker (Olsen 1994). In large epidemiological studies it may be very difficult to obtain reliable information on the time spent in each task for every individual in the study population. In addition, this approach is more suitable for frequently performed tasks since the exposure level of an individual task may be difficult to determine unless workers are monitored over various days. Disadvantages of a task-based strategy are that more tasks within a job title will increase the measurement error considerably and that a small error in estimated duration of a task with high exposure will have a profound impact on the overall estimated exposure and its associated variability.

Modelling of long-term exposure to endotoxins

An illustration of the application of modelling techniques within an epidemiological framework is the study by Preller *et al.* (1995). For each pig farmer the average endotoxin exposure was calculated based on two measurements over 8 h. A statistical model for predicting endotoxin exposure among pig farmers was constructed, as described in Section 2.2. Based on a self-administered two-week diary of daily activities, this model was subsequently used to predict long-term average exposure of each pig farmer in the study population (14 measurements). The relationship between baseline lung function (forced expiratory volume in 1 s—FEV_1) and measured and modelled endotoxin exposure was evaluated by means of a multiple linear regression analysis. The measured endotoxin exposure ($\beta = -0.03$, $p = 0.40$) did not show any relation with lung function decrease. However, when using the predicted long-term average exposure ($\beta = -0.21$, $p = 0.10$), there appeared to be a considerable decrease in lung function of about 210 ml when exposure to endotoxins (in $ng\,m^{-3}$) increased with a factor of 2.7. A larger effect ($\beta = -0.41$, $p = 0.03$) was seen among asymptomatic farmers with an estimated reduction of 410 ml in FEV_1 (Preller *et al.* 1995). The difference in health impact of measured and modelled endotoxins exposure was attributed to a strongly decreased within-worker variance for modelled exposure when compared with measured exposure. It was calculated that the variance ratio dropped from 4.7 to 1.2, which corresponded to an estimated attenuation of 70 and 8 per cent, respectively. Thus, it was concluded that the modelling approach offered the possibility to minimize the measurement effort in this epidemiological study without apparent loss of statistical power (Preller *et al.* 1995).

6.3.2   Validity of exposure prediction models

The application of prediction models for personal exposure is often legitimized by assumptions on improved accuracy in exposure estimates and less attenuation in exposure–response relationships. The validity needs to be investigated whenever possible.

A common validation method is to randomly split the available data into one set of measurements for model development and one set of measurements for model validation. The data for model development is used to identify the important determinants of exposure and to build a prediction model. Subsequently, this prediction model is used to predict a set of exposure estimates and these estimates are compared with the available measurements for model validation. The comparison may evaluate bias (average difference between the predicted and observed exposure) and precision (standard deviation of the differences) (Seixas and Checkoway 1995). An illustration of this validation method is given in a study on exposure assessment for acrylonitrile in fibre and resin companies. A deterministic modelling technique was used to predict exposure to acrylonitrile in 1977–8. For a given job-department-plant combination, this prediction was based on available measurements during 1980–3 and correction factors for major changes in process and work practice during 1977–83. Hence, more recent measurements were used to estimate more distant exposure levels. The estimates were compared with available full-shift measurements in the period 1977–8. The correlation between modelled exposure and measurements was moderate ($r = 0.6$), the bias was very small but the precision was also low (Stewart *et al.* 1998).

A slightly different validation method is one in which the prediction model is compared to measurement results from other surveys. An example of this validation method is described by Hornung *et al.* (1996). Within the framework of a mortality study among embalmers an experiment was conducted to measure the formaldehyde concentration in different combinations of ventilation rate, solution strength, and type of case. During the experiment several covariates beyond control were identified and made available for potential inclusion in the prediction model. The final prediction model involved only three terms: air exchange rate, type of case (autopsy vs. intact), and occurrence of a spill. This relatively simple model could explain 75 per cent of the variation in measured formaldehyde levels. This prediction model was compared with 15 independent measurements from other surveys. The overall accuracy showed that the estimated formaldehyde concentration was within a range obtained by multiplying and dividing the true exposure by 2.4. The validation was hampered by the fact that no information was available on occurrence of spills in the published data (Hornung *et al.* 1996).

An alternative approach in validation of exposure models is testing both the modelled exposure and the original measurements for their predictive value in the exposure–response model (Preller *et al.* 1995). The underlying assumption is that the highest effect estimate is closest to the true risk since attenuation by measurement error will be smallest. This approach does not constitute a real validation since attenuation is assumed but not proven. Nevertheless, changes in the risk estimate may provide indicative evidence as to the validity of the exposure model used (Seixas and Checkoway 1995).

A novel approach in evaluating the robustness of the exposure estimates is the bootstrap method. This method is not a formal validation technique but allows the researcher to evaluate the influence of sample size and exposure variability on the estimate of the average exposure. Bootstrapping is an empirical approach based on sampling with replacement among the measurements conducted. The sample is treated as the population by drawing randomly a large number of 'resamples' of size *n* from this original sample with replacement. This approach simulates empirically the random component of the average exposure; this technique inductively arrives at an estimate of the 'true' average exposure and its dispersion. The bootstrapping method does not require any assumption on the distribution of the data. For a practical account of this method, the reader is referred to Mooney and Duval (1993). Examples in the field of occupational and environmental exposure assessment are still somewhat difficult to find, but some good illustrations on the particular use of the bootstrap method can be found in studies on lifetime cumulative exposure to radon for California residents (Liu *et al.* 1993) and lifetime exposure to radium in drinking water (Finkelstein and Kreiger 1996).

References

Armstrong, B. G., White, E., and Saracci, R. (1992). *Principles of exposure measurement in epidemiology*. Oxford University Press, New York.

Blettner, M., Grosche, B., and Zeeb, H. (1998). Occupational cancer risk in pilots and flight attendants: current epidemiological knowledge. *Radiation and Environmental Biophysics*, **37**, 75–80.

Brody, J. G., Voruees, D. J., Melly, S. J. *et al.* (2002). Using GIS and historical records to reconstruct residential exposure to large-scale pesticide application. *J Expo Anal Environ Epidemiol*, **12**, 64–80.

Brunekreef, B., Noy, D., and Clausing, P. (1987). Variability of exposure measurements in environmental epidemiology. *American Journal of Epidemiology*, **125**, 892–8.

Burdorf, A., Lillienberg, L., and Brisman, J. (1994). Characterization of exposure to inhalable flour dust in Swedish bakeries. *Annals of Occupational Hygiene*, **38**, 67–78.

Burstyn, I. and Teschke, K. (1999). Studying the determinants of exposure: a review of methods. *American Industrial Hygiene Association Journal*, **60**, 57–72.

Burstyn, I., Kromhout, H., Kauppinen, T., *et al.* (2000). Statistical modelling of the determinants of historical exposure to bitumen and polycyclic aromatic hydrocarbons among paving workers. *Annals of Occupational Hygiene*, **44**, 43–56.

Dement, J. M., Harris, R. L. Jr, Symons, M. J., *et al.* (1983*a*). Exposures and mortality among chrysotile asbestos workers. Part I: exposure estimates. *American Journal of Industrial Medicine*, **4**, 399–419.

Dement, J. M., Harris, R. L. Jr, Symons, M. J., *et al.* (1983*b*). Exposures and mortality among chrysotile asbestos workers. Part II: mortality. *American Journal of Industrial Medicine*, **4**, 421–33.

Dosemeci, M., Stewart, P. A., and Blair, A. (1990). Three proposals for retrospective, semiquantitative exposure assessments and their comparison with the other assessment methods. *Applied Occupational and Environmental Hygiene*, **5**, 52–59.

Dodgson, J., Cherrie, J., and Groat, S. (1987). Estimates of past exposure to respirable man-made mineral fibers in the European insulation wool industry. *Annals of Occupational Hygiene*, **31**, 567–82.

Fidler, A. T., Baker, E. L., and Letz, R. E. (1987). Estimation of long term exposure to mixed solvents from questionnaire data: a tool for epidemiological investigations. *British Journal of Industrial Medicine*, **44**, 133–41.

Finkelstein, M. M. and Kreiger, N. (1996). Radium in drinking water and risk of bone cancer in Ontario youths: a second study and combined analysis. *Occupational and Environmental Medicine*, **53**, 305–11.

Glantz, S. A. and Slinker, B. K. (1990). *Primer of applied regression and analysis of variance*. McGraw-Hill, New York.

Hornung, R. W., Herrick, R. F., Stewart, P. A., *et al.* (1996). An experimental design approach to retrospective exposure assessment. *American Industrial Hygiene Association Journal*, **57**, 251–6.

Kauppinen, T. P. (1994). Assessment of exposure in occupational epidemiology. *Scandinavian Journal of Work, Environment and Health*, **20**(special issue), 19–29.

Kleinbaum, D. G., Kupper, L. L., and Muller, K. E. (1988). *Applied regression analysis and other multivariate methods* (2nd edn), PWS-Kent Publishing Company, Boston.

Kromhout, H. (2002). Design of measurement strategies for workplace exposures. *Occupational and Environmental Medicine*, **59**, 349–54.

Kromhout, H., Symanski, E., and Rappaport, S. M. (1993). A comprehensive evaluation of within- and between-worker components of occupational exposure to chemical agents. *Annals of Occupational Hygiene*, **37**, 253–70.

Lemasters, G. K., Shukla, R., Li, Y. D., *et al.* (1996). Balancing cost and precision in exposure assessment studies. *Journal of Occupational and Environmental Medicine*, **38**, 39–45.

Liu, K., Stamler, J., Dyer, A., *et al.* (1978). Statistical methods to assess and minimize the role of intra-individual variability in obscuring the relationship between dietary lipids and serum cholesterol. *Journal of Chronic Diseases*, **31**, 399–418.

Liu, K. S., Chang, Y. L., Hayward, S. B., *et al.* (1993). The distribution of lifetime cumulative exposures to radon for California residents. *Journal of Exposure Analysis in Environmental Epidemiology*, **3**, 165–79.

Mooney, C. Z. and Duval, R. D. (1993). *Bootstrapping, a nonparametric approach to statistical inference*. Sage Publications, Series 07-095, Newbury Park.

Olsen, E. (1994). Analysis of exposure using a logbook method. *Applied Occupational and Environmental Hygiene*, **9**, 712–22.

Phillips, A. N. and Smith, G. D. (1993). The design of prospective epidemiological studies: more subjects or better measurements? *Journal of Clinical Epidemiology*, **46**, 1203–11.

Preller, L., Kromhout, H., Heederik, D., *et al.* (1995). Modeling long-term average exposure in occupational exposure-response analysis. *Scandinavian Journal of Work, Environment and Health*, **21**, 504–12.

Quintana, P. J., Valenzia, J. R., Delfino, R. J., *et al.* (2001). Monitoring of 1-min personal particulate matter exposures in relation to voice-recorded time-activity data. *Environmental Research*, **87**, 199–213.

Rappaport, S. M. (1991). Assessment of long-term exposures to toxic substances in air. *Annals of Occupational Hygiene*, **35**, 61–121.

Rappaport, S. M., Symanski, E., Yager, J. W., *et al.* (1995). The relationship between environmental monitoring and biological markers in exposure assessment. *Environmental Health Perspectives*, **103**(Suppl. 3), 49–54.

Rappaport, S. M., Weaver, M., Taylor, D., *et al.* (1999). Application of mixed models to assess exposures monitored by construction workers during hot processes. *Annals of Occupational Hygiene*, **43**, 457–69.

Seixas, N. S. and Checkoway, H. (1995). Exposure assessment in industry specific retrospective occupational epidemiology studies. *Occupational and Environmental Medicine*, **52**, 625–33.

Sokal, R. R. and Rohlf, F. J. (1981). *Biometry*. Freeman and Company, San Francisco.

Stewart, P. A., Zaebst, D., Zey, J. N., *et al.* (1998). Exposure assessment for a study of workers exposed to acrylonitrile. *Scandinavian Journal of Work, Environment and Health*, **24**(Suppl. 2), 42–53.

Van Tongeren, M., Gardiner, K., Calvert, I., *et al.* (1997). Efficiency of different grouping schemes for dust exposure in the European carbon black respiratory morbidity study. *Occupational and Environmental Medicine*, **54**, 714–19.

Werner, M. A. and Attflied, M. D. (2000). Effect of different grouping strategies in developing estimates of personal exposures: specificity versus precision. *Applied Occupational and Environmental Hygiene*, **15**, 21–5.

White, E., Kushi, L. H., and Pepe, M. S. (1994). The effect of exposure variance and exposure measurement error on study sample size: implications for the design of epidemiological studies. *Journal of Clinical Epidemiology*, **47**, 873–80.

Zipprich, J. L., Harris, S. A., Fox, J. C., *et al.* (2002). An analysis of factors that influence personal exposure to nitrogen oxides in residents of Richmond, Virginia. *Journal of Exposure Analysis in Environmental Epidemiology*, **12**, 273–85.

7. Retrospective exposure assessment

Wolfgang Ahrens and Patricia Stewart

7.1 Introduction

Retrospective exposure assessment concerns the reconstruction of past exposure in epidemiological studies. It has often been applied in occupational epidemiological studies and perhaps less so in environmental epidemiological studies, and hence the methodology in the former is better developed. The quality of a study depends to a large degree on the accuracy, validity, and reliability of the exposure estimates, and these may be reduced the further back in time a study goes. A poor assessment will lead to misclassification of exposure that will decrease the power of a study to detect an association between exposure and disease (see Chapter 12).

7.2 Determination of feasibility

Little information has been provided on evaluating the feasibility of a study. There are several exposure assessment considerations, however, that should be evaluated. In a sense, a feasibility study can be thought of as a 'mini' study, that is, the same components of an exposure assessment process must also be evaluated in a feasibility study. These components are: identification of the exposure being evaluated, selection of the exposure metric (e.g. cumulative exposure), the collection and availability of exposure information (measurement and non-measurement), the development of exposure groups, the assessment of exposures, and the evaluation of the validity/reliability of the estimation process. In conceptual terms, the same components of the assessment process are present in assessment of environmental exposures as they are in industry-based studies. The exposure assessment components are presented in the following in the general order in which they are done, although there is much overlap across the components and much of the process is iterative.

If, however, it is determined that one of these components has serious deficiencies that cannot be overcome by other means (e.g. in an industry-based study job histories do not specify where individuals worked and there are few long-term workers available for interview), serious consideration should be made as to whether useful information can be obtained in the absence of an exposure assessment or in the presence of serious misclassification.

Two other issues affect the feasibility of a study. One is related to statistical power. Power should be assessed not only on the prevalence of the exposure and the number of study subjects, but also on the exposure level. If the estimates of disease risk used in the power calculation were obtained from studies that were primarily among high-exposed subjects, the study under consideration must have similar exposure levels to achieve those risks, otherwise the power will be overestimated. In addition, assumptions on the degree of misclassification may be used to simulate the loss of power in order to provide a more realistic estimate of the true power of a planned study.

A further issue is that of the representativeness of a population. The exposure experience of the study group does not have to be representative of the general population. The key to studying an unusual population, however, is to appropriately interpret the results and relate them to what would be expected in other populations.

7.3   Selection of an agent and the exposure metric

In theory, selection of the exposure and the exposure metric should be based on the toxicological mechanism of the exposure being studied. In the case of some exposures, however, the exposure to be estimated may not be the exposure of interest. For example, a sampling and analytic technique may not have been developed for the exposure of interest. There may only be historic measurement data on substances other than the substance of interest. The specific causative agent may not be known (such as the aetiologic agent in wood dust that causes respiratory function loss) or there may be multiple causative agents in the mixture (such as polycyclic aromatic hydrocarbons and lung cancer).

For most agents the exposure–disease relationship for identifying the appropriate exposure metric is not known or only poorly understood. For chronic disease, cumulative exposure is generally thought to be the best metric, but average exposure or highest exposure is sometimes evaluated. For acute diseases, such as asthma, other metrics may be more appropriate, such as the frequency of exposure above a particular threshold. If dermal route makes a significant contribution to the total exposure, this route should also be assessed (see Chapter 9). Selecting only one metric can be risky when the toxicological mechanism is not known. Different metrics often rank subjects differently and therefore will have different disease risks. It is recommended that multiple metrics be developed to allow exploration of different mechanisms.

7.4   Types of information for exposure assessment and its collection and organization

There are three major types of information that are crucial to assessing exposures: work or residential histories, measurement data, and descriptive (non-measurement) data.

7.4.1 Work and residential histories

A work history can be defined as a chronological inventory of all jobs that were performed by the subject during his or her employment in a company (in the case of industry-based studies) or lifetime (in the case of population-based studies of chronic disease). The work history is useful because it places the study subjects in an environment that provides a logical starting point for investigation. A history can be obtained from the employer (e.g. personnel records), from union records, medical records, from the study subjects themselves, or from their proxies (Bond *et al.* 1998). Obtaining work histories from the subjects is obviously more problematic if the study covers a long time period, because some of the subjects may be deceased or untraceable, possibly resulting in selection bias. The use of proxies is also problematic because they may not have complete knowledge of the subject's history. Records used must be carefully examined to ensure that they are complete, both as far as the subjects covered and the coverage of individual subjects.

Merely the presence of a work history, however, does not mean that good information on jobs is available. A recent trend in industry, but one that has existed for many years to some extent, has been to 'generalize' job titles, that is, to make them less specific to the task(s) being performed. As a result, vague terms, such as 'operator' may be used for specific jobs that in a chemical plant, for example, previously may have been called reactor operator, distillation operator, or utility operator. Even if changes in the jobs (and dates) are designated accurately, but individuals with the same title performed different tasks with different agents or exposure levels, substantial misclassification can occur. Thus, it may be necessary to collect more information by asking company personnel or workers where the individuals worked, or from records, such as foreman reports, union lists, and maintenance reports.

In population-based studies, an occupation may be characterized best by job title and branch of industry or line of business of the employer. A detailed description of each job in terms of duties and processes may improve the coding of jobs according to standard classifications and may also facilitate expert evaluations of exposure (see Section 7.4.2).

The counterpart of work histories in environmental studies are residential histories. These histories can be problematic because the subjects may have moved residences more often than jobs and the subjects may not be able to recall details, such as street and house numbers.

7.4.2 Measurements in the workplace or in the environment

Measurement data are often available for industry-based studies, but rarely for population-based studies. Measurement data can provide information both on the presence of an agent and its intensity, but without appropriate accompanying documentation on how they were taken and under what circumstances they can be misleading or useless.

It is often useful for the study investigators to take measurements of current exposures (see Chapter 5). An investigator should consider such an approach when at least some of the conditions are similar, for at least part of the period under study, to those measured. Measuring current exposures can allow comparison of measurement techniques across plants if more than one worksite is in the study; provide exposure data for jobs that had not been monitored; provide greater understanding of the variability of exposures (particularly in high variably exposed jobs such as maintenance); and confirm the historical measurements. In contrast to industry-based studies, personal exposure measurements of the general population are generally not available. Nor is it usually feasible to collect such measurements because the population is distributed over a much larger geographic area than a worksite and many worksites are no longer in existence. Routinely collected environmental measurements are sometimes available and could be used to create exposure indices. Measurements from the literature may be helpful, but their availability is generally limited. Their usefulness can be enhanced, however, by evaluation determinants of exposure (see Section 7.7). If measurement data are not available, it may be that only qualitative exposure assessments are feasible.

Environmental measurements are more 'ecologic' than measurements on occupations in the sense that there are fewer and they are used often to represent the exposures of a much larger population over extended areas.

7.4.3   Direct exposure questions

Direct exposure questions are used in case–control or cross-sectional studies where no measurement data are available. Such information is collected by either self-administered questionnaire or by interviews (see Chapter 2). Responses may be prompted by a closed format addressing specific agents or broad classes of chemicals like 'Have you ever worked with (chemical)?'. A list of specific exposures that is queried in this manner is called an exposure checklist. Such listings may contain rather general terms like 'dusts' or 'solvents' but also specific chemicals. The alternative to checklists is to ask open-ended questions such as 'What chemicals were you exposed to?'. Responses to these types of questions, however, are more vulnerable to differential recall of exposures than are prompted responses (Teschke *et al.* 2000). Furthermore, the analysis is complicated by the fact that the degree of specificity of the reported substances varies between subjects, some recalling specific chemicals and others reporting only general classes of materials. While subjects may know the common names of substances they have used, they are not likely to know the chemical names of agent exposures. As a result, it has been concluded that self-reports of occupational exposures alone, without other information, are not sufficiently accurate to warrant their sole use in most community-based studies (Ahrens 1999).

The usefulness of such questions increases if they are asked within the context of an activity. Further details about calendar time, frequency, or intensity of exposure can be questioned in order to allow an exposure–response analysis.

7.4.4   Job, process, and residential descriptions

Measurement data on its own, however, has limited usefulness. To ensure proper interpretation, the data needs to be placed within the context of the job and workplace. For example, high measurement results should be evaluated in light of tasks, controls, and other conditions. Thus, a third important type of data is descriptive data about the worksite. The job may be described in terms of services provided, products manufactured, tasks, and materials being produced, processed, or handled. A work history can be supplemented by detailed descriptions of each job task, referring to the department or process. Furthermore, each workplace may be characterized by a description of its physical layout like the type of environment (indoors/outdoors, room size, ventilation), use of protective measures, and the type of equipment or machines that were used. A short description of the activities of colleagues next to the respondent can give useful information, too.

However, three practical aspects impose severe restrictions on this need for more information. First, the ability of respondents to recall details of job tasks that have been performed in the distant past is limited. Second, broad open-ended questions may not result in responses relevant to the exposure assessment. Third, the number of specific questions that can be included in a general job history is limited by the fact that each question has to be repeated for each job. This can be time consuming since the number of job periods that can be expected in population-based studies ranges between 5 and 8 periods on average (Jöckel *et al.* 1992, 1998).

In industry-based studies, some of this information may be described in company records (e.g. job descriptions or task analyses, engineering plans, medical problems, plant layouts). In other cases, it may be necessary to interview workers. Many details, however, can be obtained by job-specific questionnaires (JSQ), administered to individuals who held a specific job or worked in an area of interest, to supplement the work histories (Joffe 1992; Tielemans *et al.* 1999). Depending on the focus of the study and on the exposure of interest, JSQs can be developed for specific job tasks, occupations, and/or industries. For example, a JSQ for welders dealt with the metals welded, preparation of metal surface (cleaners, solvents, abrasives), filler metals used, kinds of fluxes, inert gases, or electrodes in the Montreal study (Gerin *et al.* 1985). This approach was extensively used in a case–control study in Montreal covering multiple cancer sites and 294 exposures or agents (Siemiatycki *et al.* 1981; Gerin *et al.* 1985).

The JSQs in this study were meant to deal more specifically with certain manual professions that are reported frequently. The JSQs served as an aid for the interviewers to ask the technical questions relevant to the exposure assessment. In lung cancer case–control studies that were conducted in Germany between 1988 and 1996, 33 JSQs were used to assess exposure (Ahrens *et al.* 1996; Jöckel *et al.* 1998; Pohlabeln *et al.* 2000). Exposures (yes/no) and intensities (low, moderate, high) were inferred from specific job tasks and, partly, from agents or materials that were reported. The reported frequency of tasks performed was an essential basis for the quantification of exposures. Questions of a closed format were used as much as possible to reduce the laborious, costly, and less standardized task of individual coding of exposures by a team of experts. Presumed exposures of a certain job were addressed by appropriate specific and knowledge-based questions in the corresponding JSQ and were used to verify exposure or non-exposure in order to increase the specificity of the assessment.

Similarly, in studies of the environment, for example, studies of air pollution, it is crucial to collect descriptive data of the environment like industrial emission sources, traffic density, domestic heating, and weather conditions (see Chapter 3). For indoor air pollutants such as domestic radon decay products, information about the housing construction, ventilation habits, heating system, and duration of stay at home need to be recorded.

7.4.5 Biologic measurements

The advances in molecular biology have widened the scope of epidemiological research by using measurement in biological samples as indicators of internal exposure, early biological effects, or susceptibility to disease. However, many currently available biomarkers of exposure have only limited applications, because (a) they often do not reflect historical exposures due to a short biological half-life, (b) there are uncertainties as to what the biomarker is measuring, (c) they may be affected by the disease process, (d) they may be confounded and affected by problems of shipment or laboratory measurements, (e) their availability is restricted because they often require invasive procedures, for example, to obtain blood or tissue, (f) the response rate may be low, and (g) they can be very expensive (see Chapter 11).

Nevertheless, biomarkers of exposure can provide valuable quantitative information for agents that have a long persistence in humans, as in the case of certain metals that can be measured in urine or blood (Merzenich *et al.* 2001) or in the case of measurement of dioxins in blood (Flesch-Janys *et al.* 1998). In the latter study, production department-specific dose rates were derived from blood levels and working histories of a subgroup of chemical workers by applying a first-order kinetic model. These dose rates were used to estimate exposure levels for all cohort members.

Biological markers of exposure may also be used to validate exposures that were assessed in an interview and may be used to improve questionnaires (see Chapter 2). In the investigation of exposure–disease relationships biomarkers of exposure may be more suitable for prospective cohort studies, while in case–control studies of chronic diseases questionnaires still remain the primary source of exposure data.

7.5　Collection and processing of data/quality control/training

The need for standardization and documentation of the exposure assessment process has been recognized. The construction, validation, and standardization of questionnaires are often neglected and the valuable body of knowledge and experience from other sciences, such as psychiatric disorders, intelligence, or pain, is ignored. Some key issues and recommendations, which should be part of the standardization procedure, have been described by a working group of the IEA (IEA European Questionnaire Group 1998 [http://www.dundee.ac.uk/iea/EuroQuests.htm]) (see Chapter 2).

Moreover, as validated instruments are rare, the investigator should seek to adopt established instruments that have been successfully used in previous studies. Whenever possible, structured closed-ended questions and checklists rather than open-ended questions should be used. A standardized application of such instruments, including training of interviewees and development of an interviewer manual, is also important (Fink 1995). Modern technological achievements like computer-assisted interviews may help to further standardize the application of instruments, facilitate complex conditional jumps, and integrate plausibility checks and aids for interviewers for specific questions. All steps of the data collection process need to be documented and may be entered into a database immediately to allow a continuous monitoring and quality control of the data collection process.

Training of coders (see later) should also be done. Once the data has been collected, the next step is organization. Organization of data is a time-consuming but extremely important part of the exposure assessment process because of the large volume of information usually collected.

7.6 Development of exposure groups

An important component of the exposure assessment process is the development of exposure groups. One of the first steps prior to developing exposure groups is to code the jobs (and industries). To do so, in industry-based studies it is usually necessary to standardize the job titles for spelling, abbreviations and word orders to allow easy sorting and grouping. Once completed, a single 'standardized' job or department title can be used to describe all jobs (or departments) in that group. A compilation of the 'standardized' titles and the original titles is called a job dictionary.

After standardization, coding of jobs and industries is done to make direct use of this information in the epidemiologic analyses and to facilitate exposure assessment. Coding may enhance the ability to distinguish particular occupational subgroups by cross-classifying job titles and industries. In addition, coding is usually necessary to apply a job-exposure matrix (JEM) (see Chapter 8). Coding of jobs is usually done according to standard classification systems. Coding of residences is done using global positioning systems (GPS).

Assessing exposures to groups, rather than to individuals, is generally more efficient because individual assessments require multiple measurements on all or most of the study subjects (a situation rarely found) and extensive resources. Grouping also tends to be more efficient than individual assessments, because it results in less attenuation of the exposure–response relationship, unless the between-worker variability within the group is large (see Chapter 12). Exposure groups can be developed during the epidemiologic analysis or the exposure assessment phase.

The goal of developing exposure groups is to group subjects with similar exposure levels to the same agent(s). Large differences among the groups (contrast) result in less attenuation of the exposure–response relationship. Two approaches can be followed for grouping. In one, the smallest unique grouping is made. Thus, for a study of acrylonitrile workers, 3600 unique job/department/plant groups were developed across eight plants and estimates were developed for each group (Stewart *et al.* 1998). In the epidemiologic analysis, the subjects were divided into five exposure groups, which provided the contrast among the groups (Blair *et al.* 1998). Other investigators prefer to develop fewer groups with a larger number of members, but this procedure may increase the risk of heterogeneously exposed workers within the groups. To prevent this occurrence, between- and within-group variability can be evaluated by measurement data (see Chapter 6). Such an evaluation requires, however, the availability of repeat measurements, which are not always available.

In general, it is best to keep exposure groups as unique as possible (Fig. 7.1). It is recommended that various jobs be kept as separate groups rather than grouping

---

It is 'preferable to start by accumulating information in as much detail as possible; the detailed information (can) always be summarized, whereas by starting with only a comparatively coarse stratification there (is) no opportunity of breaking down the results on a more detailed basis should this later prove to be necessary' (Fay and Rae 1959).

Fig. 7.1 A lesson to be kept in the forefront of exposure assessment.

multiple jobs, because of other, unanticipated analyses. The first epidemiologic analysis may provide leads that are followed up long after the original results are published. The original exposure groups may not be appropriate for the newer analyses, because individuals within the original exposure groups may not be homogeneous for the second exposure. A new grouping of jobs would therefore be required. For example, correlation coefficients between dust and allergen levels in a bakery ranged from 0.57 to 0.86 when comparing average, cumulative, and peak exposure levels (Nieuwenhuijsen *et al.* 1995). The job title may be the unit of specificity for the exposure groups, but in some studies even more refinement may be necessary. In a study of bakeries, the job was the primary variable explaining variability of inhalable dust, whereas in the same population, the job and particular worksite (bakery) was important for wheat allergens, and the worksite alone was important for α-amylase allergens (Houba *et al.* 1997). The median between- and within-worker variability was found to be significantly different for continuous vs. intermittent processes, mobile vs. stationary workers, and general vs. local sources (Kromhout *et al.* 1993), which suggests some determinants that should be considered. Other determinants may be department, process, job assignment (e.g. board operator), area or location, tasks, equipment, craft, product, process container, batch or lot, project, production unit, controls, and sources of the contaminant. Careful consideration of these determinants of exposure (and possibly others) is likely to substantially reduce the variability of exposures within an exposure group (see Chapter 6). A description of these determinants for a job is called a job exposure profile.

In addition to the exposure determinants, the availability of measurement and descriptive data affects the grouping. For example, in a study of pneumoconiosis among coal miners, measurement data existed for some, but not all, occupation/mine/year exposure groups (Seixas *et al.* 1991). Where measurement data were available, the occupation/mine/year combinations comprised the exposure groups. Broader exposure groups (occupation/year, mine/year (within occupational group) and year (within occupational group)) were developed where data was not available.

Exposure groups are usually developed with a single or a small number of exposures in mind. This approach presupposes single agent causality. In circumstances where it is difficult to identify single agents or where multiple agents may be acting together, using a cluster analysis may be warranted. For example, workers in the semi-conductor industry study were found to have exposures to 14 chemical and physical agents, with a high correlation among the exposures (Hines *et al.* 1995). The researchers identified the exposure profile of each study subject and developed three exposure groups based on similar exposures to the 14 agents. Two other descriptions of the process of developing exposure groups have been described (Loomis *et al.* 1994; Quinn *et al.* 2001).

Evaluation of environmental exposures are based on similar concepts in that homogeneous exposure groups need to be developed. However it has been rarely applied. Use of cluster analysis should also be considered.

7.7   Quantification of exposure levels

The goal of the estimation process is to accurately develop exposure estimates for the exposure groups. Exposures can be estimated qualitatively (yes/no), semi-quantitatively (low, medium, or high; or on a scale, say, of 1–4), or quantitatively (in measurement units such as milligram per cubic metre) and can be developed for a JEM or for individuals. Qualitative assessments will not be discussed here. Typically, industry-based studies and retrospective case–control studies were based on JEMs. Recently, with the development of JSQs, assessments are being made on individuals. A decision on which approach to use is dependent on the information available. The level of detail in the work histories plays a crucial role as to how specific the estimation can be. If, for example, in an industry-based study, exposures vary considerably within department and vary little across departments, but only information on department is known of the subjects, it is inefficient to spend much time developing quantitative exposure levels. Similarly, if few measurement data are available for the period under study or some measurements are available but the effect of changes in the workplace cannot be estimated, semi-quantitative estimates may be the best the investigator can do.

In most studies investigating chronic disease, exposure levels have changed over time due to changes in technology (pollution controls), work practices, government regulations, or other reasons. In such cases, for practical reasons estimates are developed for years or even time periods (multiple years) rather than for smaller units of time, although in studies of acute or short-term adverse health effects, such as reproductive effects, smaller time units, such as months, may be appropriate. Development of time periods may be done by evaluation of the measurement data: statistically or by observation. Researchers of the dusty trades industry plotted measurement results against time (Rice *et al.* 1984). Any plot in which all measurements were higher or lower than previous or subsequent measurements was considered to represent a distinct time period if supported by descriptive data.

The measurement data may be so few, however, that other sources of information, such as engineering and production records and published emission data or interviews, are needed to identify time periods. If developing semi-quantitative estimates each exposure group is assigned a score that reflects a differing exposure level. This approach is easier and faster than the quantitative approach and is often assumed to be more credible than quantitative estimates. Caution must be taken, however, to ensure that the scores assigned to the exposure groups accurately reflect the differences in exposure to minimize misclassification; otherwise lack of an association could result from misclassification due to inappropriate scores. There are two primary disadvantages to semi-quantitative estimates. Often, the scores are not defined in terms of measurement units, so that the study's usefulness for risk assessment is limited. The second disadvantage is that because the method is less specific than the quantitative approach, it tends to encourage a superficial evaluation of exposures and little documentation of the assessment process. This disadvantage is easily overcome, of course, but it requires discipline by the assessor.

Scores have been based on a variety of exposure metrics or a combination of different metrics. Sometimes frequency of exposure has been used as the criterion (exposed 5 days a week = high, 1–3 days a week = medium, and < 1 day a week = low). Intensity, type of contact (direct, indirect), pattern of exposure (continuous or intermittent), and other types of descriptors have also been used. Well-documented studies identify the determinants evaluated and the weights assigned to these determinants to calculate scores. The weights can be estimated from measurements on the study subjects or from the literature. In a study of pesticide applicators, for example, weights from 0 to 9, developed from the literature, were assigned to tasks, application method, use of controls, work and hygiene practices, protective equipment, and the occurrence of spills and were evaluated (see Chapter 16).

Quantitative estimation can be difficult and time consuming, and the credibility of the estimates is often questioned. Moreover, usually some measurement data is required to perform quantitative assessments, although they do not have to be on the jobs or at the worksites under study. This type of assessment provides the best information for risk assessment and is more likely to allow the exploration of different exposure metrics. More care is taken when developing the estimates, because error in the estimation process is more visible.

Quantitative estimation requires several steps. The data may have to be cleaned, for example, by examining frequencies of the various data fields, standardized (e.g. spelling, abbreviations, word order), and measurements below the limit of detection treated. Summary statistics (arithmetic means and standard deviations, geometric means and standard deviations) should be developed by location and year; the duration and type of measurement (personal, area); the source of the data; the sampling and analytic method; 'representativeness' of the measurements; and so on to provide insight into the variability of the data and an overview of the exposure scenarios. For example, in a study of silica workers, different sampling and analytic methods were used. A conversion factor was applied to the results of one method to maximize comparability to the second method (Rice *et al.* 1984). In contrast, in a study of ethylene oxide workers, the authors excluded the measurements of a method with fewer measurements because the variability of the measurements differed by method (Hornung *et al.* 1994).

Examination of the measurements should be done without regard to the exposure groups because it can provide insight into how the exposure groups should be developed. Once the exposure groups and time periods have been identified, the exposure levels can be estimated for each unique exposure group/time period. Prior to assigning the exposure, first, it may be useful to develop a table of measurement means by exposure group and time to get the overall picture of the exposure scenarios. The means should then be evaluated within the context of the descriptive data and determined whether they are reasonable. If so, the measurement means or medians can be used directly as the exposure estimate. Once it is determined which means to use, the remaining empty cells (i.e. exposure group/time periods) can be completed. This is perhaps the most difficult part of the exposure assessment process.

Statistical modelling can be used to estimate exposure levels for exposure group/time periods when measurements are not available (see Chapter 6). In such approaches, determinants of exposures in the workplace, as well as those associated with measurement data, for example, personal vs. area measurements, the duration, the sampling method, and the like are identified, either through observation or questionnaires. In a study of asphalt workers the tasks of mastic laying and of oil gravel paving, and years before 1997 were significant variables for predicting bitumen fume, bitumen vapour, and benzo(a)pyrene (Burstyn *et al.* 2000). Other determinants (e.g. application temperature in non-mastic paving, type of sample (i.e. area sample), and various sampling methods) were significant for one or two of these substances.

Non-statistical deterministic modelling also can be used to estimate exposure levels. Determinants that are thought to influence exposure levels are identified from the literature, from observation, or analogy from similar situations. Each value of the determinant is assigned a weight, which is used to modify the measurement mean. In a study of flight attendants, investigators modified cosmic radiation measurement data from an existent database using taxi time, ascent and descent time, the cruise altitude, and time at the cruise altitude (Grajewski *et al.* 2002).

Unmeasured conditions can be recreated or estimated from other worksites. In a study of embalmers, historical conditions were simulated by varying the amount of formaldehyde concentration in the embalming fluid, the type of procedure (autopsied and intact), and differing levels of exhaust ventilation (Hornung *et al.* 1996). Investigators of a study of workers dealing with man-made mineral fibre used a deterministic model by identifying a set of 'job exposure elements' common to all jobs (Quinn *et al.* 2001). The elements included: distance from the source, duration of the exposure, and the intensity of the physical effort required by the job. These were used to estimate the exposures for those jobs that lacked air measurements by comparing the elements of the unmeasured job to the elements of the measured jobs.

It may be possible to use measurement data for an agent that is likely to reflect similar relative exposure levels to a second agent. In this instance two agents must be used throughout the process in the same relative quantities and be affected by the same environmental conditions to the same degree, resulting in the same ratio (between the two agents) across jobs and over time. It is important to confirm that these two assumptions are met.

In environmental studies qualitative and semi-quantitative assessments suffer the same limitations and have the same strengths as they have in industry-based studies but are generally less sophisticated in the assessment process than occupational studies. Semi-quantitative assessments have been done on distance from waste sites for solid waste contaminants (Knox 2000). Studies of air pollution have used measurement data of air contaminants from fixed sources. In some studies, recent measurements are linked to acute diseases, such as hospital admissions for respiratory disease (Atkinson *et al.* 2001). The use of current measurement data is more suitable if the disease is acute than if it is more chronic, such as birth defects, cancer, or mortality. Some investigators, however, have utilized historic measurements for air (Vena 1982; Jöckel *et al.* 1992; Pope *et al.* 2002) and water contaminants (Bove *et al.* 1995) that have approximated the time period of interest. In a study of breast cancer and triazine exposure, the level of contamination from groundwater and tap water measurements, the number of acres on which triazine application was likely, and the amount of pesticide used by applicators were scored for each county and the latter were assigned low, medium, or high exposure categories (Kettles *et al.* 1997). In an environmental study of arsenic and skin cancer around a power plant, emission levels, weather data, and topography were used to model the exposure (see Chapter 3).

As in occupational studies models can be developed based on correlation between the two substances over a known period of time to predict the exposure levels in the unknown period (Goldberg *et al.* 2001). Few environmental studies have been conducted that have incorporated environmental measurements on the study subjects (or over a small geographic area) and generally these have been indoor studies (Mahaffey *et al.* 1993; Brauer *et al.* 2001; Smedje and Norback 2001).

7.8   Accuracy and reliability

Wherever possible estimates should be evaluated for their accuracy and reliability. Evaluating the accuracy of retrospective exposure assessment is usually difficult, if not impossible, because it is rarely possible to determine what the true exposures were. Biologic measurements are limited as a gold standard not only because they usually do not exist, but also because most agents of interest have a relatively short half-life in the human body. Moreover, there may be differences in how individuals metabolize substances, and there may be non-occupational sources of exposures, or exposure to agents may have occurred in other jobs and the agents are still stored in the body. Airborne (or dermal) measurement data can result in biased estimates due to non-representative sampling. Furthermore, when measurement data are scarce it may be more efficient to use them to estimate the exposures than to use them in a validation study.

In the embalmers study mentioned previously (Hornung *et al.* 1996), measurements were collected from five funeral homes that had not been evaluated in the original study and compared to the predicted values obtained from applying the model. In the acrylonitrile study, an evaluation of the estimation methods was done prior to developing the estimates (Stewart *et al.* 1998). Job/time period combinations were identified for which measurements existed. Estimates were developed for these combinations and compared to the measurement data. The accuracy of the estimates can be evaluated by comparing the exposure estimates to measurements in other facilities, either as reported in the literature or by obtaining measurements from similar facilities. The operations, however, should be similar to those of the facility under investigation, and differences do not necessarily reflect incorrect estimates. A study of car and bus mechanics compared measurements in an inspectorate database to the exposure estimates (Plato *et al.* 1995).

Indirect validation can be done by evaluating the risk to a disease known to be caused by a particular agent using estimates developed for another investigation. For example, confidence in silica estimates developed for a lung cancer study increased when an exposure–response relationship was found with silicosis in the same population (Dosemeci *et al.* 1994). It must be noted, however, that this method does not validate the estimates if the true exposure–response relationship in the population is not known.

Validation studies require that different indicators of exposure are obtained for the same subjects. Often a detailed and more accurate exposure assessment is only possible for a subset of subjects within a study. Such information may, however, be exploited for the whole study, as in the example of a case–control study on asbestos and lung cancer, in which the intensity of exposure for a subsample of the study subjects was assessed by a panel of experts. The information on duration of exposure in the original study was combined with the expert assessment of duration and intensity using a new method called two-phase paradigm (Pohlabeln *et al.* 2002; Schill and Drescher 1997). Applying this method the efficiency of the study was increased because it gave more precise risk estimates for the expert assessment by compensating for the smaller numbers in the subsample.

Reliability, defined as the reproducibility of exposure estimates, can also be examined and together with validity of specific methods is discussed in more detail in Chapter 8.

7.9   Recommendations

Use of quantitative estimates has often been the most challenged, because of the mistaken perception that it contains more misclassification than does a semi-quantitative approach. It is not usually recognized, however, that developing a small number of exposure groups with a semi-quantitative approach (e.g. low, medium, and high, or a score of 1–4) is likely to result in much greater error than quantitative estimates. This is because the semi-quantitative approach assumes that all subjects within an exposure category have the exact same exposure level and that the relationship among the exposure levels for the subjects within each exposure category is the value assigned to the categories. Thus, all subjects assigned a score of 3 are assumed to have an exposure that is 3 times the exposure level of those subjects assigned a score of 1 and 1.5 times the exposure level of those assigned a score of 2. Usually the variability of exposures at a worksite is much greater than these differences assume. In addition, even if the relationships are correctly estimated, this approach can result in two individuals with nearly the same exposure level falling in two different categories because they are on the high end of the lower category and the low end of the higher category. Also, two individuals assigned to the same category may be on the extreme ends of the category. Therefore, semi-quantitative scores may also be interpreted as representing a rank order and be analysed accordingly, for example, using dummy variables for each level.

Quantitative assessment appears to be more prone to error than the other methods, but it should be recognized that it is unlikely that the subjects were truly exposed to the estimate assigned. Nevertheless, it is likely that the differences between the subjects' estimated exposure levels and the truth are less than for semi-quantitative estimates. Thus, we recommend that quantitative assessment be made whenever possible.

In most studies the information available varies across jobs or time periods, so that it may not be possible to use the same estimation methods for all estimates. In such a case, several methods may be used. Even when a single estimation method is used, confidence in the estimates can vary by the number of measurements, the type (area or personal), duration, or variability of the measurements, the amount of information known about the job, and other variables. Estimates of lower confidence can be a source of misclassification and therefore it is useful to assign a confidence score to each estimate. A sensitivity analysis can determine if estimates of low confidence affect the disease risk estimates.

Typically, documentation of the estimation procedure is crucial to allow others to interpret better the epidemiologic results and to increase the credibility of the study. Each of the assessment components should be discussed in the documentation in enough detail to provide the reader with an understanding of what was done and why. Examples of good documentation have been published and should include each of the steps described in this chapter (Stewart *et al.* 1998; Glass *et al.* 2000; Quinn *et al.* 2001).

References

Ahrens, W. (1999). *Retrospective assessment of occupational exposure in case–control studies.* Landsberg. ecomed Verlagsgesellschaft. 1–124. Fortschritte in der Epidemiologie.

Ahrens, W., Jöckel, K.-H., Pohlabeln, H., Bolm-Audorff, U., *et al.* (1996). Assessment of exposure to asbestos in a case–control study of lung cancer: comparison of supplementary questionnaires and an exposure check-list. *Occupational Hygiene*, **3**, 125–36.

Atkinson, R. W., Anderson, H. R., Sunyer, J., Ayres, J., Baccini, M., *et al.* (2001). Acute effects of particulate air pollution on respiratory admissions. *American Journal Respir Crit Care Med*, **164**, 1860–66.

Blair, A., Stewart, P. A., Zaebst, D. D., Pottern, L., Zey, J. N., Bloom, T. F., Miller, B., Ward, E., and Lubin, J. (1998). Mortality of industrial workers exposed to acrylonitrile. *Scandinavian Journal of Work Environment and Health*, **24**, 25–41.

Bond, G. G., Bodner, K. M., Sobel, W., Shellenberger, R. J., *et al.* (1988). Validation of work histories obtained form interviews. *American Journal of Epidemiology*, **128**, 343–51.

Bove, F. J., Fulcomer, M. C., Klotz, J. B., Esmart, J., Dufficy, E. M., and Savrin, J. E. (1995). Public drinking water contamination and birth outcomes. *American Journal of Epidemiology*, **141**(9), 850–62.

Brauer, M., Ebelt, S. F., Fisher, T. V., Brumm, J., Petkau, A. J., and Vedal, S. (2001). Exposure of chronic obstructive pulmonary disease patients to particles: respiratory and cardiovascular health effects. *Journal of Exposure Analysis and Environmental Epidemiology*, **11**, 490–500.

Burstyn, I., Kromhout, H., Kauppinen, T., Heikkila, P., and Boffetta, P. (2000). Statistical modeling of the determinants of historical exposure to bitumen and polycyclic aromatic hydrocarbons among paving workers. *Annals of Occupational Hygiene*, **44**, 43–56.

Dosemeci, M., McLaughlin, J. K., Chen, J.-Q., Hearl, F., McCawley, M., Wu, Z., Chen, R.-G., Peng, K.-L., Chen, A.-L., Rexing, S. H., and Blot, W. J. (1994). Indirect validation of a retrospective method of exposure assessment used in a nested case–control study of lung cancer and silica exposure. *Occupational and Environmental Medicine*, **51**, 136–8.

Fay, J. W. J. and Rae, S. (1959). The pneumoconiosis field research of the national coal board. *Annals of Occupational Hygiene*, **1**, 149–61.

Fink, A. (ed.). (1995). *The complete survey kit*. Thousand Oaks, London, Sage Publications, New Delhi.

Flesch-Janys, D., Steindorf, K., Gurn, P., and Becher, H. (1998). Estimation of the cumulated exposure to polychlorinated dibenzo-p-dioxins/furans and standardized mortality ratio analysis of cancer mortality by dose in an occupationally exposed cohort. *Environmental Health Perspectives*, **106**(Suppl. 2), 655–62.

Gerin, M., Siemiatycki, J., Kemper, H., Eng, B., *et al.* (1985). Obtaining occupational exposure histories in epidemiologic case–control studies. *Journal of Occupational Medicine*, **27**, 420–6.

Glass, D. C., Adams, G. G., Manuell, R. W., and Bisby, J. A. (2000). Retrospective exposure assessment for benzene in the Australian petroleum industry. *Annals of Occupational Hygiene*, **44**, 301–20.

Goldberg, M. S., Burnett, R. T., Brook, J., Bailar, J. C. III, Valois, M.-F. and Vincent, R. (2001). Associations between daily cause-specific mortality and concentrations of ground-level ozone in Montreal, Quebec. *American Journal of Epidemiology*, **154**(9), 817–26.

Grajewski, B., Waters, M. A., Whelan, E. A., and Bloom, T. F. (2002). Radiation dose estimation for epidemiologic studies of flight attendants. *American Journal of Industrial Medicine*, **41**, 27–37.

Hines, C. J., Selvin, S., Samuels, S. J., Hammond, S. K., Woskie, S. R., Hallock, M. F., and Schenker, M. B. (1995). Hierarchical cluster analysis for exposure assessment of workers in the semiconductor health study. *American Journal of Industrial Medicine*, **28**, 713–22.

Hornung, R. W., Greife, A. L., Stayner, L. T., Steenland, N. K., Herrick, R. F., Elliott, L. J., Ringenburg, V. L., and Morawetz, J. (1994). Statistical model for prediction of retrospective exposure to ethylene oxide in an occupational mortality study. *American Journal of Industrial Medicine*, **25**, 825–36.

Hornung, R. W., Herrick, R. F., Stewart, P. A., Utterback, D. F., Feigley, C. E., Wall, D. K., Douthit, D. E., and Hayes, R. B. (1996). An experimental design approach to retrospective exposure assessment. *American Industrial Hygiene Association Journal*, **57**, 251–6.

Houba, R., Heederik, D., and Kromhout, H. (1997). Grouping strategies for exposure to inhalable dust, wheat allergens and α-amylase allergens in bakeries. *Annals of Occupational Hygiene*, **41**, 287–96.

IEA European Questionaire Group (1998). Epidemiology deserves better questionaires. http://dundee.ac.uk/iea/EuroQuests.htm

Jöckel, K.-H., Ahrens, W., Wichmann, H.-E., Becher, H., *et al.* (1992). Occupational and environmental hazards associated with lung cancer. *International Journal of Epidemiology*, **21**, 202–13.

Jöckel, K.-H., Ahrens, W., Jahn, I., Pohlabeln, H., *et al.* (1998). Occupational risk factors for lung cancer: a case–control study in West Germany. *International Journal of Epidemiology*, **27**, 549–60.

Joffe, M. (1992). Validity of exposure data derived from a structured questionnaire. *American Journal of Epidemiology*, **135**, 564–70.

Kettles, M. A., Browning, S. R., Prince, T. S., and Horstman, S. W. (1997). Triazine herbicide exposure and breast cancer incidence: an ecologic study of Kentucky counties. *Environmental Health Perspectives*, **105**, 1222–7.

Knox, E. G. (2000). Childhood cancers, birthplaces, incinerators and landfill sites. *International Journal of Epidemiology*, **29**, 391–397.

Kromhout, H., Symanski, E., and Rappaport, S. M. (1993). A comprehensive evaluation of within- and between-worker components of occupational exposure to chemical agents. *Annals of Occupational Hygiene*, **37**, 253–70.

Loomis, D. P., Peipins, L. A., Browning, S. R., Howard, R. L., Kromhout, H., and Savitz, D. A. (1994). Organization and classification of work history data in industry-wide studies: An application to the electric power industry. *American Journal of Industrial Medicine*, **26**, 413–25.

Mahaffey, J. A., Parkhurst, M. A., James, A. C., Cross, F. T., Alavanja, M. C. R., *et al.* (1993). Estimating past exposure to indoor radon from household glass. *Health Physics*, **64**, 381–91.

Merzenich, H., Hartwig, A., Ahrens, W., Beyersmann, D., *et al.* (2001). Biomonitoring on carcinogenic metals and oxidative DNA damage in a cross-sectional study. *Cancer Epidemiology, Biomarkers and Prevention*, **10**, 515–22.

Nieuwenhuijsen, M. J., Lowson, D., Venables, K. M., and Newman Taylor, A. J. (1995). Correlation between different measures of exposure in a cohort of bakery workers and flour millers. *Annals of Occupational Hygiene*, **39**, 291–8.

Plato, N., Tornling, G., Hogstedt, C., and Krantz, S. (1995). An index of past asbestos exposure as applied to car and bus mechanics. *Annals of Occupational Hygiene*, **39**, 441–54.

Pohlabeln, H., Jöckel, K.-H., Brüske-Hohlfeld, I., Möhner, M., *et al.* (2000). Lung cancer and exposure to man-made vitreous fibers: results from a pooled case–control study in Germany. *American Journal of Industrial Medicine*, **37**, 469–77.

Pohlabeln, H., Wild, P., Schill, W., Ahrens, W., Jahn, I., *et al.* (2002). Asbestos fibreyears and lung cancer: a two phase case–control study with expert exposure assessment. *Occupational and Environmental Medicine*, **59**, 410–14.

Pope, C. A. III, Burnett, R. T., Thun, M. J., Calle, E. E., Krewski, D., Ito, K., Thurston, G. D. (2002). Lung cancer, cardiopulmonary mortality, and long-term exposure to fine particulate air polution. *Journal of the American Medical Association*, **287**(9), 1132–41.

Quinn, M. M., Smith, T. J., Youk, A. O., Marsh, G. M., Stone, R. A., Buchanich, J. M., and Gula, M. J. (2001). Historical cohort study of US man-made vitreous fiber production workers: VIII. Exposure-specific job analysis. *Journal of Occupational and Environmental Medicine*, **43**, 824–34.

Rice, C., Harris, R. L. Jr., Lumsden, J. C., and Symons, M. J. (1984). Reconstruction of silica exposure in the North Carolina dusty trades. *American Industrial Hygiene Association Journal*, **45**, 689–96.

Schill, W. and Drescher, K. (1997). Logistic analysis of studies with two-stage sampling: a comparison of four approaches. *Statistical Medicine*, **16**, 117–32.

Seixas, N. S., Moulton, L. H., Robins, T. G., Rice, C. H., Attfield, M. D., and Zellers, E. T. (1991). Estimation of cumulative exposures for the National study of Coal Workers' Pneumoconiosis. *Applied Occupational and Environmental Hygiene*, **6**, 1032–41.

Siemiatycki, J., Day, N. E., Fabry, J., and Cooper, J. A. (1981). Discovering carcinogens in the occupational environment: a novel epidemiologic approach. *Journal of the National Cancer Institute*, **66**, 217–25.

Smedje, G. and Norback, D. (2001). Incidence of asthma diagnosis and self-reported allergy in relation to the school environment—a four-year follow-up study in school children. *International Journal of Tuberculosis and Lung Disease*, **5**, 1059–66.

Stewart, P. A., Zaebst, D., Zey, J. N., Herrick, R., Dosemeci, M., Hornung, R., Bloom, T., Pottern, L., Miller, B. A., and Blair, A. (1998). Exposure assessment for a study of workers exposed to acrylonitrile. *Scandinavian Journal of Work Environment and Health*, **24**, 42–53.

Teschke, K., Smith, J. C., and Olshan, A. F. (2000). Evidence of recall bias in volunteered vs. prompted responses about occupational exposures. *American Journal of Industrial Medicine*, **38**, 385–8.

Tielemans, E., Heederik, D., Burdorf, A., Vermeulen, R., *et al.* (1999). Assessment of occupational exposures in a general population: comparison of different methods. *Occupational and Environmental Medicine*, **56**, 145–51.

Vena, J. E. (1982). Air pollution as a risk factor in lung cancer. *American Journal of Epidemiology*, **116(1)**, 42–56.

8. Exposure surrogates: job-exposure matrices, self-reports, and expert evaluations

Kay Teschke

8.1 Introduction

The ideal method for assessing the occupational or environmental exposures of subjects in epidemiological studies is quantitative measurement of external concentrations in the air or on the skin, or measurement of internal dose in body tissues or excreta. Unfortunately, in many study designs, this ideal is difficult or impossible to achieve, particularly in studies of a retrospective nature. Cohort studies are most often retrospective in design and historical exposure measurements are usually not available for every, or sometimes any, study subject, thus requiring other techniques for exposure estimation. Case–control studies are by nature retrospective, and these designs have almost always relied on proxy measures of exposure.

Chapter 7 presented an overview of retrospective exposure assessment methods. The purpose of this chapter is to examine more fully the promise and the pitfalls of selected exposure estimation techniques commonly used in epidemiology: job-exposure matrices (JEMs), exposures self-reported by study subjects, and exposures assessed by experts. In particular, the validity and reliability of these surrogate measures are discussed, using summary statistics such as sensitivity, specificity, predictive values, kappa, and proportions of variance explained (some of these terms are discussed in Chapters 2 and 12). Several recent reviews have examined these issues in some detail and from somewhat different perspectives (McGuire *et al.* 1998; Kromhout and Vermeulen 2001; Teschke *et al.* 2002).

While the terms 'JEMs', 'self-reported exposures', and 'expert assessments' suggest that each of these methods is clearly specified and distinct from the others, this is not the case. As will be described more fully, the techniques vary tremendously from study to study and often include elements that borrow from each other.

Some examples of studies using surrogate exposure measures are listed in Table 8.1. Although all the major epidemiological study designs are represented in Table 8.1, this is not indicative of the frequency of their use in practice. A search of the US National Library of Medicine's PubMed bibliographic database from 1966 to April 2002 indicated that case–control studies are by far the predominant users of these proxy measures. Cohort studies also use surrogate methods, but to a lesser extent and in somewhat different ways. Cross-sectional studies only rarely employ such methods of exposure assessment.

Table 8.1 Examples of epidemiological studies that include surrogate measures of occupational or environmental exposure

Author, date	Study design	Surrogate measure of exposure	Study description
Post *et al.* (1994)	Retrospective cohort	JEM	Population-based cohort in Zutphen, the Netherlands Examined associations between occupational exposure to 27 chemical agents and chronic non-specific lung disease
Laforest *et al.* (2000)	Case–control study	JEM	Tumour-registry-based study of laryngeal and other cancer cases in France. Examined associations between occupational exposure to seven substances and laryngeal cancer
London *et al.* (1998)	Cross-sectional study	JEM	Pesticide applicators and fruit farm workers in South Africa. Examined association between occupational pesticide exposure and tremor and other neurological signs and symptoms
Stick *et al.* (1996)	Prospective cohort	Self-reported exposure	Cohort of healthy infants in Western Australia Examined associations between maternal reports of smoking during pregnancy and peak tidal expiratory flow in the infants
Kamel *et al.* (2002)	Case–control study	Self-reported exposure	Population-based study of amyotrophic lateral schlerosis cases compared to population controls in the United States. Examined associations between occupational exposure to lead and ALS
Christiani *et al.* (1995)	Cross-sectional study	Self-reported exposure	Female textile workers in China. Examined associations between occupational exposure to stress and dysmenorrhea
van Loon *et al.* (1997)	Prospective cohort	Expert-assessed exposure	Population-based cohort of men in the Netherlands Examined associations between occupational exposure to four carcinogenic substances and lung cancer
Villeneuve *et al.* (2002)	Case–control study	Expert-assessed exposure	Population-based study of male brain cancer cases compared to population controls in Canada. Examined associations between occupational exposure to magnetic fields and brain cancer
Nasterlack *et al.* (1999)	Cross-sectional study	Expert-assessed exposure	Painters and construction workers in Germany. Examined associations between exposure to solvents and mood and behavioural symptoms

8.2 Occupation and industry as an occupational exposure proxy

In all occupational epidemiological designs, job and industry have been used as the most basic of exposure surrogates. Occupational data is usually collected from company personnel records in cohort studies, through job histories reported by study subjects in case–control studies, and by either technique in cross-sectional surveys. Careful consideration of exposures common to occupations or industries shown to be at elevated risk is a useful initial step towards the identification of potentially hazardous exposures. In addition, in many jobs, exposures to complex mixtures are the norm and classification by industry or occupation may be a sensible way to represent the combined exposures.

A great advantage of analyses by occupation or industry is that the data is usually reasonably accurate—both that from employment records and from self-reported employment histories (Kromhout and Vermeulen 2001; Teschke *et al.* 2002). Raw agreement between the two sources of data tends to be in the range of 70–90 per cent, with kappas for agreement beyond chance in the range of 0.65–0.82. The main problem with such analyses is that specific agents cannot be clearly identified as risk factors. For example, carpenters are exposed to wood dust, but they also have potential exposures to other agents, including solvents, formaldehyde-based resins, paints and varnishes, and bioaerosols from their own work, and many other agents, such as metal fumes and insulation materials from other trades with whom they may work closely. In addition, although finishing carpenters may be highly exposed to wood dust, framing carpenters working outdoors likely have little exposure. Therefore an elevated risk in a job only suggests risks from specific agents. In addition, if only some individuals in a job are exposed to a particular agent, its effect may be masked if no elevation in risk is observed in the heterogeneously exposed job group.

8.3 Exposure matrices: using jobs to infer occupational exposures

Job-exposure matrices list occupations and/or industries on one axis, exposure agents on the other, and the cells of the matrix indicate the presence, intensity, frequency, and/or probability of exposure to a specific agent in a specific job (Fig. 8.1). In some JEMs, the calendar period may form a third axis of the matrix.

Industry-based cohort studies have long used this matrix format, since cohort members' job histories within a company usually serve as the basis for assigning exposures. Often the data in the cells are based on measured exposure levels (Frumkin *et al.* 2001; Steenland *et al.* 2001). Where no measurement data exist or where there are data gaps, a variety of methods has been used for filling in cells, for example, expert judgement (including that of company employees and industrial hygienists), extrapolation from cells with known exposures, and empirical or deterministic modelling (Seixas and Checkoway 1995; Stewart *et al.* 1998). These JEMs are designed to be study-specific and usually assign exposure to a very detailed list of jobs identified with the industry in question.

Time period: 1991–5   Herbicides   Welding fume   Wood dust

		Exposure axis →		
		Herbicides	Welding fume	Wood dust
Agriculture	Farmer	3	1	1
	Labourer	2	0	0
	Farm manager	1	0	0
Mining	Mine manager	0	0	0
	Miner	0	1	0
	Truck driver	0	0	0
Forestry	Logger	1	0	2
	Bucker	1	0	2
	Heavy equipment op.	0	0	0
Construction	Welder	0	3	1
	Truck driver	0	0	0
	Carpenter	1	1	3
Manufacturing	Machine operator	0	0	0
	Truck driver	0	0	0
	Welder	0	3	0

(Industry/occupation axis runs vertically down the left of the exposure table.)

Fig. 8.1 Hypothetical example showing the basic elements of a JEM.

The use of the term 'JEM', however, more often refers to a type of matrix in which measured exposure data is less commonly used. Starting in the 1980s there was a movement in occupational epidemiology to develop 'generic' JEMs mainly for use in population-based case–control studies, that is, JEMs that could describe exposures across the range of jobs and industries that might be observed in the general population. The idea was to use the reasonably accurate recall by subjects of their occupational histories as the building block for inferring exposures. The JEM would allow subjects who have different jobs but the same exposures to be linked, in the hope of identifying the particular agents responsible for elevated risks.

A number of generic JEMs, which identify occupations and industries using European or American coding systems, have been made publicly available. Some were created using expert judgement, usually aided by published literature and communication with industry personnel (Hoar *et al.* 1980; Pannett *et al.* 1985; Ferrario *et al.* 1988; Orlowski *et al.* 1993; Plato and Steineck 1993; Gomez *et al.* 1994; Kennedy *et al.* 2000). Others were based on observations of potential exposure to hazardous agents in walkthrough surveys of representative samples of US worksites (Sieber *et al.* 1991). A more recent Finnish JEM used a database of exposure measurements to aid expert assessments (Kauppinen *et al.* 1998), and a Swedish JEM of magnetic field exposures was created using measurement data (Floderus *et al.* 1996).

Over the last two decades, many investigators have examined the validity of generic JEMs; the results have not promoted confidence in them. For example, Tielemans *et al.* (1999) compared the JEM of Hoar *et al.* (1980) to urinary measurements of toluene, xylene, and chromium, and found only slight agreement (kappas from 0.04 to 0.13) and low specificities (0.63–0.79) and sensitivities (0.26–0.60). Hawkes and Wilkins (1997) compared two JEMs, that of Hoar *et al.* (1980) and that of Sieber *et al.* (1991), and found that agreements for 54 job groups in the metal, wood, and chemical industries were similar to that expected by chance alone. Benke *et al.* (2001) compared the JEM of Kauppinen *et al.* (1998) to self-reports and expert assessments of exposure to five substances, and found median kappas for agreement beyond chance of 0.07 and 0.28, respectively. McNamee (1996) compared the generic JEM of Cherry *et al.* (1992) to expert-reviewed exposure self-reports and to an internal study-specific JEM. Odds ratios for the association between hydrocarbon exposure and chronic pancreatitis did not show a dose–response using the generic JEM, but did for expert-reviewed self-reported exposures, suggesting that exposure misclassification by the JEM method had obscured the exposure–effect association. Rybicki *et al.* (1997) compared the JEM of Sieber *et al.* (1991) to expert-reviewed self-reports, and found the JEM to have low sensitivities (0–0.21) but higher specificities (0.86–0.93).

Dosemeci *et al.* (1994) showed that performance of a generic JEM (Gomez *et al.* 1994) could be improved by adding features that increased the specificity of exposure assessment. Using estimates for the intensity alone of methylene chloride exposure, the odds ratio for brain cancer was 1.5; this increased to 2.5 when the analysis was restricted to those with a high probability of exposure, to 4.2 when an additional digit in the occupational coding scheme was used, and to 6.1 when a time dimension was added to the matrix. Similarly, McNamee (1996) found that a study-specific JEM out-performed the generic JEM. Kennedy *et al.* (2000) found that the performance of a JEM could be improved by ensuring that coding of jobs was checked and errors corrected.

Investigators examining the utility of generic JEMs have frequently concluded that they were not sensitive, and not in good agreement with methods in which they had more confidence. The low sensitivities of generic JEMs are understandable given the number of jobs whose exposures need to be assessed, and the often unexpected circumstances in which occupational exposures can occur. All JEMs, both generic and study-specific, suffer the inability to account for variability in exposures within a job—whether held in different plants or departments, or by different subjects with varying interactions with the agent in question. Generic JEMs often have additional limitations. The jobs or exposures under investigation may not be included in a matrix created by other investigators with different objectives in mind, or may be grouped in such a way as to obscure their impact. For example, when the geographic region under study features a major industry, which is only a small component of an existing generic JEM, its important exposures or specific jobs may be missed. While there may still be situations when generic JEMs are the only reasonable alternative, the problems discussed here have moderated the initial enthusiasm for generic JEMs and encouraged exposure assessment methods that are more study-specific.

8.4 Self-reported occupational and environmental exposures

Where studies use questionnaires, it is logical to consider questioning subjects directly about their occupational or environmental exposures as well. For example, question-naires used in population-based or nested case–control studies may ask about use of specific raw materials or tradename products, or exposures to specific agents or classes of compounds. Subjects may also be asked about tasks, equipment, locations, and control measures thought to influence exposure levels (Gérin *et al.* 1985; Stewart *et al.* 1998).

Many studies have examined the validity and reliability of self-reported occupational exposure information. For example, Rybicki *et al.* (1997) examined exposures to copper, lead, and iron and compared both a JEM and self-reports to an exposure evaluation by experts. Self-reports were more sensitive than the JEM and slightly more specific. Tielemans *et al.* (1999) compared a JEM and self-reports to measured urinary chromium, toluene, and xylene. Sensitivities were again higher using self-reports, but specificities suffered as a result, and therefore the JEM had higher positive predictive values. Self-reported exposures have also been compared to industrial hygiene measurement data. Kromhout *et al.* (1987) found that the proportions of variance in exposure explained (R^2) by self-reports of exposure to dusts or solvents varied from 0.03 to 0.56. Nieuwenhuijsen *et al.* (1997) found a Spearman rank correlation coefficient of 0.67 when farm workers self-reported inhalable dust exposures, but only 0.36 for respirable dust exposures. When considering the body of evidence as a whole, from more than 30 investigations, Teschke *et al.* (2002) concluded that the most notable feature was the variability in validity and reliability from study to study, and within studies, from agent to agent.

Fewer studies have investigated the accuracy of self-reported environmental exposures. Examples include the following studies of non-smokers' exposure to environmental tobacco smoke. Jenkins and Counts (1999) found that subjects who self-reported that they were exposed both at home and at work had higher median salivary cotinine levels (2.1 ng ml^{-1}) compared to those only exposed in the home (0.86), at work (0.37), or neither (0.19), and that 2.2–6.6 per cent of subjects would be misclassified by their self-reports. Emmons *et al.* (1994) found that self-reports of duration of exposure and numbers of smokers at home and at work predicted 29 per cent of the variance in salivary cotinine concentrations. Others have examined the validity of self-reports of exposure sources, rather than exposures themselves, for example, household appliance use (Mills *et al.* 2000), walking trips, and road crossings (Stevenson 1996).

There are characteristics that have been consistently associated with better self-reporting. Agents that are easily sensed (e.g. odiferous chemicals, visible dusts, perceptible vibrations) are more likely to be recognized by subjects and reported. Using familiar terminology promotes more accurate reporting (e.g. asking about varsol exposure, rather than its component hydrocarbons). Subjects who have been involved in choosing chemicals for workplace use are more likely to remember exposures (e.g. welders who select the welding rods and metals they use, farmers or applicators who buy pesticides), than those without this level of control or knowledge (e.g. factory labourers, farm workers). Prompting recall with a list of specific exposure agents of interest (i.e. querying whether a subject was exposed to any 'dusts, fumes, gases, or vapours'), results in higher sensitivities than open-ended questioning, without an equivalent loss in specificity. Subjects who are provided with relative or objective benchmarks against which to judge their potential for exposures do so better than those considering their own exposure in isolation. For example, Ising *et al.* (1997) asked subjects to compare noise in their workplaces to that created by machines such as typewriters, lawnmowers, and drills, and achieved a Spearman rank correlation of 0.84 between self-reports and measured exposures.

A vital consideration when exposures are self-assessed is whether reporting is influenced by disease status, and therefore might result in spuriously elevated risk estimates if cases ruminate about exposures more than healthy subjects. Where subjective measures of both exposure and disease status have been used (as has often been done in cross-sectional studies), there is evidence that recall bias may result (Fonn *et al*. 1993), perhaps because those who worry about their exposures are also most anxious about their health. However, in case–control studies, where recall bias has more typically been a concern, health outcomes are usually identified objectively (e.g. through cancer registries or hospital records). Studies investigating the validity of self-reported exposures in such studies have found little or no difference between cases and controls, except when exposures are volunteered on open-ended questioning (as opposed to structured prompting) (Rodvall *et al*. 1996; Teschke *et al*. 2000).

Overall, the quality of self-reported data on exposures is usually better than that of generic JEMs. However, although subjects can reliably and accurately report exposures in certain circumstances, the variability in results of validity studies indicate that it is also possible for subjects to provide data of such poor quality that true exposure–response relationships will be obscured or even reversed in direction (Flegal *et al*. 1986). Epidemiologists and exposure assessors who are designing questionnaires should therefore implement measures to improve subjects' reporting accuracy, including prompting about agents of interest, asking about agents that can be sensed, describing agents in terms used at worksites or in the public domain, and asking about exposures in such a way that subjects can consider their exposures in relation to those of others or in relation to identifiable exposure levels. Continued testing of questionnaire instruments is needed to further improve our understanding of factors that enhance subjects' recall and reporting.

8.5 Expert assessment of occupational and environmental exposures

In occupational cohort studies, it has been a long-standing tradition to employ industrial hygienists to use their judgement to estimate exposures, particularly to interpret the applicability of existing measurement data or fill in gaps where no data exist. In case–control studies, the use of experts to infer exposure has grown roughly in parallel with the development of generic JEMs. Not only hygienists, but chemists, engineers, occupational physicians, and industry-specific professionals (e.g. agronomists) have been engaged in exposure estimation. Experts are thought to have a better vantage point than study subjects for this task: by training, they understand the mechanisms of exposures and how to locate related information; they are likely to know the study hypotheses, and therefore which agents and what levels of exposure are important; and because they need to assign exposures to all subjects, they will have an overview of the range of jobs whose exposures need to be estimated. But these advantages are tempered by other difficulties. In retrospective cohort studies, experts may not be able to gain familiarity with all jobs and their environments throughout the time period covered by the study. In population-based studies, experts are unlikely to be acquainted with the range of industries that appear in subjects' occupational histories; and unless they have detailed reports from subjects, they cannot be aware of specific worksite characteristics.

Studies of experts' occupational exposure assessments have evaluated how these competing assets and liabilities affect their validity and reliability. For example, in the study by Tielemans *et al.* (1999), which used urinary solvent and chromium measurements as the gold standard, experts based their judgements on subject-reported job histories and job-specific questionnaires. In comparison to self-reported exposures, sensitivities were lower, but specificities and positive predictive values were higher. Kromhout *et al.* (1987) asked two hygienists to rank solvent and dust exposures in five plants, and used measured airborne levels as the reference standard. Proportions of variance explained ranged from 0.08 to 0.58, slightly higher than for subject self-reports. In a study by Cherrie and Schneider (1999), two hygienists used descriptions of jobs, tasks, work environments, and control measures to complete a structured assessment of exposures to dust, toluene, styrene, and man-made mineral fibre. Correlations to measured airborne concentrations ranged from 0 to 0.93. Benke *et al.* (1997) used three hygienists and two occupational physicians to estimate exposures to 21 chemicals and compared their estimates to 11 years of industrial hygiene survey data from the region. Sensitivities varied from 0.48 to 0.79 and specificities from 0.91 to 0.98. Thus the pattern for expert assessment of occupational exposure, though slightly better, is similar to that observed for self-reported exposures; in 20 studies, validities and reliabilities varied tremendously, between agents and studies (Teschke *et al.* 2002).

In the environmental field, expert judgements are only rarely used, and even more rarely evaluated. As an example, Walker *et al.* (2001) compared the means and 90th percentile estimates of personal benzene exposure by seven experts selected by peer nomination. Estimates of the mean varied over a 3-fold range, from 7 to 20 $\mu g\,m^{-3}$, and for the 90th percentile in a somewhat wider range, from 10 to 40 $\mu g\,m^{-3}$.

Expert assessments are often thought of as a single method, but many different evaluation structures and tools can be used. The starting points for most assessments are the job title, industry, and whatever supplementary descriptions are available, whether derived from company records or subject questionnaires. In industry-based studies, interviews with key informants may provide details about the work environment, and exposure measurements might be available from the companies involved. In population-based studies, judgement and the published hygiene literature are more frequent tools, though some experts may use measurements of similar jobs or industries available from exposure databases. In studies using questionnaires, experts' estimates can be made more subject-specific by using self-reported exposure and job duty information. Gérin *et al.* (1985) and Stewart *et al.* (1998) developed a series of occupation- and industry-specific questionnaire modules to guide expert evaluations; these include detailed questions about tasks, materials, equipment, and control measures.

A number of studies have considered the effect of these levels of data on expert assessment. Stewart *et al.* (2000) and de Cock *et al.* (1996) found little difference in the quality of the assessments when experts' were given additional information such as department, industry, date, and tasks. Segnan *et al.* (1996) and Tielemans *et al.* (1999) compared assessments based on occupational histories to assessments based on industry-specific modules; the former group found little change in sensitivities, but an increase in specificities, the latter found the reverse. Hawkins and Evans (1989) examined the effect of offering measurement data to experts, and found that initial estimates without data overestimated exposures, but with data, hygienists' estimates were less biased. When Post *et al.* (1991) gave measurement data to hygienists, their relative ranking of jobs did not improve, but their classification of jobs into quantitative exposure categories did.

A factor that has been found to affect the validity and reliability of experts' estimates is the type of agent, an effect also observed in self-reports by subjects. Well-known classes of chemicals, such as insecticides, cutting fluids, welding fumes, oils and greases, and solvents are estimated more accurately than specific agents (Segnan *et al.* 1996; Benke *et al.* 2001) as are agents that can be sensed (e.g. smelled) (Post *et al.* 1991).

In summary, there is evidence to support the view that experts are usually able to estimate exposures more accurately than study subjects, though improvements are generally small and in any case cannot be assured, underscoring the importance of testing reliability and validity. Although experts can provide reasonable exposure estimates in some situations, estimates can also be of such poor quality that true exposure–effect relationships can be obscured or even reversed in direction (Flegal *et al.* 1986). Experts' performance can be enhanced, by providing them with detailed data on work or living conditions, with exposure measurements that can be used to calibrate their estimates, and by asking them to evaluate exposures to agents that are well known to them and easily sensed.

8.6   Some additional considerations

Methods that can be used to improve the validity and reliability of occupational histories, JEMs, self-reported exposures, and expert assessments are summarized in Table 8.2. Other methodological characteristics potentially affecting exposure estimation have not yet received much attention. Although it is known that increased elapsed time since a job was held somewhat reduces the validity of an occupational history, the effect on subjects' and experts' exposure estimates has not been examined. In addition, though surrogate evaluations are often conducted by more than one expert, the optimum number of experts and the value of independent vs. consensus estimates has rarely been examined (Benke *et al.* 1997).

Factors other than the quality of the surrogate exposure assessment can affect the potential for misclassified exposures to attenuate a risk estimate. One that is relatively straightforward to control is related to the prevalence of exposure: what to do with subjects whose exposure is unknown or uncertain. Dosemeci and Stewart (1996) showed that it is best to include these subjects with the largest group—whether unexposed or exposed—so that the smaller group is not diluted with misclassified subjects. Thus in case–control studies, where exposure prevalence is likely to be low, specificity is more critical than sensitivity. This means that expert reviews of self-reported exposures should focus on reclassifying subjects who appear to have 'overestimated' their exposure in relation to others in the study. In situations where exposure prevalence exceeds 50 per cent (as is more likely to occur in cohort or cross-sectional studies), sensitivity would be more important than specificity.

Surrogate methods used to assess exposures, though often thought of as distinct from each other, are interrelated and interdependent. In addition, none of the surrogate

Table 8.2   Summary of validity and reliability of proxy measures of exposure, and methods to improve them

Type of exposure proxy	Overview of validity and reliability	Methods that may improve validity and reliability
Occupational history	Agreement between self-reported job histories and company records usually very good	Asking about more recent or longer-term jobs Having a less-complex job history Chronicling major life events to enhance recall
JEM	In comparisons usually to each other, self-reports and expert assessments, generic JEMs usually not found to be valid or reliable	Increasing the specificity of the JEM by accounting for time periods, and more clearly specifying occupation and industry Ensuring occupation and industry coding is accurate
Self-reported exposure	In comparisons to expert evaluation and measured exposures, self-reports usually better than JEMs, but there is great variability in reliability and validity estimates by agent and study	Asking about exposures that can be sensed Using terms familiar to workers Using benchmarks against which to gauge exposure levels Asking about factors related to exposures that are easier to recall (e.g. tasks)
Expert evaluation	In comparisons to measured exposures, expert assessments usually slightly better than self-reports, but again there is great variability in reliability and validity estimates by agent and study	Evaluating exposures to commonly used agents and classes of agents Evaluating exposures that can be sensed Providing measurement data, information about the properties of the agents, and detailed information about the worksite

methods is a single clearly specified technique, instead each may include a variety of methods that are combined to elicit exposure estimates. For example, JEMs may be based on experts' judgements, exposure measurements, or even subjects' self-reports. Expert assessments may use self-reported information about job histories, exposures, tasks, and the working or living environment, as well as measurement data from government, industry, or the scientific literature. Questionnaires used to gather self-reports are formulated by experts, and may include simple job or residential histories or more detailed questions about factors expected or known to be associated with exposures. The interdependencies and complex details of the methods are important to consider (and report as methods in publications), since subtle changes may affect the success of the exposure assessment.

Finally, even though the surrogate measurement techniques described in this chapter are usually envisaged as a contrast to the ideal of measured exposures, even this dichotomy is not as straightforward as it may seem. Certainly a sliding scale from measurement to qualitative assessment has long existed in retrospective cohort studies, where filling in missing values is often left to some sort of judgement process. But increasingly, as hygienists become aware of the limitations of subjective surrogate estimation techniques, methods of including measurements in the assessments have been sought. Examples include the Finnish JEM, which uses an exposure database to aid expert judgement (Kauppinen *et al.* 1998). The use of administrative exposure data or literature-reported data as components of an expert assessment has been pioneered by hygienists at the US National Cancer Institute (Stewart and Stewart 1994). More recently, exposure models (described in detail in Chapter 6) have been used as a component of questionnaire-based exposure assessments. Subjects can be asked about factors found to be related to occupational or environmental exposures in empirical models (e.g. tasks, raw materials, equipment, processes, proximity to exposure sources); the models can then be used to relate subject responses to quantitative exposure levels (Preller *et al.* 1995; Burstyn and Teschke 1999, Chapter 6). The incorporation of these more systematic and objective techniques to link qualitative and quantitative data is a positive development in epidemiological exposure assessment.

References

Benke, G., Sim, M., Forbes, A., and Salzberg, M. (1997). Retrospective assessment of occupational exposure to chemicals in community-based studies: validity and repeatability of industrial hygiene panel ratings. *International Journal of Epidemiology*, **26**, 635–42.

Benke, G., Sim, M., Fritchi, L., Aldred, G., Forbes, A., and Kauppinen, T. (2001). Comparison of occupational exposure using three different methods: hygiene panel, job exposure matrix (JEM), and self-reports. *Applied Occupational and Environmental Hygiene*, **16**, 84–91.

Burstyn, I. and Teschke, K. (1999). Studying the determinants of exposure: a review of methods. *American Industrial Hygiene Association Journal*, **60**, 57–72.

Cherrie, J. W. and Schneider, T. (1999). Validation of a new method for structured subjective assessment of past concentrations. *Annals of Occupational Hygiene*, **43**, 235–45.

Cherry, N. M., Labreche, F. P., and McDonald, J. C. (1992). Organic brain damage and occupational solvent exposure. *British Journal of Industrial Medicine*, **49**, 776–81.

Christiani, D. C., Niu, T., and Xu, X. (1995). Occupational stress and dysmenorrhea in women working in cotton textile mills. *International Journal of Occupational and Environmental Health*, **1**, 9–15.

de Cock, J., Kromhout, J., Heederik, D., and Burema, J. (1996). Experts' subjective assessment of pesticide exposure in fruit growing. *Scandinavian Journal of Work, Environment and Health*, **22**, 425–32.

Dosemeci, M. and Stewart, P. A. (1996). Recommendations for reducing the effects of misclassification on relative risk estimates. *Occupational Hygiene*, **3**, 169–76.

Dosemeci, M., Cocco, P., Gomez, M., Stewart, P. A., and Heineman, E. F. (1994). Effects of three features of a job-exposure matrix on risk estimates. *Epidemiology*, **5**, 124–7.

Emmons, K. M., Abrams, D. B., Marshall, R., Marcus, B. H., Kane, M., Novotny, T. E., and Etzel, R. A. (1994). An evaluation of the relationship between self-report and biochemical measures of environmental tobacco smoke exposure. *Preventive Medicine*, **23**, 35–9.

Ferrario, F., Continenza, D., Pisani, P., Magnani, C., Merletti, F., and Berrino, F. (1988). Description of a job-exposure matrix for sixteen agents which are or may be related to respiratory cancer. In *Progress in occupational epidemiology* (ed. C. Hogstedt and C. Reuterwall), pp. 379–82. Elsevier, Amsterdam.

Flegal, K. M., Brownie, C., and Haas, J. D. (1986). The effects of exposure misclassification on estimates of relative risk. *American Journal of Epidemiology*, **123**, 736–51.

Floderus, B., Persson, T., and Stenlund, C. (1996). Magnetic field exposures in the workplace: reference distribution and exposures in occupational groups. *International Journal of Occupational and Environmental Health*, **2**, 226–38.

Fonn, S., Groeneveld, H. T., deBeer, M., and Becklake, M. R. (1993). Relationship of respiratory health status to grain dust in a Witwatersrand grain mill: comparison of workers' exposure assessments with industrial hygiene survey findings. *American Journal of Industrial Medicine*, **24**, 401–11.

Frumkin, H., Letz, R., Williams, P. L., Gerr, F., Pierce, M., Sanders, A., Elon, L., Manning, C. C., Woods, J. S., Hertzberg, V. S., Mueller, P., and Taylor, B. B. (2001). Health effects of long-term mercury exposure among chlor-alkali plant workers. *American Journal of Industrial Medicine*, **39**, 1–18.

Gérin, M., Siemiatycki, J., Kemper, H., and Begin, D. (1985). Obtaining occupational exposure histories in epidemiologic case–control studies. *Journal of Occupational Medicine*, **27**, 420–6.

Gomez, M. R., Cocco, P., Dosemeci, M., and Stewart, P. A. (1994). Occupational exposure to chlorinated aliphatic hydrocarbons: job-exposure matrix. *American Journal of Industrial Medicine*, **26**, 171–83.

Hawkes, A. P. and Wilkins, J. R. (1997). Assessing agreement between two job-exposure matrices. *Scandinavian Journal of Work Environment and Health*, **23**, 140–8.

Hawkins, N. C. and Evans, J. S. (1989). Subjective estimation of toluene exposures: a calibration study of industrial hygienists. *Applied Industrial Hygiene*, **4**, 61–8.

Hoar, S. K., Morrison, A. S., Cole, P., and Silverman, D. T. (1980). An occupation and exposure linkage system for the study of occupational carcinogenesis. *Journal of Occupational Medicine*, **22**, 722–6.

Ising, H., Babisch, W., Kruppa, B., Lindthammer, A., and Wiens, D. (1997). Subjective work noise: a major risk factor in myocardial infarction. *Sozial-Und Praventivmedizin*, **42**, 216–22.

Jenkins, R. A. and Counts, R. W. (1999). Personal exposure to environmental tobacco smoke: salivary cotinine, airborne nicotine, and nonsmoker misclassification. *Journal of Exposure Analysis and Environmental Epidemiology*, **9**, 352–63.

Kamel, F., Unbach, D. M., Munsat, T. L., Shefner, J. M., Hu, H., and Sandler, D. P. (2002). Lead exposure and amyotrophic lateral schlerosis. *Epidemiology*, **13**, 311–19.

Kauppinen, T., Toikkanen, J., and Pukkala, E. (1998). From cross-tabulations to multipurpose exposure information systems: a new job-exposure matrix. *American Journal of Industrial Medicine*, **33**, 409–17.

Kennedy, S. M., Le Moual, N., Choudat, D., and Kauffmann, F. (2000). Development of an asthma specific job exposure matrix and its application in the epidemiological study of genetics and environment in asthma. *Occupational and Environmental Medicine*, **57**, 635–41.

Kromhout, H. and Vermeulen, R. (2001). Application of job-exposure matrices in studies of the general population: some clues to their performance. *European Respiratory Review*, **11**, 80–90.

Kromhout, H., Oostendorp, Y., Heederik, D., and Boleij, J. S. M. (1987). Agreement between qualitative exposure estimates and quantitative exposure measurements. *American Journal of Industrial Medicine*, **12**, 551–62.

LaForest, L., Luce, D., Goldberg, P., Begin, D., Gerin, M., Demers, P. A., Brugere, J., and Leclerc, A. (2000). Laryngeal and hypopharyngeal cancers and occupational exposure to formaldehyde and various dusts: a case–control study in France. *Occupational and Environmental Medicine*, **57**, 767–73.

London, L., Nell, V., Thompson, M. L., and Myers, J. E. (1998). Effects of long-term organophosphate exposures on neurological symptoms, vibration sense and tremor among South African farm workers. *Scandinavian Journal of Work, Environment and Health*, **24**, 18–29.

McGuire, V., Nelson, L. M., Koepsell, T. D., Checkoway, H., and Longstreth, W. T. Jr. (1998). Assessment of occupational exposures in community-based case–control studies. *Annual Review of Public Health*, **19**, 35–53.

McNamee, R. (1996). Retrospective assessment of occupational exposure to hydrocarbons-job-exposure matrices versus expert evaluation of questionnaires. *Occupational Hygiene*, **3**, 137–43.

Mills, K. M., Kheifets, L. I., Nelson, L. M., Bloch, D. A., Takemoto-Hambleton, R., and Kelsey, J. L. (2000). Reliability of proxy-reported and self-reported household appliance use. *Epidemiology*, **11**, 581–8.

Nasterlack, M., Dietz, M. C., Frank, K. H., Hacke, W., Scherg, H., Schmittner, H., Stelzer, O., Zimber, A., and Triebig, G. (1999). A multidisciplinary cross-sectional study on solvent-related health effects in painters compared with construction workers. *International Archives of Occupational and Environmental Health*, **72**, 205–14.

Nieuwenhuijsen, M. J., Noderer, K. S., and Schenker, M. B. (1997). The relation between subjective dust exposure estimates and quantitative dust exposure measurements in California agriculture. *American Journal of Industrial Medicine*, **32**, 355–63.

Orlowski, E., Pohlabeln, H., and Berrino, F., *et al.* (1993). Retrospective assessment of asbestos exposure-II. At the job level: complementarity of job-specific questionnaire and job exposure matrices. *International Journal of Epidemiology*, **22**, S96–S105.

Pannett, B., Coggon, D., and Acheson, E. D. (1985). A job-exposure matrix for use in population based studies in England and Wales. *British Journal of Industrial Medicine*, **42**, 777–83.

Plato, N. and Steineck, G. (1993). Methodology and utility of a job-exposure matrix. *American Journal of Industrial Medicine*, **23**, 491–502.

Post, W., Kromhout, H., Heederik, D., Noy, D., and Duijzentkunst, R. S. (1991). Semiquantitative estimates of exposure to methylene chloride and styrene: the influence of quantitative exposure data. *Applied Occupational and Environmental Hygiene*, **6**, 197–204.

Post, W. K., Heederik, D., Kromhout, H., and Kromhout, D. (1994). Occupational exposures estimated by a population specific job exposure matrix and 25 year incidence of chronic non-specific lung disease (CNSLD): the Zutphen Study. *European Respiratory Journal*, **7**, 1048–55.

Preller, L., Kromhout, H., Heederik, D., and Tielen, M. J. M. (1995). Modeling long-term average exposure in occupational exposure–response analysis. *Scandinavian Journal of Work, Environment and Health*, **21**, 504–12.

Rodvall, Y., Ahlbom, A., Spannare, B., and Nise, G. (1996). Glioma and occupational exposure in Sweden, a case–control study. *Occupational and Environmental Medicine*, **53**, 526–32.

Rybicki, B. A., Johnson, C. C., Peterson, E. L., Korsha, G. X., and Gorell, J. M. (1997). Comparability of different methods of retrospective exposure assessment of metals in manufacturing industries. *American Journal of Industrial Medicine*, **31**, 36–43.

Segnan, N., Ponti, A., Ronco, G. F., Kromhout, H., Heederik, D., De Cock, J., Bosia, S., Luccoli, L., Piccioni, P., Constantini, A. S., Miligi, L., Scarpelli, A., Mariotti, M., Scarnato, C., and Morisi, L. (1996). Comparison of methods for assessing the probability of exposure in metal plating, shoe and leather goods manufacture and vine growing. *Occupational Hygiene*, **3**, 199–208.

Seixas, N. S. and Checkoway, H. (1995) Exposure assessment in industry specific retrospective occupational epidemiology studies. *Occupational and Environmental Medicine*, **52**, 625–33.

Sieber, W. K., Sundin, D. S., Frazier, T. M., and Robinson, C. F. (1991). Development, use, and availability of a job exposure matrix based on national occupational hazard survey data. *American Journal of Industrial Medicine*, **20**, 163–74.

Steenland, K., Sanderson, W., and Calvert, G. M. (2001). Kidney disease and arthritis in a cohort study of workers exposed to silica. *Epidemiology*, **12**, 405–12.

Stevenson, M. R. (1996). The validity of children's self-reported exposure to traffic. *Accident Analysis and Prevention*, **28**, 599–605.

Stewart, P. A., Carel, R., Schairer, C., and Blair, A. (2000). Comparison of industrial hygienists' exposure evaluations for an epidemiological study. *Scandinavian Journal of Work, Environment and Health*, **26**, 44–51.

Stewart, P. A., Stewart, W. F., Siemiatycki, J., Heineman, E. F., and Dosemeci, M. (1998). Questionnaires for collecting detailed occupational information for community-based case–control studies. *American Industrial Hygiene Association Journal*, **58**, 39–44.

Stewart, P. A. and Stewart, W. F. (1994). Occupational case–control studies: II. Recommendations for exposure assessment. *American Journal of Industrial Medicine*, **26**, 313–26.

Stick, S. M., Burton, P. R., Gurrin, L., Sly, P. D., and LeSouef, P. N. (1996). Effects of maternal smoking during pregnancy and a family history of asthma on respiratory function in newborn infants. *Lancet*, **248**, 1060–64.

Teschke, K., Smith, J. C., and Olshan, A. F. (2000). Evidence of recall bias in volunteered vs. prompted responses about occupational exposures. *American Journal Industrial Medicine*, **38**, 385–8.

Teschke, K., Olshan, A. F., Daniiels, J. L., De Roos, A. J., Parks, C. G., Schulz, M., and Vaughan, T. L. (2002). Occupational exposure assessment in case–control studies: opportunities for improvement. *Occupational and Environmental Medicine*, **59**, 575–93.

Tielemans, E., Heederik, D., Burdorf, A., Vermeulen, R., Veulemans, H., Kromhout, H., and Hartog, K. (1999). Assessment of occupational exposures in a general population: comparison of different methods. *Occupational and Environmental Medicine*, **56**, 145–51.

van Loon, A. J., Kant, I. J., Swaen, G. M., Goldbohm, R. A., Kremer, A. M., and van den Brandt, P. A. (1997). Occupational exposure to carcinogens and risk of lung cancer: results from The Netherlands cohort study. *Occupational and Environmental Medicine*, **54**, 817–24.

Villeneuve, P. J., Agnew, D. A., Johnson, K. C., Mao, Y., and Canadian Cancer Registries Epidemiology Research Group. (2002). Brain cancer and occupational exposure to magnetic fields among men: results from a Canadian population-based case–control study. *International Journal of Epidemiology*, **31**, 210–17.

Walker, K. D., Evans, J. S., and Macintosh, D. (2001). Use of expert judgement in exposure assessment. Part I. Charaterization of personal exposure to benzene. *Journal of Exposure Analysis and Environmental Epidemiology*, **11**, 308–22.

9. Dermal exposure assessment

Sean Semple and John W. Cherrie

9.1 Introduction

Most epidemiological studies examining the relationship between exposure to hazardous substances and adverse health outcomes have focused on inhalation exposure. While this is appropriate for many substances and particularly for those materials having direct effects on the lung, failure to consider the importance of exposure and uptake of material deposited on the skin may lead to over or under-estimation of the risk. The skin is regarded as the largest organ of the body and plays an important role in protecting us from physical, biological, and chemical insults from our surrounding environment. With a surface area of approximately 2 m^2 the skin also provides an important route for many chemicals to enter the body. Many lipophillic chemicals can pass through the unbroken skin while others can exert important health effects locally, for example, by causing irritation or sensitization of the skin.

Dermal exposure occurs in many occupational settings. This may be a result of immersion of hands and forearms in solutions such as degreasants, or may arise from the handling of work tools or surfaces that have a thin covering layer of the contaminant. Dermal exposure can also arise from splashes or accidental spills directly onto the body or clothing, or may occur when spraying operations produce fine aerosols that are then deposited on the body. Non-occupational exposures may follow similar routes and may additionally include scenarios such as whole-body immersion (bathing), showering, washing, and direct intentional application. Examples include dermal exposure to disinfection by-products such as trihalomethanes present in the public water supply (see Chapter 15) and non-occupational exposure via the dermal route where pesticides are used to control insects or vermin in residential settings.

Solvents, pesticides, and trihalomethanes are some of the largest chemical groups where dermal exposure and uptake requires assessment in any consideration of health effects. Xylene, toluene, benzene, and carbon tetrachloride are, or have been, among the most commonly used solvents and are used either as thinners, degreasants, additives to prevent icing, or as ingredients in protective coatings. Trihalomethanes are formed during the chlorination of water and uptake occurs during showering, bathing, and swimming. Pesticides are generally non-volatile and as a result dermal exposure can often be the primary exposure route with the uptake fraction received from inhalation being low (Wolfe *et al.* 1967). Pesticides such as lindane, paraquat, and carbaryl are used extensively worldwide. In less-developed countries poor control and failure to use protective equipment during application and crop re-entry activities produces many pesticide poisoning deaths each year.

A wide variety of other materials such as mercury, tetraethyl lead additives in petrol, acrylates used in dentistry, or the nitroglycols used in explosives manufacture, are all hazardous substances that may be absorbed through the skin. Grandjean (1990) provides a useful review of chemicals that pose dermal hazards describing the typical industrial use of each.

Dermal exposure assessment is still relatively immature with only limited under-standing of the exposure process and what biologically relevant exposure metrics should be used for measurement. The importance of the dermal route in chemical risk assessment and hence in epidemiology can be traced to work carried out by Durham and Wolfe (1962). Since then interest in dermal exposure and uptake has been pioneered by researchers investigating occupational exposure to pesticides (e.g. Davis *et al.* 1983; Brouwer *et al.* 1992).

As part of the occupational exposure limit framework in many countries chemicals that could contribute substantially to total body burden by uptake via the unbroken skin and cause serious systemic health effects, may be assigned a skin notation. The UK Health and Safety Executive (HSE) currently uses a skin notation for over 120 chemicals (HSE 2001) while the American Conference of Governmental Industrial Hygienists (ACGIH) apply the 'skin' note to over 160 substances (ACGIH 2002).

The relative importance of the dermal exposure route may have increased due to developments in control technology and improved hygiene measures leading to substantial reductions in inhalation exposures over time. It has been argued that with decreasing airborne concentrations across many workplaces and environments, the relative proportion of total body uptake attributable to dermal exposure may have increased. There is however a counter-argument that control of the airborne fraction will consequentially reduce the degree of surface contamination and hence dermal exposure levels, as demonstrated by Vermeulen *et al.* (2000) in a study of changes in dermal and inhalation exposure levels in the rubber industry.

One of the main problems in developing dermal exposure assessment strategies has been the lack of a biologically relevant exposure metric. Just as with inhalation exposure it is often unknown whether it is the cumulative amount of material absorbed, the average quantity over a certain reference period, or exposure peaks that produce ill-health effects. Further, sampling methods have developed in an unstandardized manner and often without thought to how the fraction sampled relates either to exposure or to uptake. For example, when measuring the quantity of material on the skin at the end of a work shift we may simply be sampling the fraction that has not already been absorbed, or lost to the environment, over the exposure period, therefore gaining little insight into the mass uptake and hence the dermal contribution.

The relationship between exposure and uptake is a complex one for the dermal path-way. Many studies focus on the quantity of material deposited on the workers' skin as the factor regulating dermal uptake. While it is true that dermal absorption cannot phys-ically exceed the mass of material deposited on the skin, it is the concentration of the substance that drives the diffusive process (Cherrie and Robertson 1995). The mass uptake of a chemical through the skin is not necessarily a constant proportion of the mass deposited on the skin.

Often dermal exposure is viewed purely in terms of the percutaneous uptake of chemicals. It is important, however, to remember that three types of chemical–skin interactions exist and an understanding of these is vital to properly characterize the dermal exposure. First, the chemical may pass through the skin and contribute to the systemic load thereby producing systemic health effects on target organs such as the liver, kidneys, and brain. Alternatively, the chemical can induce local effects ranging from irritation to burns and degradation of the barrier properties of the skin. Last, the chemical can evoke allergic skin reactions through complex immune-system responses that can subsequently trigger dermatitis. There may often be interactions between these modes of action. For example, a chemical can irritate the skin surface thus leading to significant increases in percutaneous penetration of that, or other, chemicals. However, in each case the chemical must diffuse through the outer layers of the skin before any adverse health outcome is possible.

9.2   Understanding skin–chemical interactions

Skin is made up of an outer layer, the stratum corneum or epidermis, a water-resistant layer of dead keratinocytes, and an inner layer termed the dermis. The dermis is composed of living cells and also the microstructure of the skin including blood vessels, nerves, hair follicles, and sweat glands.

When chemicals are placed on the outer surface of the skin in contact with the epidermis a concentration gradient is generated across the 'membrane' of the skin. Assuming that the concentration of the material within the body is less than that on the epidermal surface, a diffusive mass transfer will be set up with the rate of diffusion regulated by the chemical and physical properties of the material and skin. This passive movement from outer skin to the dermis and hence to blood capillaries is governed by Fick's Law, which states that at steady-state the rate of diffusion across a barrier will be directly proportional to the concentration gradient across that barrier.

The transfer of material across the skin can be characterized by two factors. The lag time is the time it takes from application on the skin surface until the material enters the receptor medium or blood supply. The duration of the lag time can range from minutes for chemicals such as the phenoxycarboxylic herbicides 2,4 D and MCPA, to many hours for materials such as the polycyclic aromatic hydrocarbon chrysene. After the lag time is complete we have steady-state conditions with linear increments in the quantity of material passing through the skin with time, provided there is sufficient contaminant to sustain diffusion. The steady-state diffusion flux (J) is measured in units of mass per unit area per time period ($mg\,cm^{-2}h^{-1}$) and is directly proportional to the concentration gradient (C) across the skin membrane. For a given concentration gradient the rate of flux is regulated by the permeability constant (K_p) measured in units of $cm\,h^{-1}$. Knowledge of K_p for a chemical is thus essential to be able to predict or estimate the quantity or fraction of a material deposited on the skin that will be absorbed into the body.

Bowman and Maibach (2000) examined some of the factors that influence the flux of contaminant material across the skin. The region of the skin has been shown to have a large effect on the penetration of a given chemical. Differences of as much as 50-fold may be found between highly permeable areas such as scrotal skin when compared with less permeable tissue from the legs and abdomen. Occlusion, where applied material is

Table 9.1 Factors influencing
the uptake of chemicals through
the skin

Concentration
Duration
Surface area
Skin thickness
Skin location
Skin condition
Humidity
Temperature
Vehicle effects
Presence of sweat

---

covered to prevent evaporation from the surface of the skin, has also been shown to increase the quantity of absorbed material by up to five times. Gordon *et al.* (1998) demonstrated that human volunteers bathing in water containing chloroform, the main trihalomethane, absorbed some 30 times more chloroform at temperatures of 40°C when compared to 30°C. This is likely to be due to increased blood flow to the surface of the skin at higher temperatures. Experiments have also shown that irritated skin can have dermal uptake levels with an order of magnitude that is greater than in non-irritated skin. Table 9.1 lists a number of important factors that influence the uptake of chemicals through the skin.

Various groups (e.g. Sartorelli *et al.* 1998; Wilkinson and Williams 2001) have used simple diffusion cells to calculate the rate of flux across the skin for a variety of solvents, polycyclic aromatic hydrocarbons, organophosphorus insecticides, and phenoxy-carboxylic herbicides. From these and other works (Patel and Cronin 2001) it has been shown that the permeability of compounds may be modelled using quantitative structure–activity relationship (QSAR) techniques. This method employs correlation techniques to identify physicochemical properties such as the octanol/water partition coefficient (K_{ow}), the molecular weight, and the water solubility of the material that may be closely related to the permeability.

Bunge and Ley (2002) have suggested that in some circumstances solids may penetrate the skin more easily than aqueous solutions. While Kezic *et al.* (2002) have demonstrated that in some circumstances more dilute solvents may find it easier to transfer across the skin than concentrated solutions. This illustrates that our current understanding that diffusion across the skin is directly proportional to the concentration of material is a simplification and the reality may be more complex. There is still a long way to go in fully understanding the thermodynamic activity of the diffusion process of many mixtures of chemicals through skin. Differences in the experimental set-up, application methods, and measurement techniques make it difficult to compare findings across groups working in the field of percutaneous penetration and there is a need for a standardized experimental protocol that will allow the identification of vehicle, anatomical location, and other physical effects, on the rate of flux across the skin.

9.3 Measuring dermal exposure

9.3.1 What to measure

There are four key elements that are important in measuring dermal exposure: exposure intensity, surface area exposed, duration, and frequency of exposure. Exposure intensity is most often measured as a mass of material deposited over a given area. However, as described earlier, the parameter driving diffusion and hence uptake is the concentration of the material on the skin surface and so any true measure of exposure intensity should be expressed in terms of skin surface concentration. Unfortunately, no accepted sampling methods to measure concentration exist and instead the mass per unit area is often used as a surrogate. The suitability of mass as a surrogate for concentration differs in different exposure scenarios, especially between the 'finite dose' situations experienced in environmental measurements and the 'infinite dose' exposure events in occupational settings. Mass may also be an unsuitable surrogate in situations where the concentration of the contaminant changes during the measurement period, as for example, occurs when pesticides are diluted before use. Measurement of the dermal exposure intensity is often divided into 'potential exposure', the amount of material that is deposited on the worker's overalls, clothing, and gloves; and 'actual exposure', the amount of material that comes into contact with the skin.

The second element necessary to characterize dermal exposure is the surface area exposed. This can be assessed by direct visualization techniques (see later). The surface area exposed is likely to be subject to high degrees of day-to-day, between-subject and anatomical variation. Wassenius *et al.* (1998) carried out a study to examine the variability of skin exposure of machine operators exposed to cutting fluids. Using video recording of work tasks and data on fluid evaporation times this paper describes how workers' hands were wet for anything from 0 to 100 per cent of the job time. Tasks with short cycle times were more likely to have a higher degree of relative wet time but overall the degree of skin exposure was shown to be highly variable and independent of machine type or task process. A study of dermal exposure during spray painting (Lansink *et al.* 1997) demonstrated that paint overspray is not uniformly deposited over the body. More than 50 per cent of the total mass of dermal exposure was to the lower legs and less than 3 per cent to the hands. The study also found that only approximately 10 per cent of the worker's cover-all surface was covered with paint. The high degree of variation in terms of anatomical location and the amount of surface area covered will play an important role in determining the degree of systemic uptake of the chemical.

The last important parameter required is a measure of the duration and frequency of the exposure event. The duration of contact may be of little importance if the material remains on the skin or clothing for a much longer period thereafter. In these situations the time until removal (e.g. by washing, evaporation, or uptake) may be the controlling factor. However, the duration and frequency of contact may play a larger role particularly when the rate of evaporation or uptake is high. It is important that the type and frequency of sampling are chosen to reflect these factors.

Dermal exposure assessment can be achieved by either direct physical measurement of deposited material, indirect methods such as visualization and biomonitoring, or by modelling using statistical or deterministic procedures. All have advantages and disadvantages in terms of accuracy, practical considerations, expense, and what they actually tell us about dermal exposure. None of the methods are suitable for all chemical types and exposure scenarios and many suffer from a lack of standardized methodologies. Direct measurement can be further divided into surrogate skin methods and removal techniques.

9.3.2 Surrogate skin techniques

Surrogate skin includes whole-body suits and absorbent patch sampling. By using suits or patches attached to the outside of the body, both techniques aim to sample the total amount of the substance that would be deposited on the skin or clothing. This is often described as potential dermal exposure. Whole-body suits cover the entire body surface and may be augmented with a hat or hood for the head and gloves for the hands. They can be analysed in terms of body part to identify those anatomical regions receiving greatest exposure. Patches are worn at various representative locations on the body with the mass collected on each patch being extrapolated depending on the patch size relative to the size of the body area being sampled. Sampling protocols, such as the World Health Organisation (WHO) method (WHO 1982) and the Organisation for Economic Co-operation and Development (OECD) guidelines (OECD 1997) for patch sampling, vary in terms of the number of patches, their location, size, and sampling material. Even the size of each anatomical region represented by similarly placed patches differs between protocols.

One of the primary weaknesses of patch sampling is the potential introduction of large errors when the exposure is non-uniform. If a patch for a given body area is subject to a splash or spill the method will overestimate the potential dermal exposure for that body area. The converse is also true when proportionally less is deposited on the patch compared to the surrounding area. Work by Tannahill *et al.* (1996) compared exposure measurements made by whole-body sampling with those from patch sampling. In general there was a linear relationship between the two methods though the authors note that the accuracy of the patch method increased with increasing numbers of patches. In summary, when exposure is likely to be non-uniform the use and interpretation of patch sampling should be undertaken with caution.

Other difficulties with patch sampling include patch overloading and problems with detachment in highly active work situations or confined environments. Careful consideration of the quantity of chemical likely to be deposited and the absorption capabilities of the patch material should take place prior to sampling. Close observation of subjects may be required to replace patches that appear overloaded or become detached during sampling.

The use of whole-body suits, typically lightweight cotton overalls, is often used to sample potential dermal exposure among spray painters and pesticide applicators, and was recently used to collect dermal exposure data across a wide variety of exposure scenarios (van Hemmen 2002). Other investigators have also used similar suits worn by children and toddlers to investigate exposure to pesticide residues in nurseries (Cohen Hubal *et al.* 2000).

The 'reservoir' effects of clothing may also introduce error to surrogate skin measurements. Chemicals may soak into overalls or clothing and then slowly transfer to the patch or whole-body suit over time. Direct dermal exposure may occur for only a short period of the working day, but contaminated or wet clothing is often worn by workers for the remainder of the shift. In such situations interior patches or suits removed after the dermal exposure event would be likely to underestimate the true exposure.

Two other aspects of surrogate skin sampling are likely to introduce error into the exposure assessment process. First, absorbent materials such as cotton will not behave in the same manner as skin. Fluid applied to the skin will take one of three routes. It may run-off the skin, as is the case with the majority of a liquid deposited after a splash, spill, or immersion event. Alternatively, the liquid may evaporate from the warm skin surface into the surrounding air, or lastly, it may be absorbed into the stratum corneum by diffusive processes. Cotton and other similar sampling materials are more likely to absorb fluids than real skin and also the fluid is less likely to evaporate due to lower surface temperatures. Hence surrogate skin methods are likely to overestimate the amount of a chemical available for uptake through the skin. Second, and in common with most dermal measurement techniques, surrogate skin sampling measures the mass of the contaminant instead of the concentration. While mass is a useful measure and is often used as a surrogate of concentration, the mass of material deposited on the skin in occupational settings is likely to far exceed the mass uptake.

9.3.3 Removal techniques

Removal techniques can be divided into wiping, washing, or tape stripping. All of these methods aim to collect the quantity of the material present on the surface of the skin or, in the case of tape stripping, bound to the outer layer of the stratum corneum. Wiping may be carried out dry, or with absorbent material soaked in water, alcohol, or any other appropriate solvent. Wipes are usually used on the hands but may be employed to measure any area of the skin. Templates are commonly used to ensure that only a predetermined skin area is wiped. No standardized protocol exists describing the number of wipes or the amount of force that should be applied when collecting wipe samples and it is thus difficult to compare results obtained across studies.

Hand-washing methods follow similar principles with the hand being placed in a sealed bag containing a volume of water or other solvent and vigorous shaking used to remove the chemical from the surface of the skin. Brouwer *et al.* (2000) found that six different wipe sampling strategies, each with a variety of skin loadings were shown to have sampling efficiencies ranging from 41 to 104 per cent with standard deviations between 6 and 28 per cent indicating high degrees of variability. Similar variation in sampling efficiencies were evident for hand-wash sampling studies with four methods across ten pesticides at a range of skin loadings giving mean wash efficiencies from 23 to 96 per cent.

Tape stripping removes the outermost layer or layers of the stratum corneum of the skin with the aim of quantifying compounds present in the skin. This has been used extensively for the assessment of exposure to a range of chemicals (e.g. Nylander-French 2000), including acrylates, jet fuel, and epoxy components. These methods are clearly more invasive than surrogate skin and other removal techniques and suffer from error introduced by the lack of a method to standardize measurements to the quantity of stratum corneum cells removed. Recent work by Boeniger and Nylander-French (2002) aims to overcome this problem. Stripping does, however, give an indication of the amount of a substance that has already been absorbed into the skin, something that both wipe and washing methods will fail to record.

9.3.4 Visualization methods

Deposition of material onto the clothing and skin can also be assessed using direct visualization techniques. Fluorescent tracers can be added to the bulk solution of the liquid under study and the deposition of this fluid may then be visualized using ultraviolet light. This method was initially developed by Fenske *et al.* (1986) and later developed by Roff in 1994 to produce a dodecahedral illumination system (fluorescent interactive video exposure system—FIVES). Later, a similar video imaging technique to assess dermal exposure (VITAE) was employed by Bierman *et al.* (1998) to measure the exposure of agricultural workers to pesticides. By calibrating image analysis software to fluorescent intensity based on the mass per unit area, these systems are able to quantify total-body exposure at the point of image acquisition, and to also measure the skin surface area exposed, although this is often not reported. However, the system requires careful calibration and the quantity of tracer added to the bulk solution must also be closely regulated to ensure that interpretable images are produced. Issues such as timing of 'sampling' to prevent saturation of the image are similar to those relevant to surrogate skin sampling. Practical difficulties also exist in terms of expense, time to carry out the measurement, the acceptability of adding fluorescent tracers to the material being applied, and binding of the tracer to the skin preventing the same worker being measured on consecutive days.

9.3.5 Biomonitoring

Biomonitoring of blood, breath, or urine for the target substance or a metabolite (see Chapter 11) may also be employed to measure the passage of chemicals through the skin and therefore, indirectly, the degree of dermal exposure (e.g. for trihalomethane uptake). For biomonitoring to be effective the pharmacokinetics of the material must be well understood and exposure from other routes such as inhalation or ingestion should be negligible (see Chapter 10). For this reason biomonitoring remains a research tool rather than a methodology used in the field of dermal exposure assessment, although it is routinely used to assess total exposure. Chamber experiments where workers' skin is exposed to liquids (Kezic *et al.* 2001) or high concentrations of vapour (Brooke *et al.* 1998) while they are supplied with uncontaminated air to breathe, allow the measurement of the uptake of chemicals through the skin.

9.3.6 Modelling

Measuring techniques are becoming increasingly sophisticated and standardized, and advances in this field will allow greater collection of dermal exposure data across a range of industries, processes, and environmental conditions. While this is good news for future epidemiological studies that wish to incorporate the influence of dermal exposure on the risk of health effects, the situation for retrospective studies is not so positive. Few good-quality measurements of dermal exposure currently exist and those that do have often been gathered by measurement protocols that have produced exposure metrics of questionable value.

As a result, modelling dermal exposure has been the focus of much work over the past decade. The estimation and assessment of substance exposure (EASE) system developed by the UK HSE and a similar technique by the US EPA (Mulhausen and Damiano 1998) are generic models primarily used for risk assessment purposes. These procedures model likely exposure levels from information on process type and chemical used, but categorize exposure into broad ranges and so are of limited use. Initial validation work by Hughson and Cherrie (2001) has demonstrated that EASE tends to overestimate dermal exposures by up to two orders of magnitude. Additionally, from an epidemiological standpoint, it is of little value to evaluate the mass or volume of a substance that is deposited on the worker without progressing to determine the quantity absorbed into the systemic circulation. Only by estimating both deposition and uptake through the skin can we provide a 'biologically relevant' assessment of the hazard that is likely to be related to any systemic ill-health effect.

The UK HSE used a database of dermal exposure measurements to produce an empirical model and indicative distributions for a range of tasks from the pesticide and biocide application sector (Phillips and Garrod 2000). This work created a basic job-exposure matrix with four levels of potential dermal exposure and three types of profiles to reflect the degree of variability across different tasks. Deterministic modelling has also been developed. Again these models tend to be process specific. Brouwer *et al.* (2001) examined the parameters controlling the deposition of paint spray aerosol onto painters' skin and clothing. The model produced a good correlation between estimated and measured exposures.

The development of the conceptual model by Schneider *et al.* (1999) has provided a structured framework to characterize and analyse exposure scenarios by dividing them into a range of sources, compartments, and transport processes. In summary, the model focuses on sources that may emit into the work environment via four pathways, which link the source of exposure from the process or activity being undertaken to the person. Sources emit mass of contaminant material to a number of compartments: the air compartment (Air); surfaces in the environment (Su); the outside of the workers clothing (CloOut); or to the workers unprotected skin (Sk). Each compartment may then exchange contaminant substances with other compartments as illustrated in Fig. 9.1.

Emission (E) to air may be by evaporation, spraying, grinding, or some other activity. Emission to the other compartments can occur by splashing, spilling, spraying, or other mechanisms. Compartments may be defined by the mass and concentration of contaminant, the area of the compartment covered by the material, or in the case of the air compartment, its volume. The contaminant may 'flow' in or out of each compartment giving rise to increases or decreases in mass therein. For example, material may be *lost* (L) from the surface contamination layer to the air, to the outer clothing layer, or the skin contamination layer. In addition, there may be *deposition* (Dp) from the air to surfaces, or *transfer* (T) from the surface contamination layer to the skin contamination layer or the outer clothing layer.

Transfer or removal from surfaces to the skin contamination layer may be mediated by contact between the worker's body and the surface. The direction of the contaminant

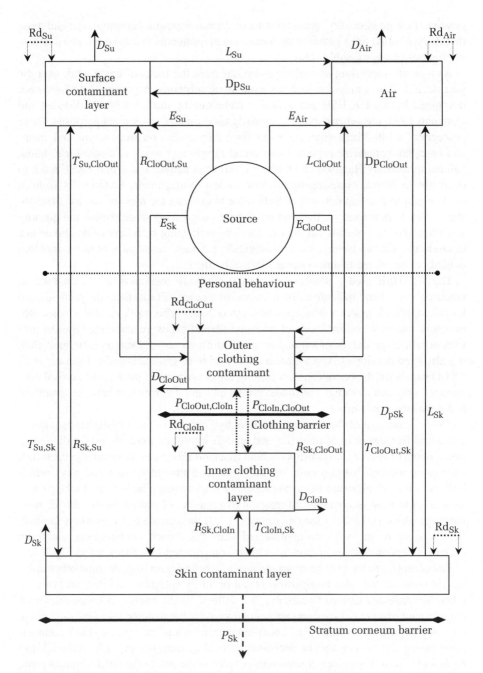

Fig. 9.1 The conceptual model of dermal exposure (for a detailed description refer to Schneider *et al.* 1999).

transfer will depend on whether there is more available contamination on the skin or the surface, the wetness of the hand, the properties of the surface, and many other factors.

In the conceptual model, clothing is recognized as an important protective measure for people handling hazardous substances. It is described by two compartments with a barrier layer that restricts the passage of substances to the skin. A substance can either permeate from the outer clothing layer (a diffusion process) or penetrate (bulk flow) to the inner layer (CloIn), or bypass the clothing and be transferred directly to the skin contamination layer.

In each compartment there are two other processes that may operate: *decontamination* (D) and *redistribution* (Rd). Decontamination, for example, by washing hands, results in the loss of some of the contaminant from the system. Redistribution is the process of modifying the pattern of contamination within a compartment, for example, by transferring some contaminant from one area of the body to another, perhaps by touching the face with dirty hands. Redistribution does not change the mass in a compartment but may alter the area covered or the contaminant concentration.

Other generic models for the estimation of dermal exposure include DREAM for occupational exposure and CONSEXPO for consumer product exposure events. DREAM (van-Wendel-de-Joode *et al.* 2003) is a new method for semi-quantitative dermal exposure assessment that may prove useful in epidemiology. The detailed questionnaire characterizes tasks and produces estimates of dermal exposure levels using the conceptual model as a framework. This system provides information on the best methods of measuring exposure and also helps target control measures. CONSEXPO (RIVM 2001) is a software-based model that enables the user to enter data on the type of exposure scenario and the chemical being used and can then provide likely dermal exposure and uptake values. Options for mean and worst-case (95th percentile) predictions are given. CONSEXPO aims to provide full multi-route exposure and uptake data and can be used to aggregate dermal, inhalation, and ingestion exposures. Modelling work has also been carried out to estimate children's residential exposure to pesticides (Zartarian *et al.* 2000) using observations of typical activity patterns and data on post-application time period, pesticide application method, etc.

9.4   Effect of personal protective equipment

The use of protective clothing and gloves to control dermal exposure is widespread in occupational settings. Most protective clothing, such as overalls, is employed to keep the worker relatively clean or prevent the workers' own clothes from becoming contaminated rather than any scientific principle of reducing dermal exposure or uptake to the chemicals in use. As a result gloves and protective clothing are rarely matched to the exposure scenario and are often poorly managed in terms of cleaning, provision of replacements, or checking when integrity is breached. In addition, while there are a variety of standards for testing protective clothing (e.g. BSI 1994), none of these tests take into account how the clothing or gloves will perform in workplace conditions. Testing does not usually include repeated exposures, temperature extremes, mechanical effects from stretching, or the effects of chemical mixtures. Work by El-Ayouby *et al.* (2002) showed that repeated use and decontamination, using alcohol, of nitrile and butyl gloves produced compromised chemical resistance to solvents after only one or two cycles.

Earlier work by Creely and Cherrie (2001) used cotton gloves to assess the effectiveness of a variety of protective glove types when used in a simulated work activity applying a pesticide. By comparing outer glove or 'potential exposure' values with inner glove 'actual dermal exposure' levels in a method similar to that employed for respiratory protective equipment, this study was able to derive 'protection factors' for the gloves used. Geometric mean protection factors between 96 and 470 were reported for three different types of glove. For all glove types protection factors were lowest when workers were classified as 'messy' or when the spray equipment was noted to leak. Similar work by Soutar *et al.* (2000) examined the effectiveness of three different types of protective overalls when spraying pesticides for timber preservation. Penetration of protective clothing was calculated using an inner sampling suit to measure how much material would normally be transferred to the skin. Inner contamination levels ranged from 0 to 36 per cent of the outside exposure quantity.

While use of protective equipment may help reduce dermal exposure when selected and used properly, there are many situations in which protective overalls or gloves may actually increase the exposure and uptake of chemicals through the skin. First, it may provide the user with a false sense of security and cause him/her to undertake exposure behaviours that they would not previously have carried out. This may be particularly problematic if the gloves or clothing have inadequate resistance to the contaminant substance. Second, there is the problem of wet overalls or gloves acting as a reservoir for contamination and thereby extending the duration of exposure. Finally, occlusion may also prevent a fluid that might normally evaporate from the skin being lost and so increase the substance available for uptake.

9.5   Use of dermal measurement and models in epidemiology

The explicit consideration of the dermal route of exposure is still rare in epidemiological studies examining the potential health effects of chemicals. A review of the literature indicates that even in studies investigating pesticide exposure, where in most scenarios the majority of the internalized dose will be from the dermal route, there are few explicit cases in which dermal exposure assessment takes place.

Most studies of pesticide exposure use simple exposure classification methods such as ever/never exposed. This data being either obtained by questionnaire or by simple job-exposure matrices (JEMs) or, in the case of non-occupational exposure, by use of geographical information systems linking residence to records of local pesticide use (Brody *et al.* 2002). Other methods use semi-quantitative surrogates of 'total exposure' such as the number of years working in agricultural industries. More advanced indices may factor in data linked to the frequency and duration of exposure by using the number of hectares where pesticide was applied, the number of animals treated, or the mass/volume of pesticide mixed.

London and Myers (1998) developed a crop and job specific JEM for retrospective assessment of long-term exposure in a study of the neurotoxic effects of organophosphates (OPs). This expert-based system allows estimation of cumulative lifetime exposure measured in kilograms of organophosphate. This study was also able to demonstrate that the generated index was significantly associated with erythrocyte cholinesterase concentrations (a biological effect marker of OP exposure) among a cohort of farmers. Earlier work by Verberk *et al.* (1990) used a number of work-related parameters such as the pesticide application method, application rate, the use of protective equipment, and the like to generate an exposure index. This general index considered both dermal and inhalation exposure elements and was used to study the health effects of pesticides in the agricultural sector in the Netherlands.

Other studies have examined the dermal exposure of farmers involved in sheep dipping operations. The use of OP-based dips has been implicated in the onset of a range of illnesses such as chronic fatigue syndrome (CFS). It is believed that a significant proportion of the biological dose received during sheep dipping comes via the dermal route. Interestingly, the study by Sewell *et al.* (1999) suggested that the primary determinant of exposure was handling or mixing sheep dip concentrate. These findings agree with the model of dermal uptake described by Cherrie and Robertson (1995), which describes concentration as the most important factor driving diffusion through the skin.

Tahmaz *et al.* (2003) also investigated CFS among farmers exposed to OP-based sheep dips. This study developed and applied a new dermal exposure metric to estimate lifetime exposure. This metric was based on the product of concentration, exposure duration, and area of skin exposed. Using questionnaire data on how often farmers carried out sheep dipping, the frequency of contact with concentrate and dilute dip and the use of protective equipment (gloves, overalls, and visors), this work demonstrated that those with higher assessed exposure to OP pesticides reported more symptoms consistent with CFS.

Determination of dermal exposure and uptake in other occupational epidemiological studies is even less common. Dick *et al.* (2000) and Chen *et al.* (2002) examined the neurological and neuropsychological effects of solvent use among painters using quantitative measures of lifetime and average annual solvent exposure that were generated using both inhalation and dermal exposure models. The dermal element utilized a predictive model developed by Brouwer *et al.* (2001) to estimate the amount of paint that would be deposited on a spray painter depending on process and environmental conditions. The degree of dermal uptake was then derived using further modelling methods (Semple *et al.* 2001) and the fraction of internalized dose received by the dermal route converted to an airborne equivalent value. This work showed that in some working conditions described by painters, where respiratory protective equipment was used and heat and humidity caused men to wear t-shirts, that the dermal route could provide the majority of absorbed solvent. More typically, however, the dermal route was found to contribute less than 10 per cent of total-body solvent in most painting conditions.

9.6 The future

Dermal exposure is clearly of importance in understanding the risk posed by many chemicals. Assessment of dermal exposure for the purposes of epidemiological investigation has been rare, with few studies employing even simple categorical exposure metrics.

However, there is now a better understanding of the parameters controlling exposure and uptake and there is a realization of the importance of measuring exposure intensity and the area of skin exposed, together with exposure duration and frequency. For prospective studies there are a range of methods capable of delivering data on these factors and attempts are being made to build up databases of dermal exposure measurements classified by industry, job, and task. We have also recognized the need to record data about the measurement conditions, skin condition, the vehicle the substance is contained within, and obtain measures of the exposure variability when gathering dermal exposure data. Advances in modelling, particularly the conceptual model developed by Schneider *et al.* (1999), have increased our understanding of how to estimate dermal exposure patterns and will prove useful for retrospective assessment purposes.

A few significant hurdles need to be overcome to ensure that the process of dermal exposure assessment improves further. Better methods are needed for measuring the concentration of material deposited on the skin rather than just mass. Pilot work presented by Robertson *et al.* (2002) on a new dermal sampler to measure solvent concentration on the skin holds promise. Appropriate exposure metrics will also be required. A metric that considers area exposed, concentration, and duration of exposure (e.g. $mg\,cm^{-3}\,cm^2\,min$) will more easily allow exposure to be linked directly to the degree of uptake. Additionally, there may be a need for a different type of metric when examining local effects. For example, in the case of irritant dermatitis, the concentration of the material may not be so important and the cyclical nature of 'wettedness' and the irritancy potential of the material may be the driving factors in development of dermatitis. There is also evidence that the ingestion route may play a significant role in exposure to materials such as pesticides, pharmaceuticals, and heavy metals using a complex path from air to skin to mouth. Future work will be required to understand the relationship between dermal exposure and ingestion uptake.

Despite these gaps in our knowledge the progress made in dermal exposure assessment has been remarkable. We have described the main parameters that should be measured to assess dermal uptake and there are many good-quality generic and process-specific models that can be used to identify the factors likely to influence potential and actual dermal exposure levels that may be used in epidemiological studies. Even if dermal exposure assessment cannot be carried out on the whole population in an epidemiological study, models could be built in a subpopulation and applied to the whole population (see Chapter 6). Future epidemiological investigations of a wide variety of skin penetrating substances, from solvents to pesticides, should now be able to incorporate detailed quantitative evaluations of dermal exposure and uptake.

References

ACGIH (2002). *Threshold limit values for chemical substances and physical agents and biological exposure indices.* American Conference of Governmental Industrial Hygienists. Cincinnati, OH, USA.

Bierman, E., Brouwer, D., and van Hemmen, J. (1998). Implementation and evaluation of the fluorescent tracer technique in greenhouse exposure studies. *Annals of Occupational Hygiene*, **42**, 467–75.

Boeniger, M. and Nylander-French, L. (2002). Comparison of three methods for determining removal of stratum corneum using adhesive tape strips. Presented at the International Conference on Occupational and Environmental Exposure of Skin to Chemicals: Science and Policy. 8–11 September 2002, Washington, DC.

Bowman, A. and Maibach, H. (2000). Percutaneous absorption of organic solvents. *International Journal of Occupational and Environmental Health*, **6**, 93–5.

Brody, J., Swartz, C., Kennedy, T., and Rudel, R. (2002). Historical pesticide exposure assessment using a geographical information system and self-report in a breast cancer study. *Epidemiology*, **13**, 726.

Brooke, I., Cocker, J., Delic, J., Payne, M., Jones, K., Gregg, N., and Dyne, D. (1998). Dermal uptake of solvents from the vapour phase: an experimental study in humans. *Annals of Occupational Hygiene*, **42**, 531–40.

Brouwer, D., Boeniger, M., and van Hemmen, J. (2000). Hand wash and manual skin wipes. *Annals of Occupational Hygiene*, **44**, 501–10.

Brouwer, D., Brouwer, E., and van Hemmen, J. (1992). Assessment of dermal and inhalation exposure to zaneb/maneb in the cultivation of flower bulbs. *Annals of Occupational Hygiene*, **36**, 373–84.

Brouwer, D., Semple, S., Marquart, J., and Cherrie, J. (2001). A dermal model for spray painters. Part I: Subjective exposure modelling of spray paint deposition. *Annals of Occupational Hygiene*, **45**, 15–23.

BSI. (1994). Protective gloves against chemicals and microorganisms. Part 3. Determination of resistance to permeation to chemicals. British Standards Institution, London (BS EN374-3:1994).

Bunge, A. and Ley, E. (2002). Dermal exposure to powdered solids and aqueous solutions: are the risks different? Presented at the International Conference on Occupational and Environmental Exposure of Skin to Chemicals: Science and Policy. 8–11 September 2002. Washington, DC.

Chen, R., Dick, F., Semple, S., Seaton, A., and Walker, L. (2002). Exposure to organic solvents and personality. *Occupational and Environmental Medicine*, **58**, 14–18.

Cherrie, J. and Robertson, A. (1995). Biologically relevant assessment of dermal exposure. *Annals of Occupational Hygiene*, **39**, 387–92.

Cohen Hubal, E., Sheldon, L., Burke, J., McCurdy, T., Beryy, M., Rigas, M., Zartarian, V., and Freeman, N. (2000). Children's exposure assessment: a review of factors influencing children's exposure, and the data available to characterize and assess that exposure. *Environmental Health Perspectives*, **108**, 475–86.

Creely, K. and Cherrie, J. (2001). A novel method of assessing the effectiveness of protective gloves-results from a pilot study. *Annals of Occupational Hygiene*, **45**, 137–43.

Davis, J., Stevens, E., and Staff, D. (1983). Potential exposure of apple thinners to azinphos-methyl and comparison of two methods for assessment of hand exposure. *Bulletin of Environmental Contamination and Toxicology*, **31**, 631–8.

Dick, F., Semple, S., Chen, R., and Seaton, A. (2000). Neurological deficits in solvent-exposed painters: a syndrome including impaired colour vision, cognitive defects, tremor and loss of vibration sensation. *Quarterly Journal of Medicine*, **93**, 655–61.

Durham, W. and Wolfe, H. (1962). Measurement of the exposure of workers to pesticides. *Bulletin of the WHO*, **26**, 75–91.

El-Ayouby, N., Gao, P., Wassell, J., and Hall, R. (2002). Effect of cycles of contamination and decontamination on chemical glove performance. Presented at the International Conference on Occupational and Environmental Exposure of Skin to Chemicals: Science and Policy. 8–11 September 2002, Washington, DC.

Fenske, R., Wong, S., and Leffingwell, J. (1986). A video imaging technique for assessing dermal exposure: II, fluorescent tracer testing. *American Industrial Hygiene Association Journal*, **47**, 771–5.

Gordon, S. M., Wallace, L. A., Callahan, P. J., Kenny, D. V., and Brinkman, M. C. (1998). Effect of water temperature on dermal exposure to chloroform. *Environmental Health Perspectives*, **106**, 337–45.

Grandjean, P. (1990). *Skin penetration: hazardous chemicals at work*. Taylor & Francis, London.

HSE. (2001). *EH40/2001. Occupational exposure limits 2001*. HSE Books, Sudbury, UK.

Hughson, G. and Cherrie, J. (2001). Validation of the EASE expert system for dermal exposure to zinc. *Arbete Och Halsa*, **10**, 17–19.

Kezic, S., Mohammadi, N., Jakasa, I., Kruse, J., Monster, A., and Verberk, M. (2002). Percutaneous absorption of neat and water solutions of 2-butoxyethanol in man. Presented at the International Conference on Occupational and Environmental Exposure of Skin to Chemicals: Science and Policy. 8–11 September 2002, Washington, DC.

Kezic, S., Monster, A., van de Gevel, I., Kruse, J., Opdam, J., and Verberk, M. (2001). Dermal absorption of neat liquid solvents on brief exposures in volunteers. *American Industrial Hygiene Association Journal*, **62**, 12–18.

Lansink, C., van Hensgstum, C., and Brouwer, D. (1997). Dermal exposure due to airless spraying. TNO Report V97.1057.

London, L. and Myers, J. (1998). Use of a crop and job specific exposure matrix for retrospective assessment of long term exposure in studies of chronic neurotoxic effects of agrichemicals. *Occupational and Environmental Medicine*, **55**, 194–201.

Mulhausen, J. and Damiano, J. (1998). *A strategy for assessing and managing occupational exposures*. Appendix II. Dermal exposure assessments. American Industrial Hygiene Association, Fairfax, VA, USA.

Nylander-French, L. A. (2000). A tape stripping method for measuring dermal exposure to multifunctional acrylates. *Annals of Occupational Hygiene*, **44**, 645–51.

OECD. (1997). Environmental health and safety publications series on testing and assessment No. 9: guidance document for the conduct of studies of occupational exposure to pesticides during agricultural application. OECD/GD(97)148y. OECD, Paris.

Patel, H. and Cronin, M. (2001). Determination of the optimal physico-chemical parameters to use in a QSAR-approach to predict skin permeation rate. Final report: CEFIC-LRI project No. NMALRI-A2.2UNJM-0007. Liverpool John Moores University, Liverpool, UK.

Phillips, A. and Garrod, A. (2000). Assessment of dermal exposure-empirical models and indicative distributions. *Annals of Occupational Hygiene*, **16**, 323–8.

RIVM. (2001). CONSEXPO 3.0, consumer exposure and uptake models. RIVM Report 612810011. National Institute of Public Health and the Environment, The Netherlands.

Robertson, A., Lindsay, F., and Cherrie, J. (2002). Measuring dermal exposure: Practical and scientific considerations. Presented at the International Conference on Occupational and Environmental Exposure of Skin to Chemicals: Science and Policy. 8–11 September 2002, Washington, DC.

Roff, M. (1994). A novel lighting system for the measurement of dermal exposure using a fluorescent dye and an image processor. *Annals of Occupational Hygiene*, **38**, 903–19.

Sartorelli, P., Aprea, C., Cenni, A., Novelli, M., Orsi, D., Palmi, S., and Matteucci, G. (1998). Prediction of percutaneous absorption from physiochemical data: a model based on data of *in-vitro* experiments. *Annals of Occupational Hygiene*, **42**, 267–76.

Schneider, T., Vermeulen, R., Brouwer, D., Cherrie, J., Kromhout, H., and Fogh, C. (1999). A conceptual model for assessment of dermal exposure. *Occupational and Environmental Medicine*, **56**, 765–73.

Semple, S., Brouwer, D., Dick, F., and Cherrie, J. (2001). A dermal model for spray painters. Part II: estimating the deposition and uptake of solvents. *Annals of Occupational Hygiene*, **45**, 25–33.

Sewell, C., Pilkington, A., Buchanan, D., Tannahill, S., Kidd, M., Cherrie, B., and Robertson, A. (1999). *Epidemiological study of the relationships between exposure to organophosphate pesticides and indices of chronic peripheral neuropathy, and neuropsychological abnormalities in sheep farmers and dippers. Phase 1. Development and validation of an organophosphate uptake model for sheep dippers*. IOM Report TM/99/02a. Institute of Occupational Medicine, Edinburgh, UK.

Soutar, A., Cherrie, B., and Cherrie, J. (2000). *Field evaluation of protective clothing against non-agricultural pesticides*. IOM Report TM/00/04. Institute of Occupational Medicine, Edinburgh, UK.

Tahmaz, N., Soutar, A., and Cherrie, J. (2003). Chronic fatigue syndrome and organophosphate pesticides in sheep farming: a retrospective study amongst people reporting to a UK pharmacovigilance scheme. *Annals of Occupational Hygiene* (in press).

Tannahill, S., Robertson, A., Cherrie, B., Donnan, P., MacConnell, E., and Macleod, G. (1996). *A comparison of two different methods for assessment of dermal exposure to non-agricultural pesticides in three sectors.* IOM Report TM/96/07. Institute of Occupational Medicine, Edinburgh, UK.

Van Hemmen, J. (2002). Riskofderm: Risk assessment for occupational dermal exposure. Presented at the International Conference on Occupational and Environmental Exposure of Skin to Chemicals: Science and Policy. 8–11 September 2002, Washington, DC.

van-Wendel-de-Joode, B., Brouwer, D., Vermeulen, R., van Hemmen, J., Heederik, D., and Kromhout, H. (2003). DREAM: a method for semi-quantitative dermal exposure assessment. *Annals of Occupational Hygiene*, **47**, 71–87.

Verberk, M., Brouwer, D., Brouwer, E., Bruyzeel, D., Emmen, H., Van Hemmen, J., Hooisma, J., Jonkman, E., Ruijten, M., and Salle, H. (1990). Health effects of pesticides in the flower-bulb culture in Holland. *Medicina del Lavoro*, **81**, 530–4.

Vermeulen, R., Heideman, J., Bos, R., and Kromhout, H. (2000). Identification of dermal exposure pathways in the rubber manufacturing industry. *Annals of Occupational Hygiene*, **44**, 533–41.

Wassenius, O., Jarvholm, B., Engstrom, T., Lillienberg, L., and Medling, B. (1998). Variability in the skin exposure of machine operators exposed to cutting fluids. *Scandinavian Journal of Work, Environment and Health*, **24**, 125–9.

WHO. (1982). *Field survey of exposure to pesticides. Standard protocol: VBC/82.1.* World Health Organisation, Geneva.

Wilkinson, S. and Williams, F. (2001). *In vitro dermal absorption of liquids.* Contract Research Report for HSE (350). HSE Books, Sudbury, UK.

Wolfe, H., Durham, W., and Armstrong, J. (1967). Exposure of workers to pesticides. *Archives of Environmental Health*, **14**, 622–33.

Zartarian, V., Ozkaynak, H., Murke, J., Zufall, M., Rigas, M., and Furtaw, E. (2000). A modelling framework for estimating children's residential exposure and dose to chlorpyrifos via dermal residue contact and nondietary ingestion. *Environmental Health Perspectives*, **108**, 505–14.

10. Physiologically based pharmacokinetic modelling

George Loizou and Martin Spendiff

10.1 Introduction

Exposure estimates in epidemiological studies tend to be based on environmental and personal measurements and models, that is, concentrations outside the body. Generally little information is available on the concentrations or 'dose' reaching target organs such as the liver and kidney. Yet tissue concentrations may be much more accurate estimates of exposure, particularly when the factors that constitute human variability can be quantified and incorporated, and can contribute to the reduction of exposure measurement error. In this chapter we present physiologically based pharmacokinetic (PBPK) modelling and propose how this technique may be used to improve chemical exposure estimates in epidemiological studies.

Pharmacokinetics is the study of the absorption, distribution, metabolism, and elimination of exogenous chemicals in biological systems. By studying the fate of an exogenous chemical, such as a drug, or an environmental or occupational pollutant, it is possible to relate the target tissue response to the concentration profile of the pollutant in that tissue (Clewell and Andersen 1985; Krewski *et al.* 1994; Krishnan and Andersen 1994). Various types of mathematical models have been used to describe the pharmacokinetic behaviour of xenobiotics. The models simplify biological complexity by subdividing the body into discrete subelements, referred to as compartments. Two general types of compartmental models have been used for pharmacokinetic modelling: data-based or empirical and PBPK models (Clewell and Andersen 1985). A typical data-based compartmental model attempts to relate the blood or tissue concentration profile of the parent chemical or metabolite to the administered dose of the parent chemical using a set of mathematical equations. The parameters for these equations are determined from experiments following the time course of the chemical in body fluids and occasionally in specific tissues. A typical, simple model might consist of only two compartments (rarely more than three) within which chemicals are assumed to distribute homogeneously: a central compartment in equilibrium with the blood and a peripheral compartment whose concentration can be related to the central compartment by rate constants describing uptake from, and elimination to, the blood (Fig. 10.1). The volumes of the compartments and the values of the rate constants are adjusted to fit the experimental data—hence the term data-based compartmental models. After the values of the rate constants have been adjusted, the model can be used for interpolation

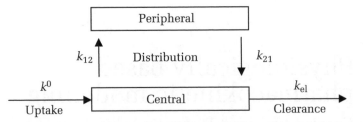

Fig. 10.1 Schematic of data-based compartmental model. The composite rate constants, k_{12} and k_{21}, describe the movement of chemical to and from the central compartment, k^0 describes uptake into the central compartment, and k_{el} describes clearance from the central compartment including metabolism (adapted from Clewell and Andersen 1985).

(Clewell and Andersen 1985), although they should not be used for extrapolation beyond the range of doses, dose routes, and species used in the study on which they were based (Krishnan and Andersen 1994).

In contrast, PBPK models divide the body into realistic compartments connected by the arterial and venous blood flow pathways (Fig. 10.2). Instead of compartments defined by the experimental data themselves, actual organ and tissue groups are described by weight and blood perfusion rates obtained from the literature (ICRP 1975; Brown *et al.* 1997). Instead of composite rate constants determined by fitting the data, actual chemical-specific parameters such as partition coefficients (tissue retention of chemicals related to solubility in biological media and binding to specific proteins) and metabolic constants are used. The result is a model that predicts the qualitative behaviour of the experimental time course without being based on it (Clewell and Andersen 1985). The model may be refined to incorporate additional insights gained from comparison with experimental data, which produces a model that can be used for quantitative extrapolation well beyond the range of experimental conditions (Clewell and Andersen 1985). Indeed, the predictive power of these models has led to a proliferation of PBPK-based chemical-risk assessments (Andersen *et al.* 1987; Krishnan and Andersen 1991; Krewski *et al.* 1994; Andersen 1995).

It is the use of fundamental metabolic parameters that makes possible the extrapolation of dose over ranges where saturation of metabolism occurs. Also, chemical kinetics can be modelled in any species by simply replacing the appropriate physiological and anatomical parameters of one organism with those of another (Andersen *et al.* 1987, 1991; Clewell III and Andersen 1994; Clewell *et al.* 2001). Inhalation, dermal, and oral routes of exposure can be simulated easily as can different exposure scenarios, for example, single 4 h exposure, 6 h per day, 5 days per week and pulsatile exposures. Perhaps the most desirable feature of a PBPK model is that it provides a conceptual framework for conducting the scientific method. Hypotheses can be described in terms of the known biological processes, predictions made on the basis of model description, and hypotheses revised on the basis of comparison with experiment (Clewell and Andersen 1985).

Inevitably, the increased number of parameters and equations, which confer the greater predictive potential of PBPK models, has led to the criticism that they are 'data

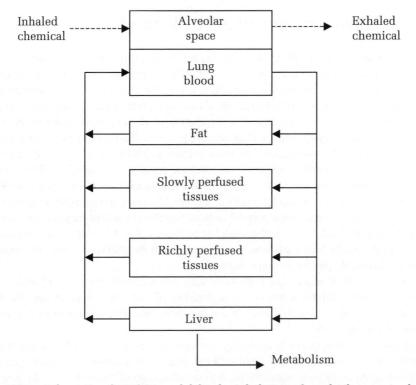

Fig. 10.2   Schematic of a PBPK model for the inhalation of a volatile organic chemical. The compartments represent organs or groups of organs defined with respect to their volumes, blood flows, and partition coefficients for the test chemical. The uptake of vapour is determined by alveolar ventilation, cardiac output, blood:air partition coefficient and the concentration gradient between arterial and venous pulmonary blood. Equilibrium between arterial blood and alveolar air is assumed. Metabolism occurs in the liver and is described by the kinetic constants V_{max}, which is the maximum rate of metabolism and K_m, which is the concentration of chemical at half-maximum rate of metabolism (adapted from Krishnan and Andersen 1994).

hungry' and resource intensive. However, the physiological and anatomical parameters pertinent to any model are already available in the literature (ICRP 1975; Arms and Travis 1988; Brown *et al.* 1997). Techniques for the prediction of compound-specific partition coefficients using tissue composition-based algorithms have shown potential (Poulin and Krishnan 1996*a,b*). There are even quantitative structure–activity studies, that promise the prediction of metabolic rate constants from molecular orbital energy parameters such as ionization potential and calculated energy of hydrogen abstraction (in preparation: Lewis *et al.* 2002). These computer-based, parameter-predicting techniques have the potential to rapidly provide all the parameters necessary to build a model and ameliorate the reservations people may have about the time and effort required to construct a PBPK model.

10.2   Development of a PBPK model

When developing a PBPK model, the organism is represented as a network of compartments, each of which is physically, physiologically, and biochemically characterized. Conceptual representation of a PBPK model for a chemical requires an understanding of the anatomical and physiological characteristics of the organism of interest, as well as the pathways of uptake and disposition of the chemical under study. The organism should be represented mathematically in terms of a set of *mass balance* equations. More precisely, maintaining the mass balance in PBPK models requires that the *total blood flow* (i.e. cardiac output) in the model is equal to the *sum* of the flows to the tissue compartments of the model. Only tissues that receive chemical via blood flow need be represented in the model. Further, it is not necessary to represent all tissues as individual compartments, some may be lumped together, provided they are kinetically homogeneous and total flow in the model is accounted for. Kinetically homogeneous tissues have similar blood perfusion rates and metabolic capacities (e.g. the slowly perfused and richly perfused compartment).

In a typical PBPK model, the body is divided into n compartments; m of which are non-metabolizing. Given a known concentration of the compound in the air, the concentration of the compound in each compartment over time is governed by a set of mathematical equations.

Pulmonary exchanges are modelled by assuming instantaneous equilibrium between alveolar air, venous blood, and arterial blood. Since the amount of substance in the alveoli is assumed to be in equilibrium, the rate of change of the amount in the lung is zero, that is,

$$Q_P(C_{inh}(t) - C_{exh}) + Q_C(C_V - C_{art}) = 0, \tag{10.1}$$

where Q_P is the pulmonary flow, Q_C is the cardiac output, Q_{exh} is exhaled concentration, C_V is the venous concentration, and C_{art} is the arterial concentration. Exposure is determined by the function $C_{inh}(t)$, which represents the inhalation concentration of the compound at a given time. It is also assumed that the concentration of chemical in exhaled air is the same as the concentration on the alveoli, therefore the arterial concentration, C_{art}, is given by,

$$C_{art} = C_{exh}P_b, \tag{10.2}$$

where P_b is the blood:air partition coefficient. Thus, the concentration of the chemical in arterial blood can be determined,

$$C_{art} = \frac{P_b(Q_C C_V + Q_P C_{inh}(t))}{P_b Q_C + Q_P}. \tag{10.3}$$

The non-metabolizing compartments are governed by the first-order ordinary differential equation,

$$\frac{dC_S}{dt} = \left(C_{art} - \frac{C_S}{P_S}\right)\frac{Q_S}{V_S}, \tag{10.4}$$

which describes the rate of change of the concentration C_S of the compound in each compartment, S, as a function of blood flow, Q_S, volume, V_S, arterial blood concentration, C_{art}, and partition coefficient P_S. Compartments that incorporate metabolic clearance of the compound are described by

$$\frac{dC_S}{dt} = \left(C_{art} - \frac{C_S}{P_S} \right) \frac{Q_S}{V_S} - \sum_{i=1}^{k} \frac{V_{max,i} C_S}{K_{m,i} + C_S},$$ (10.5)

where $V_{max,i}/(K_{m,i} + C_S)$ is the intrinsic metabolic clearance for the ith metabolic process. Finally, Eqs (3)–(5) are linked by the concentration for venous blood, C_V, which is given by

$$C_V = \frac{1}{Q_C} \sum_{i=1}^{m} \frac{Q_S C_i}{P_i}.$$ (10.6)

This defines the full system of governing equations that constitute a PBPK model. Due to the non-linear metabolism term, algebraic solution of the system is not feasible and numerical methods must be employed. Fortunately, many computer packages are available that can quickly and accurately solve these equations. Solutions of our conceptual representation of the physiology can then be used to improve our understanding of key biological mechanisms, to determine the critical factors in reaction to a compound, and to perform population modelling.

10.3   Applications of PBPK modelling

Although a PBPK model for diethyl ether was published back in 1924 (Haggard 1924) this remained a theoretical exercise due to the unavailability of the computing power required to solve simultaneously the differential equations comprising the model. More PBPK models began to appear in the 1970s, which paralleled the availability of computing power (for more references see Andersen *et al.* 1993*a*). An early application of a PBPK model to a chemical of occupational and environmental interest is the styrene model of Ramsey and Andersen (1984). This may also be regarded as a seminal work, since it is frequently cited as the model on which most subsequent models, with appropriate modifications, are based. The model described blood and tissue concentrations and hepatic metabolism of the parent chemical following inhalation of styrene vapours at a variety of concentrations. The intravenous and intragastric routes of administration were also incorporated. The compartments described were the lung, as the site of uptake, fat, as a storage depot, liver, as the principle site of metabolism, richly perfused tissues, which included the viscera, kidney, and brain, and slowly perfused tissues, which included muscle, skin, bone, and cartilage. Non-linear, kinetic behaviour, that is, the problem of extrapolation from a high dose to a low dose, was described by including the well-known Michaelis–Menten equation for metabolism in the liver compartment using realistic, experimentally determined constants for V_{max}, the maximum rate of metabolism, and K_m, the substrate concentration that gives half the maximum rate of metabolism, which may also be regarded as a measure of the enzyme binding affinity for styrene. Interspecies extrapolation was conducted by dividing the rat tissue:air partition coefficients by a human blood:air partition coefficient to give surrogate human-tissue:blood partition coefficients. Tissue volumes were considered proportional to body weight and tissue perfusion rates proportional to body weight raised to the 0.7 power (such calculations are known as allometric scaling; for more discussion see Ings 1990; Bachmann *et al.* 1996). Lastly, styrene metabolism was scaled by assuming that K_m did not change from species to species and V_{max}, like basal metabolic rate, was proportional to body weight raised to the 0.7 power. Existing blood and organ concentration data were adequately described by the model for intravenous, inhalation, and intragastric doses of styrene (Ramsey *et al.* 1980). Metabolism was saturable at inhalation exposures above 200 ppm for 6 h in mice, rats, and humans. The fit of the model was sensitive to changes in the fat:blood partition coefficient and V_{max}. Recently, the increased availability of human hepatic microsomes and other tissues has led to the *in vitro* determination of metabolic rate constants and partition coefficients and their incorporation into PBPK models thus ensuring that more models are *a priori*.

The first example in which an agency used a full PBPK model in a chemical-risk assessment was the US EPA's risk assessment of dichloromethane (EPA 1987). The metabolism of dichloromethane proceeds via two pathways: oxidation by the mixed function oxidase enzyme, cytochrome P-450 2E1, and conjugation by glutathione transferase enzymes. The model was based on that by Andersen *et al.* (1987), which focussed on metabolism by these two pathways in the liver and lung, the two target sites in the mouse for dichloromethane carcinogenicity. Metabolic rate constants for these enzymes were introduced into the lung and liver tissue compartments (Reitz *et al.* 1988, 1989) and they accurately predicted the pharmacokinetic behaviour of dichloromethane and its metabolite, carbon dioxide, in rats, mice, and humans (Andersen *et al.* 1987, 1991). Accurate descriptions of the dose–response relationships for flux through each metabolic pathway has implied that metabolites generated by the glutathione pathway are involved in tumour induction.

Different groups of workers modify and often improve existing PBPK models to meet the intended application. The uptake, distribution, and metabolism of chloroform ($CHCl_3$) was initially described by a model based on the styrene model of Ramsey and Andersen (1984) and subsequently modified to describe multiple routes of administration (Corley *et al.* 1990). The model was modified to include a kidney, as well as a liver, compartment and further validated against experimental data after *in vitro* metabolic rate constants, determined using human tissue, were also incorporated. Later, the model was again modified in order to consider the known biochemical mechanisms of $CHCl_3$ toxicity, rates and routes of metabolism, cell dynamics, and physiological differences between animals and man (Reitz *et al.* 1990). The latter model was capable of describing the metabolism and induction of cytotoxicity in liver tissue following inhalation, gavage, and drinking water exposures (Reitz *et al.* 1990). The induction of cytotoxicity, which is a pharmacodynamic response, was a description of the rate of cell death as a consequence of $CHCl_3$ metabolism. In order to derive an equation capable of quantitatively describing the rate of cytotoxicity, compensatory cellular regeneration was measured in the liver of mice. This was achieved by measuring the incorporation of [^{3}H]thymidine into DNA isolated from liver and kidney at various time points during 5–6 h exposures to varying concentrations of $CHCl_3$ vapour (Reitz *et al.* 1990).

The selection of PBPK models described thus far was chosen to demonstrate that they may be formulated to estimate tissue levels of the parent chemical (styrene), rates of metabolism to reactive metabolites (dichloromethane), and cytotoxicity as a consequence of rate of metabolism ($CHCl_3$). Other models could also have been included, for example, to describe regional protein induction over time after exposure to 2,3,7,8-tetrachlorodibenzo-*p*-dioxin and tissue interaction with specific macromolecules (methotrexate) (for more references see Krewski *et al.* 1994). The incorporation of this type of toxicodynamic and toxicokinetic information is considered necessary for quantitative risk assessment, which requires the definition of a toxicologically relevant measure of dose known as a dose surrogate.

10.4 Dose surrogates

The term 'dose surrogate' or 'dose metric' is used to describe the different ways of expressing a target tissue-dose estimate calculated using a PBPK model. The ability to use any dose surrogate in chemical-risk assessment ultimately depends on knowledge of the relationship between the measure of tissue dose and cellular response involved in a toxic endpoint. There have been many attempts at incorporating pharmacokinetic data in risk assessments that have used a measure of dose, such as peak blood concentration of parent chemical (C_{max}) or total amount metabolized, but without proffering a rationale for the relationship between the selected dose surrogate and pharmacodynamic response. In the model for $CHCl_3$, two dose surrogates were calculated with the PBPK model for use in risk assessment; the average amount of $CHCl_3$ metabolites covalently bound to biological macromolecules per litre of liver per day (AVEMMB), and the fraction of liver cells killed per day as a result of $CHCl_3$ exposure (PTDEAD) (Reitz *et al.* 1990). The calculated dose surrogates were tested for any correlation with liver tumour incidences in rats and mice reported in the NCI carcinogenesis bioassay study (NCI 1976). There was some correlation between predicted AVEMMB levels and development of liver tumours across species and dose when only bolus gavage studies were considered. No significant differences were observed between the predicted binding for no observed tumorigenic and tumorigenic doses. Also, no correlation was observed between predicted AVEMMB and liver carcinogenicity following $CHCl_3$ exposure through drinking water. The conclusion was that AVEMMB for $CHCl_3$ risk assessment would probably be more reliable than use of the administered dose, but nonetheless, was still too simple and did not consider other factors important in $CHCl_3$ liver carcinogenesis (Reitz *et al.* 1990). In contrast to AVEMMB, remarkable differences were obtained between tumorigenic and non-tumorigenic doses of $CHCl_3$ when PTDEAD levels were calculated. Predicted levels in PTDEAD were also consistent with the relative carcinogenicity of $CHCl_3$ administered to mice in drinking water or by bolus gavage. Further, the predicted values of PTDEAD in rats and mice receiving $CHCl_3$ by gavage were consistent with the relative sensitivity of these two species to induction of liver tumours. Consequently, the authors proposed the use of PTDEAD as likely to provide the most reliable estimates of the risk of liver cancer following exposure to $CHCl_3$ (Reitz *et al.* 1990).

Recently, the risk of cancer from household exposure to chloroform was examined using a PBPK model (Levesque *et al.* 2002). The routine daily exposure of 18 men through inhalation, oral, and dermal routes was assessed. Exposures to $CHCl_3$ in cold water (for drinking), indoor air, and during and following a shower were measured. Two

Table 10.1   Covalent binding of CHCl$_3$
reactive metabolites to target organ
macromolecules predicted by a PBPK model
for various exposure scenarios

	μg CHCl$_3$ equivalent/kg tissue/24 h	
Exposure scenario	Liver	Kidneys
Shower only	0.0091	0.0119
Average multi-route	0.1155	0.0568
Worst-case multi-route	0.4118	0.1991

scenarios were tested. The first was called an 'average-exposure scenario' where the following assumptions and CHCl$_3$ concentrations were made: 1.5 l of water containing 25 μg l^{-1} were drunk per day, inhalation of 9 μg m^{-3} in household air for 19 h per day, and dermal exposure during a 10-min shower to 25 μg l^{-1} in the water and 147 μg m^{-3} by inhalation in the shower stall. The second 'worst-case scenario' involved identical activities except that it was assumed that 2.4 l of water containing 54 μg l^{-1} were drunk per day, inhalation of 28 μg m^{-3} in household air for 24 h per day, and dermal exposure during a 10-min shower to 54 μg l^{-1} in the water and 259 μg m^{-3} by inhalation in the shower stall. The PBPK model was used to predict the amounts of CHCl$_3$ metabolites bound to hepatic and renal macromolecules over a 24-h period for the different exposure scenarios and activities. The data is reproduced in Table 10.1 (Levesque *et al.* 2002).

In the worst-case exposure scenario the model predicted 0.412 μg CHCl$_3$ equivalent/kg tissue, which was 3.5-fold higher than that for the 'average-exposure scenario'. However, this level of covalent binding is still approximately 6400 times smaller than the no-effect level (NOTL) (2.6 mg CHCl$_3$ equivalent/kg tissue) for liver tumours (Reitz *et al.* 1990). Therefore, the model predictions suggest a very large margin of safety for cancer effects from exposure to CHCl$_3$ by all relevant routes.

The pharmacokinetic dose metrics most commonly applied to characterize the exposure of a tissue to a chemical are C_{max} and the area-under-the-curve (AUC). However, there are other possible forms for dose metrics that might be useful for describing non-linear processes, for example, time above a critical concentration (TACC) has been suggested as an appropriate dose metric for the effects of compounds whose toxicity demonstrates a strong dependence on dose rate (Dedrick 1975). Another non-linear dose metric recently discussed for receptor-mediated effects is based on average receptor occupancy (Andersen *et al.* 1993*b*). Unfortunately, it is more difficult to collect the data necessary for the use of dose metrics that involve pharmacodynamic events.

In the process of dose metric selection, the underlying principle, is the use of the most up-to-date knowledge on the mode of action of the chemical at the cellular and sub-cellular level. For example, the neurological effects of short-term exposure to solvents such as trichloroethylene are rapidly reversible. This suggests that the parent chemical may disrupt normal lipophilic cellular membrane function via a physico-chemical effect. An appropriate dose metric for such an effect would be the C_{max} or AUC for the parent chemical in the brain. Since tissue–blood partition coefficients are relatively uniform across species, C_{max} in the blood can be used as a surrogate. As will be discussed later, the choice of the best dose-surrogate is fundamental to the development of population PBPK models, which in turn, can improve the design and analysis of epidemiological studies.

10.5 PBPK modelling of human variability in risk assessment

It is well known that individuals do not respond in the same way following exposure to the same concentration of chemical under identical conditions. The broad range of susceptibilities to the biological effects of chemical exposure is due to the heterogeneity of the human population. Sources of inter-individual variability include exposure, hereditary factors, such as enzyme polymorphisms and physiology, and environmental factors, such as diet and lifestyle. The reader is directed to some excellent reviews for more details (Hattis and Silver 1994; Hattis 1996; Hattis *et al.* 1999; Pacifici and Pelkonen 2001). As with research into the mechanisms involved in inter-individual and inter-ethnic variability in drug metabolism, which has the promise of improving the quality of drug therapy by using individualized dosing schedules; so it is with exposure to industrial and environmental chemicals. The quantification and incorporation of such differences should allow risk assessments that are more focussed on groups, which due to their particular difference may be more susceptible to any given chemical or mixture of chemicals (Pacifici and Pelkonen 2001).

The current emphasis in risk assessment research in the UK is the quantification of inter-individual variability, which, it may be argued, is contrary to the practice of trying to minimize variability in experimental work. For example, variability in the subjects of experimental or clinical studies is reduced as much as is feasible since the greater the variability, the larger the sample size required to demonstrate differences between effects of experimental and control exposures at an acceptable level of statistical confidence (Hattis 1996). Yet, the quantification of variability is a growing trend only made possible by the application, relatively recently, of various mathematical techniques in biological research (Bois *et al.* 1996; Gelman *et al.* 1996; Johanson *et al.* 1999). The US National Research Council has promulgated the use of measurements and models of intermediate parameters to 'break open the black box' between exposures and disease and the development of a variety of 'biological markers' as indicators of various processes along the exposure–dose–response continuum (Hattis 1996). A toxicity/susceptibility database is under construction, which will store parameter types that encompass different portions of the pathway from external exposure to the production of biological responses (Hattis *et al.* 1999). In fact, most of the parameters listed for incorporation into the database are exactly those that are described in most PBPK models, for example, breathing rates per body weight, uptake or absorption as a fraction of breathing rate, general systemic availability (e.g. initial blood concentration per mg/kg uptake), systemic elimination, active site concentration per systemic blood or plasma concentration, and even changes in parameters as a result of exposure to a chemical (Hattis *et al.* 1999). Thus, it is no surprise that PBPK models are particularly suited to the quantification of inter-individual variability and parameter uncertainty exactly because of the greater number of parameters they contain. In fact, one of the little recognized capabilities of PBPK modelling in risk assessment is the ability to quantify pharmacokinetic uncertainty and variability.

10.6   Uncertainty and variability

Uncertainty and variability affects all experimental biological data. Uncertainty is a consequence of a lack of knowledge about a parameter. In the context of PBPK modelling, uncertainty is defined as the possible error in estimating the 'true' value of a parameter for a representative (average) animal or human. Variability, however, is considered to represent true inter-individual differences in characteristics among individuals (inter-individual variability) or across time within a given individual (inter-occasion or intra-individual variability) (Bois 2001). These differences may stem from genetic differences, lifestyles, physiological status, age, and so on. Experimental toxicology studies are generally designed to obtain specific types of data from a few individuals and the results are extrapolated to a larger and obviously different, population. This, however, requires careful consideration. Unlike clinical pharmacokinetic studies most toxicokinetic studies aim at deriving information about 'average' pharmacokinetic behaviour in sensitive populations, age groups, and even an entire country. They also seek to quantify the variability in such kinetics (Bois 2001). Uncertainty may be reduced, by conducting further, optimally designed experiments to maximize the amount of information one can extract or to better understand the underlying biology. This potentially represents considerable effort and resource. On the other hand, variability is inherent in animal and human species and cannot be reduced. Unfortunately, the presence of uncertainty hinders the precise assessment of variability. However, quite sophisticated Bayesian statistical 'population' models have been developed in an attempt to 'disentangle' uncertainty and variability (Johanson *et al.* 1999; Bernillon and Bois 2000; Bois 2001).

10.7   Monte Carlo analysis

The variability of the parameters that contribute to human inter-individual variability in susceptibility to chemical exposure can be estimated using Monte Carlo analysis. A PBPK model is run with parameter values sampled from distributions that reflect the observed variation in each pharmacokinetic parameter in the human population. For example, the coefficients of variation for various mixed-function oxidase enzymes such as the various isoforms of cytochrome P450 can be based on reported variations (Bois *et al.* 1996; Thomas *et al.* 1996*a*). The distributions of partition coefficients for many compounds have been reported (Gargas *et al.* 1989). The distributions of physiological and anatomical parameters are also readily available (ICRP 1975; Arms and Travis 1988; Brown *et al.* 1997). Each time the model is run with a sampled set of parameter values, effectively representing a single hypothetical human being, the appropriate dose metric for the toxicity of interest is output. The process is repeated a large number of times (typically 500–1000) to generate a distribution of the dose metric for a simulated population.

10.8 Population modelling

Population models provide a methodology that allows us to use individual data to derive a quantitative description of variability in the response to a compound within a population. It is based on the assumption that the same PBPK model can describe the temporal behaviour of a compound and its metabolites for each population member, given the relevant parameters for that individual. Extrapolations to populations may be made, provided the factors responsible for heterogeneity are incorporated into the PBPK model.

The use of a hierarchical model structure, which distinguishes between individual and population variability, enables us to describe inter-individual variability in response to a compound. Typically, we define two levels of parameters, population and individual subject parameters. Inter-individual variability is accounted for by defining a multivariate population distribution from which the subject-level parameters are independently sampled. This population distribution has population parameters reflecting (and separating) the degrees of uncertainty and variability. For example, for metabolic parameters, we may suspect that the variability within our population is relatively small whilst there is a large amount of uncertainty regarding its true population mean. The population framework allows us to express these uncertainties in our analysis (for a detailed discussion, see Bernillon and Bois 2000). In order to utilize this framework, we require a statistical technique suited to our non-linear models and the small datasets typically involved in exposure studies. Bayesian techniques are an ideal candidate for such work.

10.9 Bayesian analysis

A variety of methods exist for performing population modelling. These fall into two categories, parametric and non-parametric. Non-parametric methods are best suited to situations where there is a sufficient amount of experimental data to estimate the entire parameter distribution—including its shape. Parametric methods assume that parameters have specific distributions (e.g. normal), and the data is used to estimate the characteristics of these distributions (e.g. mean and standard deviation). Bayesian analysis is a statistical technique that is appropriate for population modelling using PBPK models since it combines prior knowledge of the PBPK model parameter values and experimental data, leading to a modification of existing beliefs in the form of updated prior knowledge, known as the *posterior distribution*. Bayes' Theorem states that the posterior probability distribution of the model parameters, given the experimental data, is proportional to the product of the likelihood function and the prior parameter distribution. Here we take the likelihood function for a dataset to be the conditional distribution, that is, the distribution given our model and parameter set, for the observed data. This is well suited to PBPK modelling because the distribution of many model parameters within a population are known *a priori* and experimental datasets are relatively small. The technique yields both predicted distributions for tissue dosimetry and updated distributions for model input parameters, which may be used as prior beliefs in subsequent simulations.

10.10   Markov Chain Monte Carlo

When using Bayesian analysis to generate posterior distributions for model parameters a problem is encountered. Due to the non-linearity of PBPK models, there is no explicit formula for the probability of the model parameters given the experimental data. This was a major sticking point until the recent application of Markov Chain Monte Carlo (MCMC) methods. In short, MCMC methods use an iterative sampling scheme to provide samples of parameters from the posterior distribution despite the fact that there is no analytical expression that can be used to determine this conditional probability. Thus, MCMC methods facilitate the use of Bayesian analysis of population models by rendering the calculation of posterior distributions mathematically tractable (technical details are beyond the scope of this chapter; see Gilks *et al.* (1998) for an excellent overview of these methods).

Although MCMC is a Monte Carlo-based technique, it should not be confused with the Monte Carlo analyses more commonly applied to PBPK model predictions (Thomas *et al.* 1996*a,b*). Regular Monte Carlo techniques are more often used to estimate variability in model output, whereas MCMC is fundamentally a parameter estimation technique (Jonsson *et al.* 2001*a*).

10.11   PBPK modelling in epidemiology

Epidemiological studies require accurate, precise, and biologically relevant exposure estimates (Nieuwenhuijsen *et al.* 2000). Inaccurate and imprecise exposure estimates may lead to loss of power and precision and attenuation in health-risk estimates (Chapter 12) (Thomas *et al.* 1993; Nieuwenhuijsen 1997; Armstrong 1998; Nieuwenhuijsen *et al.* 2000). In a review of the uptake of the by-products of chlorinated disinfectants Nieuwenhuijsen *et al.* (2000) discuss what would be an efficient exposure assessment study design. Would a study with a small number of subjects and a very accurate exposure estimate, for example, a biomarker in urine, be as efficient and informative as a study with a large number of subjects and with a less-accurate exposure estimate? It has been suggested that personal uptake of trihalomethanes is needed to interpret, or improve the interpretation of, health-risk estimates because of possible exposure misclassification (Swan and Waller 1998). Conversely, others maintain that the use of individual estimates of uptake, in addition to variability in lifestyle, may lead to measurement error and, consequently, attenuation of health-risk estimates (Armstrong 1998). Repeated measurements within a subset of the population have been proposed in order to improve intra- and inter-individual variability and exposure estimates (Armstrong 1998). However, no epidemiological studies involving repeated measurement of a validated biomarker have been reported (Nieuwenhuijsen *et al.* 2000).

The estimation of individual body burden in every subject in an epidemiological study is prohibitive in terms of time and cost. However, study power must be optimized by balancing sample size and exposure approximation or accuracy (Armstrong 1996). A significant contribution to the optimization of epidemiological studies can be made using PBPK models. As described previously, a population PBPK model quantitatively describing the variability of the kinetics of a compound within a larger population can be developed by extracting data from individual subjects of a much smaller sample (Bois 2001). By merging prior knowledge with new data, Bayesian statistical and MCMC techniques can be used to estimate and reduce the uncertainty around PBPK model parameters to produce 'posterior distributions'. These revised parameter distributions can, in turn, be used in regular Monte Carlo analysis of a PBPK model to estimate the variability in model output (Bois *et al.* 1996; Bois 2001; Jonsson *et al.* 2001*b*; Jonsson and Johanson 2001, 2002). The required sample size in an epidemiological study can be estimated using the variance around the estimated uptake or other dose metric predicted by a population PBPK model. This approach is likely to reduce the costs of such studies as well as increase the accuracy, precision, and confidence in estimation in health-risk assessment.

References

Andersen, M. E. (1995). Development of physiologically based pharmacokinetic and physiologically based pharmacodynamic models for applications in toxicology and risk assessment. *Toxicology Letters*, **79**, 35–44.

Andersen, M. E., Clewell III, H. J., Gargas, M. L., Smith, F. A., and Reitz, R. H. (1987). Physiologically based pharmacokinetics and the risk assessment process for methylene chloride. *Toxicology and Applied Pharmacology*, **87**, 185–205.

Andersen, M. E., Clewell, I., H. J., Gargas, M. J., MacNaughton, M. G., Reitz, R. H., Nolan, R. J., and McKenna, M. J. (1991). Physiologically based pharmacokinetic modelling with dichloromethane. Its metabolite, carbon monoxide, and blood carboxyhemoglobin in rats and humans. *Toxicology and Applied Pharmacology*, **108**, 14–27.

Andersen, M. E., Krewski, D., and Withey, J. R. (1993*a*). Physiological pharmacokinetics and cancer risk assessment. *Cancer Letters*, **69**, 1–14.

Andersen, M. E., Mills, J. J., Gargas, M. L., Kedderis, L., Birnbaum, L. S., Neubert, D., and Greenlee, W. F. (1993*b*). Modeling receptor-mediated processes with dioxin: implications for pharmacokinetics and risk assessment. *Risk Analysis*, **13**, 25–36.

Arms, A. D. and Travis, C. C. (1988). *Reference physiological parameters in pharmacokinetic modeling*. Office of Health and Environmental Assesment, US EPA, Washington, DC. NTIS PB88-196019.

Armstrong, B. G. (1996). Optimizing power in allocating resources to exposure assessment in an epidemiologic study. *American Journal of Epidemiology*, **144**, 192–7.

Armstrong, B. G. (1998). Effect of measurement error on epidemiological studies of environmental and occupational exposures. *Occupational and Environmental Medicine*, **55**, 651–6.

Bachmann, K., Pardoe, D., and White, D. (1996). Scaling basic toxicokinetic parameters from rat to man. *Environmental Health Perspectives*, **104**, 400–7.

Bernillon, P. and Bois, F. Y. (2000). Statistical issues in toxicokinetic modeling: a Bayesian perspective. *Environmental Health Perspectives*, **108**, 883–93.

Bois, F. Y. (2001). Applications of population approaches in toxicology. *Toxicology Letters*, **120**, 385–94.

Bois, F. Y., Jackson, E. T., Pekari, K., and Smith, M. T. (1996). Population toxicokinetics of benzene. *Environmental Health Perspectives*, **104**(Suppl. 6), 1405–11.

Brown, R. P., Delp, M. D., Lindstedt, S. L., Rhomberg, L. R., and Beliles, R. P. (1997). Physiological parameter values for physiologically based pharmacokinetic models. *Toxicology and Industrial Health*, **13**, 407–84.

Clewell, H. J. and Andersen, M. E. (1985). Risk assessment extrapolations and physiological modeling. *Toxicology and Industrial Health*, **1**, 111–31.

Clewell III, H. J. and Andersen, M. E. (1994). Physiologically-based pharmacokinetic modeling and bioactivation of xenobiotics. *Journal of Toxicology and Industrial Health*, **10**, 1–24.

Clewell, H. J., Gentry, P. R., Gearhart, J. M., Allen, B. C., and Andersen, M. E. (2001). Comparison of cancer risk estimates for vinyl chloride using animal and human data with a PBPK model. *Science of the Total Environment*, **274**, 37–66.

Corley, R. A., Mendrala, A. L., Smith, F. A., Staats, D. A., Gargas, M. L., Conolly, R. B., Andersen, M. E., and Reitz, R. H. (1990). Development of a physiologically based pharmacokinetic model for chloroform. *Toxicology and Applied Pharmacology*, **103**, 512–27.

Dedrick, R. L. (1975). Pharmacokinetic and pharmacodynamic considerations for chronic hemodialysis. *Kidney International Supplement*, 7–15.

EPA (1987). Update to the health assessment document and addendum for dichloromethane (methylene chloride): pharmacokinetics, mechanism of action, and epidemiology. External Review Draft.

Gargas, M. L., Burgess, R. J., Voisard, D. E., Cason, G. H., and Andersen, M. E. (1989). Partition coefficients of low-molecular weight volatile chemicals in various liquids and tissues. *Toxicology and Applied Pharmacology*, **98**, 87–99.

Gelman, A., Bois, F., and Jiang, J. M. (1996). Physiological pharmacokinetic analysis using population modeling and informative prior distributions. *Journal of the American Statistical Association*, **91**, 1400–12.

Gilks, W. R., Richardson, S., and Spiegelhalter, D. J. (eds) (1998). *Markov chain Monte Carlo in practice: interdisciplinary statistics*. Chapman & Hall/CRC, Boca Raton.

Haggard, H. W. (1924). The absorption, distribution and elimination of ethyl ether. II. Analysis of the mechanism of the absorption and elimination of such a gas or vapor as ethyl ether. *The Journal of Biological Chemistry*, **59**, 753.

Hattis, D. (1996). Human interindividual variability in susceptibility to toxic effects: from annoying detail to a central determinant of risk. *Toxicology*, **111**, 5–14.

Hattis, D. and Silver, K. (1994). Human interindividual variability—a major source of uncertainty in assessing risks for noncancer health effects. *Risk Analysis*, **14**, 421–31.

Hattis, D., Banati, P., Goble, R., and Burmaster, D. E. (1999). Human interindividual variability in parameters related to health risks. *Risk Analysis*, **19**, 711–26.

ICRP (1975). *Report of the task group on reference man*. Pergamon Press, New York.

Ings, R. M. J. (1990). Interspecies scaling and comparisons in drug development and toxicokinetics. *Xenobiotica*, **20**, 1201–31.

Johanson, G., Jonsson, F., and Bois, F. (1999). Development of new technique for risk assessment using physiologically based toxicokinetic models. *American Journal of Industrial Medicine*, supplement 1, 101–3.

Jonsson, F. and Johanson, G. (2001). A Bayesian analysis of the influence of GSTT1 polymorphism on the cancer risk estimate for dichloromethane. *Toxicology and Applied Pharmacology*, **174**, 99–112.

Jonsson, F. and Johanson, G. (2002). Physiologically based modeling of the inhalation kinetics of styrene in humans using a Bayesian population approach. *Toxicology and Applied Pharmacology*, **179**, 35–49.

Jonsson, F., Bois, F., and Johanson, G. (2001*a*). Physiologically based pharmacokinetic modeling of inhalation exposure of humans to dichloromethane during moderate to heavy exercise. *Toxicological Sciences*, **59**, 209–18.

Jonsson, F., Bois, F. Y., and Johanson, G. (2001*b*). Assessing the reliability of PBPK models using data from methyl chloride-exposed, non-conjugating human subjects. *Archives of Toxicology*, **75**, 189–99.

Krewski, D., Withey, J. R., Ku, L. F., and Andersen, M. E. (1994). Applications of physiologic pharmacokinetic modeling in carcinogenic risk assessment. *Environmental Health Perspectives*, **102**(Suppl. 11), 37–50.

Krishnan, K. and Andersen, M. E. (1991). Physiological modeling and cancer risk assessment. In *New trends in pharmacokinetics* (ed. A. Rescigno and A. K. Thakur), pp. 335–54. Plenum Press, New York.

Krishnan, K. and Andersen, M. E. (1994). Physiologically based pharmacokinetic modeling in toxicology. In *Principals and Methods of Toxicology* (ed. A. W. Hayes), pp. 149–88. Raven Press Ltd., New York.

Levesque, B., Ayotte, P., Tardif, R., Ferron, L., Gingras, S., Schlouch, E., Gingras, G., Levallois, P., and Dewailly, E. (2002). Cancer risk associated with household exposure to chloroform. *Journal of Toxicology and Environmental Health*, A **65**, 489–502.

Lewis, D. F., Sams, C., and Loizou, G. D. (2002). A quantitative structure–activity relationship (QSAR) analysis on a series of alkyl benzenes metabolized by human cytochrome P450 2E1 (CYP2E1). *Journal of Biochemical and Molecular Toxicology*, **17**(1) (in press).

NCI (1976). *Carcinogenesis bioassay of chloroform*. National Technical Information Service, Bethesda, MD.

Nieuwenhuijsen, M. J. (1997). Exposure assessment in occupational epidemiology: measuring present exposures with an example of a study of occupational asthma. *International Archives of Occupational and Environmental Health*, **70**, 295–308.

Nieuwenhuijsen, M. J., Toledano, M. B., and Elliott, P. (2000). Uptake of chlorination disinfection by-products; a review and a discussion of its implications for exposure assessment in epidemiological studies. *Journal of Exposure Analysis and Environmental Epidemiology*, **10**, 586–99.

Pacifici, G. M. and Pelkonen, O. (eds) (2001). *Interindividual variability in human drug metabolism*. Taylor & Francis, London.

Poulin, P. and Krishnan, K. (1996*a*). A mechanistic algorithm for predicting blood: air partition coefficients of organic chemicals with the consideration of reversible binding in hemoglobin. *Toxicology and Applied Pharmacology*, **136**, 131–7.

Poulin, P. and Krishnan, K. (1996*b*). A tissue composition-based algorithm for predicting tissue: air partition coefficients of organic chemicals. *Toxicology and Applied Pharmacology*, **136**, 126–30.

Ramsey, J. C. and Andersen, M. E. (1984). A physiologically based description of the inhalation pharmacokinetics of styrene in rats and humans. *Toxicology and Applied Pharmacology*, **73**, 159–75.

Ramsey, J. C., Young, J. D., Karbowski, R., Chenoweth, M. B., McCarty, L. P., and Braun, W. H. (1980). Pharmacokinetics on inhaled styrene in human volunteers. *Toxicology and Applied Pharmacology*, **53**, 54–63.

Reitz, R. H., Mendrala, A. L., Park, C. N., Andersen, M. E., and Guengerich, F. P. (1988). Incorporation of in vitro enzyme data into the physiologically-based pharmacokinetic (PB-PK) model for methylene chloride: implications for risk assessment. *Toxicological Letters*, **43**, 97–116.

Reitz, R. H., Mendrala, A. L., and Guengerich, F. P. (1989). In vitro metabolism of methylene chloride in human and animal tissues: use in physiologically based pharmacokinetic models. *Toxicology and Applied Pharmacology*, **97**, 230–46.

Reitz, R. H., Mendrala, A. L., Corley, R. A., Quast, J. F., Gargas, M. L., Andersen, M. E., Staats, D. A., and Conolly, R. B. (1990). Estimating the risk of liver cancer associated with human exposures to chloroform using physiologically based pharmacokinetic modeling. *Toxicology and Applied Pharmacology*, **105**, 443–59.

Swan, S. H. and Waller, K. (1998). Disinfection by-products and adverse pregnancy outcomes: what is the agent and how should it be measured? *Epidemiology*, **9**, 479–81.

Thomas, D., Stram, D., and Dwyer, J. (1993). Exposure measurement error: influence on exposure-disease. Relationships and methods of correction. *Annual Review of Public Health*, **14**, 69–93.

Thomas, R. S., Bigelow, P. L., Keefe, T. J., and Yang, R. S. H. (1996*a*). Variability in biological exposure indices using physiologically based pharmacokinetic modeling and Monte Carlo simulation. *American Industrial Hygiene Association Journal*, **57**, 23–32.

Thomas, R. S., Lytle, W. E., Keefe, T. J., Constan, A. A., and Yang, R. S. H. (1996*b*). Incorporating Monte Carlo simulation into physiologically based pharmacokinetic models using advanced continuous simulation language (ACSL): a computational method. *Fundamental and Applied Toxicology*, **31**, 19–28.

11. Biological monitoring

Mark J. Nieuwenhuijsen and Pierre Droz

11.1 Introduction

Biological monitoring is the analysis of human biological samples, which may include, for example, exhaled breath, urine, or blood for a particular substance of interest and/or its metabolite(s) to provide an index of exposure and/or dose. Measurement of concentrations of potentially harmful substances in a critical organ such as the brain, liver, kidney, or skeleton are rarely possible. Ideally, biological monitoring mirrors the concentration of a (hazardous) substance in the critical organ. This may depend on various factors including absorption, distribution, and transformation of the substance. Biological monitoring may also be used to assess susceptibility and/or early health effects, but this will not be discussed in this chapter. Some advantages of biological monitoring compared to personal exposure monitoring of, for example, airborne substances are:

(1) Routes of exposure other than inhalation may exist. This depends on the nature of the exposure and the chemicals to which subjects are exposed. Biological monitoring enables estimation of uptake though all exposure routes, while this would not be possible by air monitoring.

(2) Workers often use personal protective equipment and their efficiency cannot be estimated by air monitoring, but could be with biological monitoring.

(3) Physical activity is known to increase pulmonary ventilation and thus uptake of chemicals. This is not reflected in air monitoring results, but is reflected in biological monitoring results.

(4) Exposure may fluctuate widely over time, for example, from day to day. This would require repeated air sampling to estimate the average long-term exposure. This may not be the case for biological monitoring as it could provide information on long-term exposure when the biological half-life is sufficiently long.

(5) Individual differences are known to exist between subjects, such as build of body or ability to metabolize chemicals. This will have an impact on the level of active species at the site of action, which could be reflected in biological monitoring results, but not in air monitoring results (see also Chapter 9).

The use of biological monitoring can, at least partly, overcome these limitations. Biological monitoring consists of taking measurements of chemicals or their metabolites in body fluids, and therefore it takes into account all routes of exposure, inhalation, dermal and oral, (the protection afforded by) personal protections, influence of physical exercise on uptake, individual differences in the handling of chemicals, and in some situations it reduces the uncertainties produced by the day-to-day exposure variability.

The use of biological monitoring should be considered when there are several pathways and routes of exposure and good laboratory methods exist or can be developed. Examples include exposure to solvents, pesticides, and some chlorination by-products. The issues that need to be considered are the feasibility of the sampling, that is, how easy is it to collect samples, biological half-life of the substance of interest, sensitivity of the method, and the cost. Some of these may have restricted the use of biological monitoring in occupational and environmental epidemiological studies. Furthermore, some generic issues such as sampling strategy that must be addressed are described in Chapters 5 and 6.

11.2   Types of biological samples

The range of biological samples that can be obtained and analysed includes blood, urine, exhaled breath, hair, nail, milk, faeces, sweat, saliva, and semen (Aw 1995) (Table 11.1). The choice of biological sample depends on the substance of interest, its characteristics (e.g. solubility, metabolism, transformation, and excretion), and how invasive the method is. Knowledge of the distribution of a substance, the products of its biotransformation within the body, and the time course of these processes is essential when designing a sampling strategy (see Chapter 10). It is important to consider the timing of sampling when interpreting data: a blood sample may represent 10 s of blood flow; a urine sample may represent 10 h of collection in the bladder; while a hair sample of 10 cm in length may represent 10 months of hair growth.

11.2.1   Urine

Urine samples can be used to determine exposure by detecting the amount of parent compounds present, for example, metals such as lead, mercury, or cadmium. It can also identify the amount of metabolites of specific chemicals, for example, organic solvent such as benzene, (which produces phenol in the urine), toluene (hippuric acid), xylene (methyl hippuric acid), and styrene (mandelic acid). Organophospate pesticides are metabolized to alkylphosphates, which can be detected in the urine. Inorganic arsenic is metabolized in the body by the process of methylation. Inorganic and organic methylated arsenic species can be detected in the urine. This appears to depend upon, for example, arsenic burden and individual differences. Urine samples are often favoured as they are relatively easy to collect compared to blood or other biological samples. Samples are generally collected over a 24-h period or, for more practical reasons, the first void sample in the morning or at the end of the work shift. Subjects are less likely to decline to cooperate when asked to produce a urine sample rather than blood and it does not require a medically trained person or involve any discomfort. However, urine samples are more prone to external contamination than other biological samples and precautions need to be taken to prevent this. Several factors should be considered before deciding on using urine samples over other biological samples for biological monitoring. For example, whether the specific chemical of interest is organic or inorganic, its valency state, as well as the period and duration of exposure. For example, for metallic

Table 11.1 Types of biological samples and analytes

Urine	
Parent compounds	Heavy metals, e.g. organic lead, mercury, cadmium, chromium
	Metalloids, e.g. arsenic
	Ketones, e.g. methyl ethyl ketone and methyl isobutyl ketone
	Disinfection by-products, e.g. trichloroacetic acid
	Herbicides such as 2,4 D and mecoprop
Metabolites	Aromatic compounds, e.g. phenol for benzene and phenol, hippuric acid for toluene, methyl hippuric acids for xylenes, mandelic acid for styrene and ethyl benzene, 1-hydroxypyrene for PAHs
	Chlorinated solvents, e.g. trichloroacetic acid for trichloroethylene and 1,1,1-trichloroethane
	Dialkylphosphates for organophosphates
	Cotinine for nicotine
	MMA and DMA for inorganic arsenic
	Thiocyanate for tobacco smoke
Blood	
Parent compounds	Heavy metals, e.g. inorganic lead, mercury, and cadmium
	Aromatic compounds, e.g. toluene
	Chlorinated solvents, e.g. trichloroethylene, perchloroethylene, and 1,1,1-trichloroethane
	Chlorination by-products, e.g. trihalomethanes
Metabolites	Carboxyhaemaglobin for methylene chloride and carbon monoxide
	Trichloroethanol for trichloroethylene
Exhaled breath	
Parent compounds	Aromatic compounds, e.g. benzene, toluene, ethyl benzene
	Chlorinated solvents, e.g. trichloroethylene, perchloroethylene, 1,1,1-trichloroethane, and methylene chloride
	Chlorination by-products, e.g. trihalomethanes
	Carbon monoxide
Hair and nail	Arsenic and mercury
Fat	Polychlorinated biphenyls

Source: Adapted from Aw (1995).

mercury, urine is the biological choice for assessing long-term (3–4 weeks) exposure. For recent, acute exposure (1–2 days) blood mercury gives a better indication of exposure. In the case of exposure to inorganic lead, blood lead is preferred over urinary lead, as it reflects long-term exposure, the latter being more affected by recent exposure. However for exposure to organic lead compounds the situation is reversed, with urinary lead being a better index of exposure than blood lead. With exposure to chromium compounds, metabolism results in chromium being excreted in the urine in the trivalent form, regardless of whether exposure and absorption includes hexavalent as well as trivalent forms. Hence total chromium in the urine will not indicate the relative exposures to different chromium species (Aw 1995). Furthermore, urine sampling may become more complicated where metabolites of some substances are the same as the substance of interest. For example, the chlorination by-product trichloroacetic acid in drinking water is the same as the metabolite of chlorinated solvent such as trichloro-ethylene, perchloroethylene, and 1,1,1-trichloroethane. Thus when trying to determine the uptake of trichloroacetic acid through ingestion of tap water, exposure to chlorinated solvents should also be estimated and taken account of.

The concentration of a substance in urine is influenced by a number of factors: the degree of dilution, the kidney function, the body burden of the substance, the metabolic and kinetic pathways, and current and past exposure. Urine is produced continuously by the kidneys as part of a complex process of water and electrolyte control. The kidney's glomeruli produce at a rate of 125 ml min^{-1} an ultra-filtrate (the primary urine) consisting of water, salts, and small molecules. A total blood volume of about 300 l is filtered everyday. If the glomerular filtration (GFR) is decreased, the capacity for eliminating toxic substances also decreases. In such cases, the concentration of a substance in the urine will become lower while the body burden increases. This is the case for aluminium, a pollutant that is normally excreted in the urine, but which accumulates in the body of those suffering from severe renal impairment (Berglund *et al.* 2001). In order to maintain the water balance of the body, water may be reabsorbed. In this process other xenobiotics may be reabsorbed either actively or passively. This is notably the case for lipophilic substances that can cross membranes easily, such as unchanged organic solvents. This reabsorption will affect the concentration of substances in urine. To evaluate the concentration of a substance in urine it is often necessary to consider the degree of concentration of the urine. The composition of urine is usually compatible with maintenance of body water and solute content within physiological limits. A short time after consumption of a large volume of fluid, the urine will become diluted, with a low solute content. When water is evaporated, for example, due to perspiration as a result of high environmental temperature or hard physical work, the urine concentration increases. The concentration of a substance can be related to creatinine (a metabolic product of the muscles excreted in the urine in fairly constant quantities) or specific gravity to compensate for the degree of dilution. The excretion rate is higher in males: muscular individuals and those who eat a lot of meat. The substance can therefore be reported in micrograms (or mole) per gram (or mmole) creatinine. The other way to compensate for the degree of dilution is to adjust for a specific gravity. If a urine sample has specific gravity of 1.012, which is fairly diluted urine, and is to be adjusted to represent urine with a more normal specific gravity (1.022), the following calculation can be made:

The concentration in the urine sample $\times (1.022 - 1.000)/(1.012 - 1000)$.

The factor of 1000, which is the specific density of water, must be subtracted from both the numerator and denominator (Berglund *et al.* 2001). Sometimes the concentration of the substance is not adjusted for and expressed simply as the measured concentration (μg/l). This is mainly the case for passively reabsorbed substances, such as solvents. In rare situations, biomarkers levels are expressed as rates of excretion (amounts per unit of time) as, for example, mmol min^{-1}.

11.2.2 Blood

Blood is a transport medium. After absorption in the gastrointestinal tract or the lungs, substances are transported via the bloodstream to different tissues and organs where they are stored, accumulated, or metabolized. Substances that have been absorbed by tissues will be released and degraded by normal tissue metabolism, transported in the blood, and eventually eliminated from the body. The blood concentration of a substance is influenced by the exposure and concentrations in the tissues (body burden). The relative importance of these two factors varies according to the substance in question and the exposure level (Berglund *et al.* 2001). A substance in blood is bound to red cells or to plasma proteins. For most essential metals such as iron, copper, and zinc, the body has special transport proteins such as transferring, ceruplasmin, and alpha-2-microglobulin. Certain non-essential and toxic substances, metals in particular, bind preferentially to red cells. Cadmium and lead are almost completely bound to red cells. Sometimes it may be necessary to adjust for the haemoglobin concentration or hematocrit, when comparing the metal concentration between individuals or groups. The concentration of contaminants in plasma is of particular interest since it constitutes the fraction of the substance in blood that is readily available for transport in and out of tissues. However, for many toxic substances concentrations are so low that they are very difficult to measure. Highly lipophilic compounds, for example PCBs, should be adjusted for cholesterol, triglyceride, or low-density lipid concentration (Berglund *et al.* 2001).

Blood samples can be collected to identify parent compounds or their metabolites. Heavy metals such as lead, mercury, and cadmium can be measured in blood. In the UK, lead blood concentrations are routinely measured for compliance reasons in the workplace. For organic solvents such as perchloroethylene and trichloroethylene, the solvents themselves can be identified in blood, while for other solvents their metabolites can be detected in blood (e.g. free trichloroethanol for exposure to trichloroethylene). Very low levels of chlorination by-products such as chloroform and chlorodibromomethane can also be detected in blood at apparently lower levels than in exhaled breath (Nieuwenhuijsen *et al.* 2000) (see Chapter 15).

The disadvantage of using blood samples for biological monitoring include poorer cooperation because of the discomfort of the procedure, especially if venepuncture is required on a regular basis. Some individuals may faint during venepuncture or even at the thought of the procedure. Facilities have to be in place to deal with this possibility. For those with veins that are not prominent, a degree of skill and experience is required to successfully collect a suitable quantity of blood.

Care must be taken to prevent external contamination of the blood sample, especially when the parent compound is determined. The site of venepuncture has to be adequately cleaned. For determining chromium levels in blood, the use of chromium-free needles have been suggested. For trihalomethanes, the containers need to be processed to expel compounds that are present in the containers (Aw 1995). Concentrations of chemicals measured in blood samples are expressed in amounts per unit volume, in some cases whole blood is considered and in other situations only plasma is taken into account.

11.2.3 Exhaled breath

Biological monitoring of exhaled breath involves breathing out into a direct reading instrument or into a sampling bag or other collection device before dispatching the collected sample to a laboratory for analysis. It is preferable to obtain a sample of alveolar breath rather than all the exhaled breath, since it is appears to be the best indicator for blood levels. Special devices have been developed to obtain this fraction

(Dyne *et al.* 1997). The advantages of exhaled breath sampling are that the collection of samples is non-invasive, and repeated samples can be taken within a short period of time. The disadvantages include current lack of agreement on how samples have to be collected, standardization on the type of collection device used, and laboratory methods for analysis. Furthermore, the method may not be as sensitive as blood sampling, which appears to be the case for trihalomethanes (see Chapter 15). Exhaled breath sampling is suitable for the detection and determination of, for example, benzene, toluene, carbon monoxide, ethyl benzene, *n*-hexane, carbon tetrachloride, perchloroethylene, trichloroethylene, and trihalomethanes (Aw 1995). Concentrations in exhaled breath are expressed in ppm or mmol l^{-1}. It should always be mentioned which fraction of the exhaled breath the data refers to: mixed exhaled, alveolar, or end-expired air.

11.2.4   Hair and nail

Analysis of hair and nail samples has been used to assess exposure to arsenic and mercury. The rationale for this is that as nail and hair growth occurs, absorbed arsenic and mercury are incorporated into a portion of the hair and nail. The analysis of hair and nail can provide a measure of exposure over a longer time period, although varying growth rates during the exposure period may need to be taken into account. This may be difficult. External contamination of the hair and nail may give an erroneous indication of the amount absorbed systematically, and certain washing procedures need to be carried out to prevent this. Contamination may occur from, for example, consumer products such as the use of hair dye and shampoo and may affect the subsequent analysis. Procedures to wash and clean the samples before analysis may not adequately remove contaminants absorbed onto the surface of samples. The difference between the concentration of substances measured in head vs. pubic hair or in fingernail vs. toenail samples may indicate the extent of surface contamination. There are limitations in the interpretation of the results obtained, particularly for individuals rather than groups (Aw 1995).

11.2.5   Other media

Samples of body fat have been used for determining the extent of exposure to polychlorinated biphenyls (PCBs). Substances such as PCBs are not easily biodegradable and therefore persist in the environment and in adipose tissue. Fat samples are obtained by needle biopsy or surgical excision. The quantity of fat required for the assay of PCB content is several hundred grams. The amount of PCB determined is in parts per billion or parts per trillion quantities. It is not practical to collect fat samples periodically nor does it attract many volunteers. Therefore its use is somewhat limited (Aw 1995).

Analysis of breast milk has been very useful for following time-trend in human exposure to lipophilic chemicals, such as organochlorine contaminants. Monitoring breast milk has generally been carried out to estimate the exposure of the child, rather than that of the mother, but the content of lipophilic substances in the milk also represents the body burden of the contaminants in the adipose tissue of the mother. Breast milk is a useful medium since most newborn children obtain all their nutrition from their mother's milk. The concentration of a contaminant is a function of parity, age, body mass, time of sampling, nutritional status, lactation period, and fat content of the milk

(Berglund *et al.* 2001). Biological monitoring of semen, tooth enamel, faeces, and skeleton has been carried out but to a much lesser extent.

11.3   Biological half-life

The biological half-life of a substance refers to the time required for clearance of 50 per cent of the substance from the medium. Biological half-lives vary substantially (Table 11.2) and this needs to be taken into account in the sampling strategy. For example, in the case of the exposure assessment of chlorination by-products in drinking water, chloroform, generally the main volatile by-product, has a biological half-life of approximately 30 min and can be measured in blood and exhaled breath. Trichloroacetic acid, generally the main non-volatile by-product, can be measured in urine and has a half-life of 70–120 h. It is therefore essential that chloroform monitoring takes place very quickly after activities associated with chloroform uptake, such as ingestion of, showering and bathing with, and swimming in chlorinated water. Chloroform levels in exhaled breath and blood fall rapidly and the actual uptake may be underestimated the longer the period between exposure and sampling. This, however, is much less of a concern for trichloroacetic acid for which the main route of uptake is ingestion. A concern for the measurement of trichloroacetic acid is that other chlorinated solvents have trichloroacetic acid as their metabolite. People may be exposed to these kinds of activities repeatedly during the day or during the week and this may be reflected in the biological samples.

Table 11.2   Examples of biological indicators and their half-lives

Biological indicator	Approximate $T_{1/2}$ (h)
Solvent in breath/blood ES	0.5–2
Solvents in breath/blood PS	20–70
Chloroform in breath/blood	0.3–0.5
Trichloroacetic acid in urine	50–120
Dichloroacetic acid in urine	<2
Trichloroethanol in urine	12
Mandelic acid in urine	5
Phenol in urine	3.5
Hippuric acid in urine	1–2
Carbon monoxide in breath/blood	5
Lead in blood	900
Chromium in urine	15–40
Cadmium in urine	10–30 years
Mercury in blood	100
Haemoglobin adducts	3000[a]
Albumin adducts	400[a]

ES = end of work shift sample; PS = prior to work shift sample.
[a] $T_{1/2}$ of haemoglobin/albumin, adducts $T_{1/2}$ may be lower.
Source: Adapted from Droz and Wu (1991).

Since variability is inherent in biological monitoring, even more so than in, for example, personal air sampling, it is important to identify the main categories of variability. Figure 11.1 illustrates the effects of variable exposure. The time profiles of two hypothetical biological indicators, behaving according to a one-compartment kinetic model, are indicated: one with a half-life of 5 h and the other, 50 h. As shown in Table 11.2 many indicators have half-lives in this range. In Fig. 11.1(a), there is no variability in exposure at all, and after a certain time, which depends on the half-life, the biological indicator reaches a steady-state level. Sampling after this point would completely define the exposure situation and the health risk if the exposure–response relationship were known. In Fig. 11.1(b), a typical work schedule is taken into account: 8 h exposure per day with a 1 h break, 5 days per week, week after week. In this case the biological sampling becomes a little more complex. The concentration in the

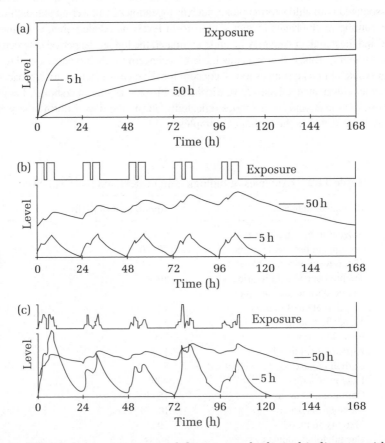

Fig. 11.1 Effects of air exposure variability on two biological indicators with half-lives of 5 and 50 h. Ordinate is an arbitrary scale. Graph (a) constant continuous exposure; (b) constant industrial exposure (8 h day^{-1}, 1-h break, 5 days/week); (c) fluctuation industrial exposure (1-h air concentrations sampled from a lognormal distribution with $\sigma_g = 2.0$).

biological sample will depend on the sampling time with respect to the work shift for the biological indicator with a half-life of 5 h, and with respect to the work shift and the day of the week for the biological indicator with a biological half-life of 50 h. In Fig. 11.1(c), the exposure is not steady any longer; rather it fluctuates from hour to hour according to a lognormal distribution (geometric standard deviation of 2.0). The concentration in the biological samples is more variable, especially for the 5-h biological indicator. This suggests that biological indicators with a short half-life are more sensitive to fluctuations in exposure from day to day and even within one day (Droz and Wu 1991). The biological half-life of a substance may differ from person to person, depending on, for example, age, diet, stress, metabolic polymorphism, and disease. These factors may have to be considered when conducting a study. Upto a certain extent variation in biological half-life can be incorporated in a sampling strategy using physiologically based pharmacokinetic (PBPK) modelling (see Chapter 10).

11.4   Autocorrelation

Depending on what kind of sampling strategy is chosen, repeated samples may be required (see Chapters 5 and 6). Airborne exposures are usually considered as following approximately a lognormal distribution. Although short-term air samples (e.g. 15 min sampling duration) are generally considered to be autocorrelated, there is very little evidence for autocorrelation between 8-h samples in the workplace. The latter can therefore be treated as being random. The situation is different for biological indicators, which are themselves autocorrelated due the finite rates of biological elimination. This can probably be described by using a first-order autoregressive process according to the following model:

$$Y_t = \mu(1 - b_1) + b_1 Y_{t-1} + a_t,$$

where Y_t is the biological indicator on day t, Y_{t-1} the biological indicator on day $t - 1$, μ the long-term mean of the biological indicator, b_1 the first lag autoregressive coefficient, and a_t is a term describing random variation in exposure and individual variability. The autocorrelation coefficient can furthermore be expressed as a function of the half-life ($T_{1/2}$) of the biological indicator:

$$b_1 = e^{-24k} \quad \text{with } k = 0.693/T_{1/2}.$$

This is the autocorrelation coefficient of lag 1 (one day). Coefficients of higher lags can be calculated, for example, for lag n: $b_n = (b_1)^n$.

As could be expected, the longer the half-life of the biological indicator, the larger the autocorrelation coefficient. If $b_1 < 0.10$, it may be assumed that any autocorrelation is negligible, thus one can see that

(1) at $T_{1/2}$ smaller than 5 h, days may be considered as uncorrelated;
(2) at $T_{1/2}$ between 5 and 50 h, weeks may be considered as uncorrelated;
(3) at $T_{1/2}$ between 50 and 200 h, months may be considered as uncorrelated.

A strategy for biological monitoring is easier to establish if the results are unlikely to be autocorrelated. Therefore, the time of sampling should be chosen in order to minimize autocorrelation. For biological indicators belonging to case (2), for example, sampling frequency should be restricted to once a week and for case (3) to once a month. For case (1), sampling can be as frequent as once a day (Droz and Wu 1991).

11.5   Damping of exposure variability

As already seen in Fig. 11.1 sampling of biological indicators with long half-lives is likely to introduce some damping of the exposure variability. That is, if one compares the distribution of the biological monitoring results with that of, for example, air sampling results, the variance will be lower. For biological indicators with half-lives smaller than 5 h, this damping effect will be negligible. In this case essentially all the variability of the environmental concentrations is expected to be transmitted to the biological indicators. For indicators with half-lives of 40 h and above, less than 50 per cent of the variability will be transmitted. However for estimating the mean exposure, or the mean target site concentration, biological indicators with long half-lives may be more useful, as they are less sensitive to exposure fluctuations (Droz and Wu 1991).

Results from biological monitoring of similarly exposed subjects are subject to intra- and inter-subject variation. Factors that have been taken into account in the interpretation of results include:

(1) those related to the individual (age, sex, body mass index, genetic differences in the metabolism of the compounds, pregnancy, exercise and physical activity, smoking, medication, consumption of alcohol and dietary factors, and the presence of existing lung, liver, or kidney disease or other illness);

(2) those related to exposure (timing and intensity of exposure in relation to timing of collection of the biological sample, mixed exposures that may affect the metabolism of the compounds absorbed, and route of exposure);

(3) those related to the chemical of interest (half-life, where and how it is metabolized and excreted (Aw 1995).

11.6   Variability

Exposure variability may also have implications for the choice of the appropriate measure of exposure, since different measures may be associated with different patterns of exposure variability. A theoretically superior measure of exposure with expected high variability may be less attractive in an epidemiological study than a more proximal measure of exposure with less inherent variability (see Chapter 12). This also governs the applicability of markers of exposure in biological monitoring. Although theoretical arguments may be in favour of biological monitoring, it has to be considered whether biomarkers of exposure can be measured with higher accuracy and precision than environmental agents. Few studies have been published on the utility of markers of exposure in relation to within- and between-subject variability in these markers. Hence, the choice between environmental exposure measurements and measurement of markers of exposure in human material partly depends on the variability in the parameter of interest (see Chapter 6 for further discussion).

The strengths and weaknesses of both measurement approaches were explored in a longitudinal study among boat workers exposed to styrene (Rappaport *et al.* 1995). The exposure assessment consisted of full-shift personal measurements of styrene exposure per worker carried out over one year on seven occasions. Sister chromatid exchanges (SCEs) was used as a marker of exposure. This was measured in lymphocytes from two venous blood samples taken from each worker obtained during the measurement surveys. The correlation between styrene exposure and SCEs was low (11% explained variance). A within- and between-subject variance ratio of 0.33 for styrene exposure was observed and of 2.21 for SCEs. If attenuation of the health risk estimates would be restricted to 10 per cent, three measurements per person would be required for airborne styrene exposure vs. 20 measurements per person for SCEs. This latter value would be impossible in epidemiological studies due to the invasive character of the technique and the associated costs. So although intuitively biological monitoring would have been the preferred option for an epidemiological study, detailed analysis showed that this is not the case and that it would be more efficient to obtain air samples. Obviously, this is just one specific example and may not be applicable to all studies or situations.

11.7   Models and determinants

Feasibility issues, cost, and time may restrict biological monitoring in epidemiological studies and it is rare that biological samples can be obtained from the entire study population, particularly when it is large. However, biological monitoring could be useful to build dose and/or exposure models in a subpopulation, which subsequently could be applied to whole population after information is obtained in this population on particular determinants, for example, by questionnaire (see Chapter 6). For example, Harris *et al.* (2002) measured 2,4-dichlorophenoxyacetic acid (2,4 D), 2-(4-chloro-2-methylphenoxy) propionic acid, MCPP (mecoprop) and 3,6-dichloro-*o*-anisic acid (dicamba) in urine (two consecutive 24-h periods) collected from a group of 98 professional turf applicators from 20 companies across southwestern Ontario. The group also filled out questionnaires to acquire information on all known variables that could potentially increase or decrease pesticide exposure to the amount handled to build models for epidemiological studies. They used linear regression to assess the relationship between the concentration of the substances in urine and the questionnaire data. They found that the volume of pesticide (active ingredient) applied was only weakly related to the total dose of 2,4 D absorbed ($R^2 = 0.21$). Two additional factors explained a large proportion of the variation in measured pesticide exposure: the type of spray nozzle used and the use of gloves while spraying. Individuals who used a fan type nozzle had significantly higher doses than those who used a gun type nozzle. Glove use was associated with significantly lower doses. Job satisfaction and current smoking influenced the dose but were not highly predictive. In the final multiple regression models predicting absorbed dose of 2,4 D and mecoprop, approximately 63–68 per cent of the variation in doses could be explained by the small number of variables identified (Table 11.3). Biological monitoring in this case was important to be able to determine the true effect of wearing protective equipment such as gloves. This study provided extremely useful information for epidemiological studies, which could focus on obtaining information on these particular variables.

Table 11.3   Regression models predicting the log of total dose of mecoprop and 2,4 D in 94 volunteers (after Harris *et al.* 2002)

Variable	Estimate	SE	p-value	Partial R^2
2,4 D ($R^2 = 0.64$)				
Intercept	−1.09	0.01	0.29	
Log spray	0.96	0.12	0.001	0.44
Nozzle	1.37	0.23	0.001	0.29
Glove wear	−1.50	0.25	0.001	0.29
Satisfaction	−0.39	0.17	0.021	0.06
Smoke	0.51	0.22	0.02	0.06
Mecoprop ($R^2 = 0.67$)				
Intercept	−1.44	0.98	0.14	
Log spray	1.05	0.11	0.001	0.50
Nozzle	1.12	0.22	0.001	0.23
Glove wear	−1.63	0.25	0.001	0.34
Satisfaction	−0.40	0.16	0.02	0.07
Smoke	0.63	0.22	0.005	0.09

Spray: ln (ml product over week + 900); glove wear: if sprayer and not wearing gloves or mixer/loader then glove wear = 0; if sprayer and wearing gloves then glove wear = 1; nozzle type: 1 = fan and 0 = gun; job satisfaction: 1 highly satisfied, 2 satisfied, 3 neither satisfied nor unsatisfied, 4 unsatisfied; smoker 1 = yes and 0 = no.

Another example is arsenic for which uptake is most likely through inhalation and digestion of soil and house dust, including hand to mouth contact, but also through ingestion of contaminated vegetables, fish and water, and smoking. Soil represents an important pathway of exposure, through handling of soil materials (e.g. during play or work), through contact with soil-derived dust, and through foodstuffs. Exposures to arsenic have attracted particular concern, and several studies have suggested an association between soil arsenic and cancer of, for example, the skin, lung, and bladder. This is mainly attributed to the inorganic form of arsenic, although other forms may be as toxic. Inorganic arsenic is reduced by methylation in humans, forming monomethylarsonic acid (MMA) and dimethylarsinic acid (DMA).

Arsenic and its species can be measured in soil, house dust and by biomonitoring in hair, urine, blood, and toenails. Mining and smelting have left certain areas of southwest England with high arsenic levels in soil. There has been considerable concern about these high levels, although it was unclear how much was taken up by the residents. Kavanagh *et al.* (1998) measured arsenic levels in soil, house dust, and urine of residents in three areas: two exposed areas (Gunnislake and Devon Great Consols) and one unexposed area (Cargreen) (Table 11.4). High levels of arsenic were found in the soil and, to a lesser extent, in house dust. Marked variations were evident, however, between the different areas. Concentrations of As in the soil were up to 122 times greater in areas with high exposure compared to non-exposed areas. For house dust, concentrations were up to 24 times higher. In urine, there was only a 2-fold difference in arsenic levels between the areas. This suggests that the actual uptake of arsenic from soil and house dust is relatively low. Moreover, biological monitoring needs to be

Table 11.4 Arsenic (As) in soil, house dust, and urine in the southwest of England (after Kavanagh *et al.* 1998)

Ratios between sites	Cargreen	Gunnislake	Devon GC
Soil (μg g^{-1}) $1:10:122$	37	365	4500
House dust (μg g^{-1}) $1:4:24$	49	217	1167
Urine (μg g^{-1} creatine)			
Total As $1:2:2$	4.7	9.2	10.0
Arsenite (As III)	<LOD	1.7	0.9
Arsenate (As V)	<LOD	0.9	1.3
DMA	4.7	5.6	8.5
MMA	<LOD	0.3	0.7

<LOD, below limit of detection; GC, great consols; DMA, dimethylarsinic acid; MMA, monomethylarsonic acid.

undertaken to obtain good estimates of personal arsenic uptake, since soil or house dust samples cannot be relied upon to provide a reliable dose estimate. The study also suggested that arsenic speciation is very important, for inorganic arsenic levels in the control village were below the detection limit, while in the other two areas they were measurable.

11.8 Quality control

Normal quality control procedures apply to the sampling, storage, and laboratory analysis of biological samples (Armstrong *et al.* 1992; Weber 1996, chapter 1). The measured concentrations are often very low and therefore caution needs to be taken to avoid contamination of the sample by, for example, environmental concentrations and containers, and degradation during storage.

References

Aw, C. (1995). Biological monitoring. In *Occupational hygiene* (ed. J. M. Harrington and K. Gardiner, 2nd edn). Blackwell Science, Oxford.

Armstrong, B. K., White, E., and Saracci, R. (1992). *Principles of exposure measurement in epidemiology.* Oxford University Press, Oxford.

Berglund, M., Elinder, C.-G., and Jarup, L. (2001). *Human exposure assessment.* World Health Organisation, Stockholm, http://www.imm.ki.se.

Dyne, D., Cocker, J., and Wilson, H. K. (1997). A novel device for capturing breath samples for solvent analysis. *Science of the Total Environment,* **199**, 83–9.

Droz, P. O. and Wu, M. M. (1991). Biological monitoring strategies. In *Exposure assessment for epidemiology and hazard control* (ed. S. M. Rappaport and T. J. Smith). Lewis Publishers, Michigan.

Harris, S. A., Sass-Kortsak, A. M., Corey, P. N., and Purdham, J. T. (2002). Development of models to predict dose of pesticides in professional turf applicators. *Journal Exposure Analysis and Environmental Epidemiology,* **12**, 130–44.

Kavanagh, P., Farago, M. E., Thornton, I., Goessler, W., Kuehnelt, D., Schlagenhaufen, C., and Irgolic, K. J. (1998). Urinary arsenic species in Devon and Cornwell residents, UK. *The Analyst*, **123**, 27–30.

Nieuwenhuijsen, M. J., Toledano, M. B., and Elliott, P. (2000). Uptake of chlorination disinfection by-products: a review and a discussion of its implications for epidemiological studies. *Journal Exposure Analysis and Environmental Epidemiology*, **10**, 586–99.

Rappaport, S. M., Symanski, E., Yager, J. W., *et al.* (1995). The relationship between environmental monitoring and biological markers in exposure assessment. *Environmental Health Perspectives*, **103**(Suppl 3), 49–54.

Weber, J. P. (1996). Quality in environmental toxicology measurements. *Therapeutic Drug Monitoring*, **18**, 477–83.

12. Exposure measurement error: consequences and design issues

Ben Armstrong

12.1 Introduction

This chapter is concerned with the effects of inaccuracy in exposure assessment (including misclassification of exposure) on results of epidemiological studies. Most readers will be aware that such error adversely impacts on studies, but fewer will be aware in just what way. Does it add to uncertainty in estimates of measures of effect? If so, is this extra uncertainty reflected in the usual statements of uncertainty, such as confidence intervals? Under what circumstances does it cause bias in a result, and can the direction and extent of bias be known, or even corrected for? Does it compromise the power of the study?

The chapter will summarize, in a manner accessible to the non-statistician, what is known about the effects of measurement error on the results of a study. The chapter is organized in three sections. The first covers the types and contexts of measurement error and how to describe them formally. The second describes the effects of error according to its type, first qualitatively and then where possible quantitatively; it also includes an introductory discussion of methods of correcting for these effects. Finally, the chapter addresses issues in designing epidemiological studies in the presence of measurement error—the resources to be utilized for exposure measurement, and the extent of validity or reliability studies.

12.1.1 Terms and notation

The term relative risk (RR) is used here in the statistical tradition, generically to include rate ratios, odds ratios, prevalence ratios, and the like. (This usage is standard in statistics. Some epidemiologists restrict the meaning of RR to be the ratio of cumulative incidence.) The term effect measure is used to denote a summary of the association between exposure and outcome, for example, RR or regression coefficient. The true exposure is denoted as T, the approximate measure X, and the error E, with

$X = T + E.$

The standard deviation of T, X, and E are written as σ_T, σ_X, and σ_E, respectively.

12.2   Describing measurement error

The effects of measurement error critically depend on its context and type.

12.2.1   Error in measuring what?

There are three categories of explanatory variables that may be measured with error:

(1) a variable of interest (environmental or occupational exposure);
(2) a potential confounder (active smoking, socio-economic status);
(3) a potential effect-modifier (markers of vulnerability to the effects of the variable of interest, e.g. age).

12.2.2   Differential or non-differential?

(1) Error is called differential if it varies according to the health outcome. The classic example of this is recall bias in case–control studies, in which cases may recall exposure with error that is different from controls.
(2) Non-differential error does not depend on health outcome. This can usually be assumed if exposure is measured before outcome is known, or deduced from written records, for example using work histories and a job-exposure matrix.

12.2.3   Scale of measurement of the variable(s) with error

(1) Categorical (qualitative), comprising:
   - dichotomous ('exposed' vs. 'not exposed');
   - polytomous ('high', 'medium', 'low');
(2) numerical (concentration of particles in air in milligram per cubic metre, number of cigarettes smoked per day).

When occurring in categorical variables, measurement error is termed misclassification—study subjects may be classified incorrectly. Numerical variables can be grouped, thus becoming categorical variables. Conversely ordered polytomous variables can sometimes be treated as numerical.

Two further distinctions apply to error in numerical variables:

12.2.4   Random or systematic?

- Systematic (e.g. all exposures overestimated by 2 units or by 20%),
- random—some exposures overestimated, some underestimated (the mean error is zero).

Error often has some systematic and some random component. This chapter concentrates on the random component because effects of systematic error are easier to infer by commonsense reasoning. Furthermore, if measurement is known to be subject to systematic error, it can be corrected.

12.2.5   Classical or Berkson?

This distinction is not well known and is a little tricky to understand, but it has major implications for the effects of the error.

(1) Classical: The average of many replicate measurements of same true exposure would equal the true exposure.
(2) Berkson: The same approximate exposure ('proxy') is used for many subjects; the true exposures vary randomly about this proxy, with mean equal to it.

Example: A study investigates the relationship of average lead exposure up to age ten with IQ in ten-year-old children living in the vicinity of a lead smelter. IQ is measured by a test administered at age ten. Consider two study designs for assessing exposure:

Design 1: Each child has one measurement made for blood lead, at a random time during their life. The blood lead measurement will be an approximate measure of average blood lead over life. However, if the investigators were able to make many replicate measurements (at different random time-points), the average would be a good indicator of lifetime exposure. This measurement error is thus classical.

Design 2: The children's place of residence at age ten (assumed as known exactly) are classified into three groups by proximity to the smelter—close, medium, and far. Random blood leads, collected as described in Design 1, are averaged for each group, and this group average is used as a proxy for lifetime exposure for each child in the group. Here the same approximate exposure ('proxy') is used for all subjects in the same group, and true exposures, though unknown, may be assumed to vary randomly about the proxy. This measurement error is thus a Berkson error.

Often error has both classical and random components, although one usually predominates. Exposures estimated from observed determinants using an exposure prediction model have predominantly Berkson error. Indeed if the determinants are measured without error, it is entirely a Berkson error.

The two types of error are defined statistically as:

(1) Classical: $X = T + E$, with E independent of T and mean$(E) = 0$;
(2) Berkson: $T = X + E$, with E independent of X and mean$(E) = 0$.

12.2.6   Describing the magnitude of error

Effects of measurement error usually depend on its magnitude. With random error this will vary from measurement to measurement, so more properly one says that the effects of measurement error depend on its distribution. Error distributions are important conceptually, even if there is no data for inference. However, it makes this section less abstract if data from a validity study is assumed to be available. A validity study is a study in which for a sample of subjects exposure is measured accurately as well as by the approximate method to be used in the main study. Alternatively, but less usefully, investigators may have data from a reliability study, in which for a sample of subjects exposure is measured two or more times, each time independently. If the same method is used each time, this is called an intra-method reliability study. Otherwise it is an inter-method reliability study. There is more about estimation of magnitude of error from validity and reliability studies later in the chapter, but basic summaries of error magnitude are introduced here.

Categorical variables

The likely extent of misclassification of categorical variables is usually specified as probabilities of misclassification. For dichotomous variables, it is conventional to

Table 12.1 Describing misclassification of a dichotomous
exposure variable

		True	
		Exposed n(%)	Unexposed n(%)
According to	Exposed	40 (80%)	20 (40%)
misclassified	Unexposed	10 (20%)	30 (60%)
variable			
	Total	50	50

express these through the sensitivity (the probability of correctly classifying a truly
exposed subject as exposed) and the specificity (the probability of correctly classifying
a non-exposed subject as non-exposed) of the classification. In the exposure classification illustrated in Table 12.1, sensitivity is 80 per cent (0.8) and specificity is 60 per cent
(0.6); so the probability of misclassifying an exposed subject as non-exposed is
$1 - 0.8 = 0.2$, and the probability of misclassifying a non-exposed subject as exposed is
$1 - 0.6 = 0.4$.

Sensitivity and specificity cannot easily be estimated from a reliability study,
although construction of a table of agreement similar to Table 12.1 is often useful.
There are various ways of summarizing agreement between the measurements, the most
popular being the kappa (κ) statistic, which takes the value 1 if there is complete agreement and 0 if there is no more agreement than can be explained by chance (Armstrong
et al. 1992). However for a validity study, data sensitivity and specificity are usually a
more useful summary than kappa. The calculation of kappa from the data in Table 12.1
is illustrated below. If the four cell counts are labelled clockwise from top left as n_{00},
n_{01}, n_{11}, and n_{10}, the row totals $n_{0.}$ and $n_{1.}$, and the column totals $n_{.0}$ and $n_{.1}$, then

$$\hat{\kappa} = \frac{2(n_{00}n_{11} - n_{01}n_{10})}{n_0 n_{.1} + n_1 n_{.0}} = \frac{2(40 \times 30 - 20 \times 10)}{60 \times 50 + 40 \times 50} = 0.4.$$

For categorical variables of more than two levels, many different sorts of misclassification can occur, which can be specified in a matrix of misclassification probabilities that
take the same form as Table 12.1, but with more than two columns and rows. An example
is shown in Table 12.2 in which the only misclassification is from the 'very near' to
'quite near' group. The example will be referred to later. Similar tables of agreement can
be assembled from reliability studies, but column percentages can no longer be
described as misclassification probabilities, because column classification is not by true
level. Summaries (such as a κ-statistic) are possible, but often are more complex when
there are more than two levels, because some types of disagreement are usually more
important than others. For example, misclassification into adjacent categories is usually
less important than other misclassification. This can be reflected in summaries if
different degrees of misclassification are weighted.

Table 12.2 Describing misclassification of a polytomous exposure variable

		According to true variable		
		Very near n (%)	Quite near n (%)	Far n (%)
According to	Very near	80 (80)	0 (0)	0 (0)
misclassified	Quite near	20 (20)	100 (100)	0 (0)
variable	Far	0 (0)	0 (0)	200(100)
	Total	100	100	200

Numerical variables

The important aspect of the distribution of random errors (classical or Berkson) in numerical variables are their standard deviation (σ_E) or variance (σ_E^2). This can be estimated directly from a validity study as the sample standard deviation of the observed values of *X–T*. However other summaries are used often, sometimes because they are more easily obtained, and sometimes because they are more convenient in deducing consequences of error or correcting epidemiological results for error. Classical error is generally described by its coefficient of reliability, which can be defined as the correlation of independent repeated measurements of exposure (ρ_{XX}), such as might be estimated from a reliability study. In theory (in large samples) this may be shown as being equal to the square of the coefficient of validity, which is the correlation between the true and approximate measurements (ρ_{XT}), such as might be estimated from a validity study. The coefficient of reliability is also theoretically equal to several expressions involving standard deviation of errors (σ_E), true exposures (σ_T), and observed approximate exposures (σ_X^2) as follows:

$$\rho_{XX} = \rho_{XT}^2 = \sigma_T^2/\sigma_X^2 = (\sigma_X^2 - \sigma_E^2)/\sigma_X^2 = \sigma_T^2/(\sigma_T^2 + \sigma_E^2)$$
$$= 1/(1 + \sigma_E^2/\sigma_T^2) = 1/[1 + (\sigma_E/\sigma_T)^2].$$

These values are only theoretically equal (i.e. in large samples, when the classical error model is correct). When they are estimated from validity or reliability data exact values will differ. Choice of which summaries to use is discussed further in the following, after discussion of which are important in describing consequences of error.

12.3 The consequences of measurement error in exposure

This section begins with and focuses mainly on the effects of non-differential error or misclassification in the exposure of interest, first on effect measures followed by the results of significance tests. A brief discussion on effects of errors on confounder control and the investigation of interaction as well as on effects of non-differential errors concludes this section.

12.3.1   Consequences of error in the exposure of interest for effect measures

In general, random measurement error or misclassification leads to bias in effect measures (RRs, regression coefficients, differences in means). This bias is usually downwards (towards the null) but there are important exceptions. The extent of bias can be estimated with information on magnitude of measurement error and exposure variability (or prevalence).

Exposure measured on a dichotomous scale

Non-differential error always biases the effect measure towards the null value (there is a technical but unrealistic exception when the sum of sensitivity and specificity of exposure classification is less than 1, implying measurement that tends to reverse exposed and unexposed categories!)

Example: A study of lung cancer in relation to proximity of residence to a coke oven classifies subjects (cases and populations) by distance of residence from the oven at the time of follow-up: NEAR = <4 km from oven; FAR = 4–10 km. The incidence rate is compared in the two groups. Here there is misclassification due to migration—not all persons living NEAR the oven at time of follow-up will have lived there at the etiologically relevant time. Thus if the true RR for subjects living in these areas throughout their lives were 1.5, the observed RR would tend to be less.

The extent of bias is dependent on and can be calculated from the sensitivity and specificity of the classification and the proportion of truly exposed in the non-diseased. This calculation may be by first principles, calculating number of cases and non-cases expected to move between cells of a two-by-two table, or by a formula:

$$OR_{Obs} = [p_D \times (1 - p_N)]/[p_N \times (1 - p_D)],$$

where

$$p_D = \text{sensitivity} \times P_D + (1 - \text{specificity}) \times (1 - P_D),$$
$$p_N = \text{sensitivity} \times P_N + (1 - \text{specificity}) \times (1 - P_N)$$

and 'P' and 'p' are the true and observed proportion exposed, respectively, 'D' indicates diseased, and 'N' indicates non-diseased.

Suppose misclassification (migration) in the foregoing example was such that 10 per cent of the NEAR group was in fact FAR at the time of relevant exposure, and vice-versa (i.e. sensitivity = specificity = 0.9), and that 50 per cent of the population overall lived in the NEAR area. The observed RR would then be 1.38.

Further examples are given in Table 12.3. Notice that where exposure is less common than not (<50%) poor specificity biases the odds ratio much more than poor sensitivity.

There is also an approximate formula using the κ-statistic for agreement between two independent classifications with the same instrument (see section 'Analysing validity and reliability studies') to link the observed naïve and the true odds ratio (Armstrong 1992, p. 109):

$$OR_{Obs} \approx (OR_T - 1) \times \kappa + 1.$$

Table 12.3 The effect of non-differential misclassification on RRs in two groups

Exposure sensitivity	Exposure specificity	Proportion of exposed in the population	Observed RR
1.00	1.00	Any	2.00
0.90	0.90	0.01	1.08
0.90	0.90	0.50	1.72
0.90	0.99	0.01	1.47
0.90	0.99	0.50	1.82
0.99	0.90	0.01	1.09
0.99	0.90	0.50	1.89
0.99	0.99	0.01	1.50
0.99	0.99	0.50	1.97

Table 12.4 The effect of non-differential misclassification on RRs in three exposure groups—example

	RR		
	Very near	Quite near	Far
True	2.0	1.3	1.0
Misclassified	2.0	1.42	1.0

For example, if a repeat classification gave $\kappa := 0.7$, and $OR_T = 1.5$, then

$$OR_{Obs} \approx (1.5 - 1) \times 0.7 + 1 = 1.35.$$

Exposure measured on a polytomous scale

Non-differential error biases downwards estimates of trend across ordered groups, but comparisons between specific categories can be biased in either direction.

Example: Assume that in the foregoing example the NEAR group was split into two: VERY NEAR, and QUITE NEAR, with true RRs, relative to FAR, of 2.0 and 1.3. If there is 20 per cent migration from VERY NEAR to QUITE NEAR, but not otherwise (as in Table 12.2), observed risks for VERY NEAR group relative to the FAR group is unchanged on average, but that for the QUITE NEAR group is increased by contamination by the VERY NEAR migrants. The specific value of the misclassified RR was calculated assuming that the NEAR group was divided into two equal-sized groups (25% of total population each), so the misclassified RR is a weighted mean of 1.3 and 2, with weights $w_1 = 25$ and $w_2 = 0.2 \times 25 = 5$ (the migrants from VERY NEAR). Thus RR = $\{1.3 \times 25 + 2 \times 5\}/\{25 + 5\}) = 1.42$. The RR is increased by misclassification (Table 12.4).

Exposure measured on a numerical scale

Classical errors bias regression coefficients (RRs per unit exposure) towards zero. The association is described as attenuated. In fact, for linear regression the bias factor is equal to the coefficient of reliability (ρ_{XX}); with the observed regression coefficient. Thus if

$$Y = \alpha_T + \beta_T.T;$$

then

$$Y = \alpha_{Obs} + \beta_{Obs}.X \quad \text{with } \beta_{Obs} = \rho_{XX} \times \beta_T.$$

The parameter β_{Obs} is sometimes called the 'naïve' regression coefficient.

Lead-IQ example—design 1: Suppose that a regression of IQ on true lifetime average blood lead has a regression with coefficient -2 (IQ reduces by 2 points per $\mu g \, dl^{-1}$ blood lead). With classical measurement error with coefficient of reliability 0.5, this would be attenuated, on average, to $0.5 \times -2 = -1$.

From the alternative expressions for the coefficient of reliability ($\rho_{XX} = 1/[1 + (\sigma_E/\sigma_T)^2]$), bias in β depends on the average magnitude of measurement error relative to the average magnitude of the true exposure (σ_E/σ_X). This implies that measurement error will have lesser effects if the true exposures are more spread out (σ_X is greater). Table 12.5 gives attenuation bias as the function of the ratio of the standard deviation of errors to that of true exposures (σ_E/σ_X). This is quite reassuring—error has to be relatively big to give serious bias.

For logistic and log-linear (Poisson) regression coefficients the same qualitative result is true, and the quantitative one approximately so, with the approximation being good except for large error and large RRs. For logistic and log-linear regression RR is linked to the regression coefficient by the formula $RR = \exp(\beta)$, thus

$$RR_{Obs} = (RR_T)^{\rho_{xx}}.$$

If, in the children exposed to blood lead, investigators were to use as an outcome a child having IQ below 80, and if the RR (odds ratio) increment per 10 $\mu g \, dl^{-1}$ true blood lead (from logistic regression) was 1.5, then the observed RR is given by:

$$RR_{Obs} = 1.5^{0.5} = 1.22.$$

Table 12.5　The attenuation bias due to exposure measurement error in linear regression

Error σ_E/σ_X	0.0	0.1	0.2	0.3	0.4	0.5	0.75	1.0	1.5	2.0
Attenuation*	1.0	0.99	0.96	0.92	0.86	0.80	0.64	0.50	0.31	0.20

*Attenuation is the factor by which the naïve regression slope will underestimate the true slope.

Berkson errors, however, lead to no bias in linear regression coefficients, and little or no bias in logistic or log-linear regression coefficients. The distinction between classical and Berkson error is thus important.

Lead-IQ example—design 2: In this grouped design the error is of Berksonian, so there is no bias in the regression coefficient. However, precision would be lost (width of confidence interval would be wider), and power would not be as great as without measurement error, or as in the biased Design 1.

12.3.2 Consequences for significance tests and power

All types of non-differential random measurement error or misclassification reduce study power—the chance that a study will find a statistically significant association if one is truly present. This is true for Berkson as well as classical error, and for misclassification. The extent of power loss can be quantified if magnitude of measurement error and exposure variability (or for a dichotomous measure prevalence) are known.

Example: A cohort study is designed to have 80 per cent power to detect a RR of 2.0 between truly exposed and truly unexposed persons (80% of similar-sized studies would find the association), by inclusion of sufficient subjects (equal numbers exposed and unexposed) to expect 20 cases in each group under the null hypothesis (Breslow and Day 1987). If approximate measurements were used, the power would be less. If the measure of exposure has sensitivity = specificity = 0.9 and 10 per cent of the population are exposed, then a true RR of 2.0 would be attenuated, on average, to 1.48. Power to detect this reduced RR is only 30 per cent (Breslow and Day 1987). To restore 80 per cent power would require a study about four time bigger.

For numerical exposure variables (and approximately for dichotomous exposures if coded as 0 and 1) power loss is based on the result that the effective loss in sample size is equal to the coefficient of reliability of the measure (Lagakos 1988).

Example: A study with exposure measured with a coefficient of reliability 0.5 will have similar power to one with accurate exposure assessment and half the number of subjects.

Despite the bias and power loss, the *p*-values obtained by using the usual methods on data, subject to random error or misclassification, are valid. Spurious 'significant' results (where there is in fact no association) are no more likely with than without measurement error.

Example: A study finds an association between dust and loss of lung function, with $p = 0.02$, but dust measurements were known to be subject to error. Provided the error is non-differential, the low *p*-value cannot be attributed to the measurement error.

12.3.3 Confounders

Errors in confounders

The general rule is that errors in confounders compromise our ability to control for their effect, leaving 'residual' confounding. The effect measure adjusted using the approximate confounder will on average lie between the crude, unadjusted effect measure and the effect measure adjusted using the true (unknown) confounder. The validity of significance tests on the effect of exposure is compromised.

Example: A study of the relationship of lung cancer to air pollution adjusts for smoking using a crude estimate of pack-years for each subject. Any confounding of the RR for lung cancer vs. air pollution will be only partially controlled. For example, if crude $RR_{(crude)} = 1.50$ (95% CI 1.20–1.88; $p < 0.001$), and $RR_{(adjusted\ for\ true\ pack-years)} = 1.04$ (95% CI 0.86–1.24; $p = 0.67$), then the partially adjusted $RR_{(adjusted\ for\ approximate\ pack-years)}$ will in general lie between 1.50 and 1.04 and the partially adjusted p-value will lie between 0.001 and 0.67.

The degree of residual confounding depends on the coefficient of reliability of the measure of the confounder. A coefficient of reliability of 0.5 will imply that about half the confounding present will be controlled, in the sense that the observed log(RR) (more generally the regression coefficient) will on average lie about halfway between the crude unadjusted log(RR) and the fully adjusted log(RR).

Continuing the same example, if the coefficient of reliability of measured pack-years is 0.5, then $\log(RR_{(adjusted\ for\ approximate\ pack-years)})$ will lie about halfway between $\log(RR_{(crude)})$ and $\log(RR_{(adjusted\ for\ true\ pack-years)})$, which gives $RR_{(adjusted\ for\ approximate\ pack-years)} = 1.25$ (95% CI 1.03–1.52; $p = 0.03$).

There are a few exceptions. Entirely systematic error (everyone under-reporting their smoking by 20%) will not usually compromise control of confounding. In special situations (when the effects of the confounder and the exposure of interest are strictly additive) Berkson error (e.g. use of group mean rather than individual pack-years of smoking) also leaves no residual confounding. Most importantly, if the variable suspected of confounding is in fact not associated with the exposure of interest (smoking is not associated with air pollution) then there is no confounding or residual confounding, however strongly the variable is associated with the outcome (however bad the smoking data, the observed association of lung cancer with air pollution is not biased).

Correlation between errors in measuring confounders with errors in measuring the exposure of interest or with exposure itself further complicates the situation, although the same broad conclusion—that error compromises control of confounding—remains.

Presence of confounders measured without error

Having to control for confounders, whether measured with error or not, somewhat increases the effect of error in the variable of interest on the RR of interest. The formulae for the simple situation without confounders can be extended to cover this situation by replacing each of the coefficients with their value conditional on the presence of the confounder (Armstrong 1989, p. 1179; Carrol 2000, p. 538). For example, the reliability coefficient of an exposure measure conditional on age is the partial correlation between independent repeat measures after control for age, which is typically lower.

12.3.4 Effect modifiers

An effect modifier is a variable that modifies the effect of the exposure of interest (e.g. identifying subgroups vulnerable or resistant to the exposure). In statistical terms, this is described as an interaction between the effect modifier and the exposure.

Error in the effect modifiers

Error in measuring effect modifiers tends to diminish effect modification. Vulnerable subgroups are thus harder to identify.

Lead-IQ example. Suppose diet modified the effect of lead on IQ, children with vitamin-deficient diets have a regression slope of -3 and others a slope of -1. If diet is measured with error (misclassified), the apparent modification will tend to be less, for example, the slope in vitamin-deficient children might be -2.5 and that in others -1.5.

Error in the exposure of interest

Even if the putative effect-modifier is measured without error, error in the variable of interest can distort effect modification, and even create spurious modification. This may happen because the magnitude of error, and hence bias, depends on the putative modifier. Even if this is not the case, the variation of exposure may depend on the putative modifier, in which case the bias due to measurement error will again depend on the putative modifier.

Lead-IQ example. Suppose now that interest is in modification of the effect of lead on IQ by sex, which is measured without error, but lead is again measured with (classical) error. Suppose also that although the average error was the same for boys and girls, boys had more varied lead exposures than girls (σ_T is higher in boys than in girls). In this case, if the true regression slope of IQ on lead is -2 for both boys and girls, the estimated slope will tend to be more attenuated for girls (say to -0.5) than for boys (say to -1.5). (For girls the standard deviation σ_T is lower, and hence the attenuation bias σ_E^2/σ_T^2 is greater.) Thus sex appears to modify the effect of lead on IQ, but does not in fact do so.

12.3.5 Differential error

Differential error can cause bias in the effect measure either upwards or downwards, depending on whether adverse outcomes are associated with over or underestimation of exposure. Significance tests are not valid in the presence of differential error. For dichotomous exposure, the bias can be quantified if the sensitivity and specificity of the approximate classification are known.

Example: The association of exposure to VDU use with spontaneous abortion is investigated by means of a case–control study in which women are interviewed after a live birth or abortion, and asked about the number of hours per week that they spent using a VDU. The RR of spontaneous abortion in women using VDUs for 15 or more hours per week was 1.20 (95% CI 1.06–1.34). Due to media attention to the hypothesized association, women who had experienced spontaneous abortions may have been more likely to recall their VDU use fully. In this case, some or all of the excess of VDU users in the cases relative to the controls would be spurious, so that the true RR would be less than 1.20, possibly 1.00.

12.3.6 Correcting for measurement error

If there is information on the magnitude and type of error it is possible (but not always easy!) to allow for it in estimating the effect measure, at least for reasonably simple forms of measurement error. Sometimes, it is sufficient to invert the formulae for deriving the effects of measurement error, for example

$$\beta_T = \beta_{Obs}/\rho_{XX}, \quad RR_T = (RR_{Obs})^{(1/\rho_{XX})}.$$

In the Lead-IQ study, if investigators had observed a regression coefficient (β_{Obs}) of -1, and known that the coefficient of reliability of measurement (ρ_{XX}) was 0.5, then they could estimate

$$\beta_T = -1/0.5 = -2.$$

Similarly, if investigators observed an increment in RR of low IQ per 10 $\mu g dl^{-1}$ observed blood lead: $RR_{Obs} = 1.22$, then approximately

$$RR_T = 1.22^{(1/0.5)} = 1.5.$$

Corrections will not in general affect the *p*-value of a test of the null hypothesis of no association, nor will the power of the test be improved. Confidence intervals will however normally get wider.

In the lead-IQ study mentioned earlier, suppose the regression coefficient of -1 had a 95 per cent CI $(-1.8, -0.2)$, with $p = 0.01$. Assuming coefficient of reliability 0.5, the corrected coefficient is -2, the 95% CI $(-3.6, -0.4)$, and $p = 0.01$, as before. If there was uncertainty in the coefficient of reliability, then the a more sophisticated approach that reflected this would give a wider confidence interval, but its lower limit would remain below zero, consistent with the *p*-value, for which a correction is not required.

Other methods are available that refine and generalize this approach. The aim of these more sophisticated methods is usually to use other sorts of information on measurement error, more precisely to eradicate bias, or to reflect in the estimate and confidence intervals uncertainty as to the magnitude of the error. A review is given by Carrol (2000).

   Probably the most popular group of methods is called regression calibration. In general, these seek to correct an observed effect measure by applying to it a calibration factor, typically obtained from a validity or reliability study. For example, from validity study data one can estimate the calibration factor λ as the regression coefficient of true accurate exposure (*Y* variable) on approximate exposure (*X* variable)—this estimates the average change in the accurate exposure corresponding to unit change in the approximate variable. Observed regression coefficients from the main study are divided by λ to obtain an unbiased estimate of the true coefficient: $\beta_T = \beta_{Obs}/\lambda$. Using the formulae given earlier with ρ_{XX} or ρ_{XY} estimated from reliability of validity studies are also examples of regression calibration.

Example: Zeger *et al.* (2000) applied the regression calibration method when correcting estimates of increased mortality per $\mu g m^{-3}$ PM_{10} from a time-series mortality study in Riverside, California, which used a central site monitor to estimate exposure. The study found mortality to increase by 0.84 per cent per 10 $\mu g m^{-3}$ PM_{10} (95% CI -0.06, 1.76). A validity study had been carried out in which 49 people from Riverside had worn personal monitors for a total of 178 sampling days. Regressing personal measure (*Y* variable) on ambient exposure (*X* variable) gave a regression calibration slope of 0.60 (SE 0.08). (Thus each 1 $\mu g m^{-3}$ change in PM_{10} in ambient exposures was on average reflected in a 0.6 $\mu g m^{-3}$ change in personal levels.) This allowed the observed regression slope of 0.84 to be corrected by dividing by 0.60: true regression slope $= 0.84/0.60 = 1.40$. Confidence limits were be obtained by applying the same correction to the naïve limits, thus $(-0.11, 2.95)$. These confidence limits are slightly too narrow, because they do not reflect uncertainty in the calibration factor. As Zeger discusses, the measurement error in this situation is a mixture of the Berkson and classical types. Regression calibration making direct use of the calibration slope provided a way of correcting for bias without having to assume either all-Berkson or all-classical error.

The 'method of moments' estimator is an alternative correction procedure. For this, one estimates just the variance of the error distribution—(σ_E^2) from a reliability study (half the variance of differences in measurements) or validity study. This estimate can be transported to the main study with fewer assumptions than needed for λ, ρ_{XX}, or ρ_{XY} (see below). The variance of observed exposures (σ_X^2) is then estimated from the main study and the naïve regression slope is corrected using the expression $\rho_{XX} = (\sigma_X^2 - \sigma_E^2)/\sigma_X^2$.

For an example showing two methods of correction for measurement error applied to occupational epidemiology, see Spiegelmann and Valanis (1998).

Limitations of corrections for measurement error

Information on the magnitude of measurement error is needed. This requires reliability studies (a sample of repeated independent measurements) or validity studies (a sample of gold standard measurements in parallel with the approximate measurements). These are not often available, and even if they are, much uncertainty remains unless they are large. If corrections are carried out on the basis of incorrect information on error magnitude, bias may be increased, rather than decreased. 'Corrections' for attenuation can also magnify confounding or other information bias, rather than a true association. Researchers should give the 'naïve' effect measure (using the approximate exposure in a regular analysis), even if including effect measures corrected for measurement error. Also worth considering is the calculation of corrections under a variety of assumptions, in the spirit of a sensitivity analysis.

12.4   Design issues

12.4.1   What resources should be utilized for estimating exposure?

Random exposure measurement error reduces the power of a study and (except Berkson error) biases effect measures. To avoid these problems it is desirable to design studies with minimum measurement error. However, making exposure measurement more accurate may be costly and must be considered against alternative uses for the resources. Thus the practical question is usually 'What proportion of resources should be put into exposure measurement in order to improve accuracy?'.

Where a study aims to add to evidence as to whether an exposure causes an outcome, study power is the main consideration. For these studies, Lagakos's result cited previously can be used to address this question, by justifying the principle:

To maximize study power, resources should be spent on improving accuracy until the proportional increase in the square of the validity coefficient (ρ_{XT}^2) is less than the proportional increase in total study costs per subject that is required to achieve it.

For example, if it is possible to increase ρ_{XT}^2 from 0.6 to 0.9 (i.e. by a factor of 1.5) by spending 30 per cent more per subject, it is worth it. If it costs 100 per cent more, it is not—the money would be better spent recruiting more subjects. As usual in such design decisions, input information (ρ_{XT}^2 or equivalent) may have to be obtained from pilot studies if it is not available. More details and examples are given by Armstrong (1996).

Deciding on the number of repeat exposure measurements

A special case in this problem occurs where increase in precision is possible by making independent repeat measurements of exposure for each study subject, and the question is 'How many replicates?' With costs of each exposure measurement C_Z, other marginal study costs per subject (e.g. outcome measurement) C_I, and the reliability of the measurement ρ_{XX}, the forementioned principle yields the optimal number n of replicates:

$$n = \frac{C_I(1 - \rho_{XX})}{C_Z \rho_{XX}}.$$

For example, if ρ_{XX} is 0.6, C_Z is \$20, and C_I is \$100, then $n = 100(1 - 0.6)/(20 \times 0.6) = 40/12 = 3.3$; that is, about three repeat exposure measurements per subject. The square of the validity coefficient, or another of the equivalent expressions can be substituted for reliability coefficient in this expression.

Limitations to designing for maximum power

Where a study aims not only to add evidence to whether an exposure causes an outcome, but also to quantify how much risk is consequent to a measured level of exposure (the absolute dose–response relationship), then the bias in effect measure assumes an added importance, and power is an inadequate criterion for choice of resources to go into exposure measurement. Increasing the sample size does not reduce measurement error bias—although it does increase power. Formal approaches to this problem require more assumptions. Less formal trade-offs between bias and power, perhaps informed by the power criterion, are likely to be necessary. The sections that follow address this situation.

12.4.2   Designing for Berkson rather than classical error

If bias in effect measure is the major consideration (rather than study power), there is sometimes scope to design exposure measurement to utilize the fact that Berkson error causes little bias. This can be achieved through two ways:

(1) By using mean exposure over groups of subjects. The lead-IQ study can provide an example. Using each child's blood lead measurement gave rise to classical error, biasing the regression coefficient, but if investigators group children according to proximity to smelter, this error was changed to mainly Berkson type, not biasing the coefficient. (Mainly rather than entirely Berkson, because any error in the mean as an estimate of true group mean remains classical, but this will be small unless the number of measurements per group is small.) Using the group mean thus eliminates or greatly reduces bias. Remaining bias can be reduced by making groups larger. However, this procedure does not improve power. In fact, using group means in this way usually reduces power. Thus, there is a choice between retaining power and reducing bias.

(2) By using a prediction model. This is a generalization of the grouping method. Individual measures are used to estimate coefficients of a model for predicting exposure given some easily measured predictor variables. Then, predicted values from the

prediction model are used in place of the individual measures when investigating the association of exposure with outcome. The resulting error is again mainly Berksonian. Some classical error will remain if the sample in the prediction model is small, as when using group means, and also if the predictor variables are measured with error. Again, bias will be reduced, but usually at the cost of power.

In fact, both grouping and prediction models are usually used when not all subjects in the study have individual exposure measures, so their use is forced and there is no choice. Nevertheless it may be useful when deciding between strategies to be aware that the resulting primarily Berkson-type error will bias effect measures little if at all, but will reduce power. The use of grouping and of prediction models is discussed further in Chapter 6.

12.4.3 Validity, reliability, and two-stage studies

As an alternative to or in addition to improving exposure assessment for every study subject investigators can use a cheap approximate method for the main study and supplement this by a smaller validity study (a sample of gold standard measurements in parallel with the approximate measurements) or reliability substudy (a sample of repeated independent approximate measurements). In this section we discuss analysis of such substudies, and how parameters estimated from the substudy can be used to inform interpretation of the main study and sometimes to correct the effect measure in the main study for measurement error. It is usually best if the validity or reliability study samples can be drawn from among the main study subjects. This is partly to improve portability of error parameters (see section 'Portability'), and partly so that the additional information on exposure in the subsample can be used to improve the power of the main study (see section 'Two-stage studies').

Analysis of validity and reliability studies

Data from a validity or reliability substudy should be analysed first to describe agreement, rather than immediately focussing on estimation of parameters required for correction of attenuation of exposure–response relationships under specific assumptions. A few key features of standard analysis of agreement between two numerical measurements are given here. Fuller treatment is available in Shoukri (2000) and in Bland and Altman (1986).

(1) The mean (and CI) of differences between numerical measurements displays the extent to which one instrument measures consistently higher than another.

(2) The standard deviation of the differences in measurements displays the extent of variation in agreement (random error). The mean and standard deviation can be brought together to define 'limits to agreement', for example, mean ± 1.96SD estimates the limits within which the difference will lie 95 per cent of the time. In a validity study, the standard deviation of differences estimates the standard deviation of measurement error σ_E. In an intra-method reliability study, the standard deviation estimates $(\sqrt{2})\sigma_E$. (The variance of differences estimates twice the variance of errors.)

(3) Various plots can be used to explore whether agreement depends on other factors. For example, plotting differences against the mean or sum of the two measurements identifies whether agreement varies according to the magnitude of exposure, and will suggest departure from additivity if present.

(4) With data from a validity study, classical and Berkson error can be distinguished by examining whether differences are correlated with true or approximate measurements, for example, by plotting.

These analyses allow evaluation of some assumptions of measurement error models and correction techniques (additivity, Berkson/classical distinction). Also, most investigators will wish to be aware of features of error, for example, additive bias, even if it does not affect study power or bias effect measures. Once a general description of agreement is obtained, it is reasonable to focus on the parameters that determine the extent of attenuation due to measurement error, and hence are needed to correct it. The standard deviation (σ_E) or variance of errors (σ_E^2) may be the most useful parameter for this purpose (see discussion in the section 'Portability'). However, the parameters most directly related to attenuation are the validity and reliability coefficients.

If there are two repeats of each measurement the validity or reliability coefficient can be estimated directly as the Pearson correlation coefficient from the paired measurements. However, it is more efficient to estimate them as 'intra-class' correlation coefficients (ICC) or equivalently from variance components. When there are several repeat measurements, the ICC/variance component method is the only one.

The ICC can be expressed as a function of the ratio of variances within (σ_W^2) to between (σ_B^2) pairs (or triplets, etc.): ICC $= 1/[1 + (\sigma_W^2/\sigma_B^2)]$ (Armstrong *et al.* 1992; Shoukri 2000), if these variances are estimated from the measurements in the substudy as 'variance components'. Variance components and ICC are obtainable from most statistical software. Interpretation of the ICC will depend on context. With data from a reliability study, the ICC estimates the reliability coefficient ρ_{XX}, which in simple models is the attenuation factor and loss in effective sample size and hence power (see Section 12.3). With data from a validity study, the ICC estimates the validity coefficient, which estimates the square root of the reliability coefficient. If the mean for a subject is the true exposure, and repeated measurements are taken on a sample of subjects, the variance components become those between- and within-subjects. If the main study relating exposure to outcome uses just one exposure measure per subject, the formula for ICC again estimates reliability coefficient and attenuation. If means of exposures from m repeats are used in the main study, the attenuation reduces to $1/[1 + (\sigma_W^2/\sigma_B^2)/m]$ (Liu *et al.* 1978). Variance components are discussed further in Chapter 6.

In general, it is not possible to use measures of agreement from inter-method reliability studies to estimate the bias that use of either method might produce in an epidemiological study. The problem is in apportioning the lack of agreement between the two methods. However, the regression calibration method can be used if the errors of the two measures are independent (Wacholder and Armstrong 1993).

Portability of coefficients from substudies to main studies

Using results from a validity or reliability substudy to inform a main study requires 'transporting' estimates of agreement, for example, a validity coefficient from one to the other. This should be done cautiously, with a view to possible factors that might make the underlying values of the coefficients different in the two contexts. For example, a reliability coefficient depends not only on the variance of the error distribution, but also on the variance of true exposures. Thus even if the measurement instrument used in the main and reliability studies are identical, if the distribution of true exposures differ the reliability coefficient is not portable. The same applies to calibration regression coefficients and to κ-statistics.

This problem can be minimized by randomly choosing the reliability or validity sample from the main study subjects. Alternatively, more portable coefficients can be used. For example, the method of moments correction requires only the variance of the error from a validity or reliability study, which is usually more portable than the reliability coefficient.

Sample size of validity and reliability studies

Given that the motivation for conducting validity and reliability studies usually goes beyond their use for correcting exposure–response relationships, it is useful to consider simple general-purpose aids to decide their sample size. Perhaps most important is the following frequently misunderstood point:

Sample size determinations for identifying the presence of an association (e.g. by a χ^2-test, or test of a correlation being zero) are of no interest when determining sizes of validity or reliability studies.

Such tests merely assess evidence for the two measurements being associated. This would not advance us much—even very poor measurements are associated somewhat with the true exposure. The requirement is to quantify the strength and features of the association. Depending on the context, the parameter or parameters of interest may be any of many, for example, sensitivity and specificity (proportions), validity of reliability coefficients (correlation coefficients), a regression coefficient, a mean difference, or a κ coefficient. Usually, the most straightforward and adequate approach is to show how the precision of an estimate to be made from the proposed study depends on the sample size, choosing a sample size reflects the trade-of between the advantages of a precise estimate and the cost of obtaining it.

For example, a validity coefficient of 0.5 estimated from a validity study would have confidence intervals depending on sample size as displayed in Table 12.6. The method of estimating confidence intervals is given in most intermediate-level statistical methods textbooks, and they may be obtained from many statistical software (e.g. stata's. 'ci2' command). The results are quite sobering, suggesting that with less than say 100 pairs of measurements the validity coefficient would be rather imprecisely estimated. Of course,

Table 12.6 Effect of reliability study sample size on estimate of reliability coefficient

Sample size (pairs)	10	25	50	100	250	500
Confidence interval	−0.19, 0.86	0.13, 0.75	0.26, 0.69	0.34, 0.63	0.40, 0.59	0.43, 0.56

investigators do not know that the correlation coefficient will be 0.5, but the pattern of widths of confidence intervals does not usually depend very strongly on such guessed values. To check, the calculations can always be repeated using a range of values.

Two-stage studies

Epidemiological studies with more accurate exposure assessment on a subsample are sometimes called 'two-stage' studies. Careful choice of which subjects to include in the subsample can improve precision and power, although analysis to achieve this becomes more complicated (Zhao and Lipsitz 1992). The optimal design of two-stage and other studies with validation substudies has been discussed by Greenland (1988), who concludes that unless the cost of the better measurement is many times that of the approximate one, a 'fully validated' study (using the better measure or replicate measures on all subjects) is frequently the optimal one. Where differential error is a concern, validation studies must be particularly large.

12.5   Issues not covered in this chapter

For simplicity of presentation some assumptions and points of interpretation have been passed over. The most important of these are described here.

Outcomes. This chapter has not dealt with errors in measuring outcomes. Where outcomes are numerical (e.g. lung function) these do not cause bias in effect measures, but do cause loss of power and precision. Where outcomes are categorical, misclassifying them non-differentially (with respect to exposure) biases effect measures towards the null. All our results have assumed that errors in measuring exposure are unrelated to errors in measuring outcome. Such associations can cause bias in any direction.

Bias. Many of the results concern bias in an effect estimate. Bias is an average effect if the study were to be repeated many times. In a large study the effect of measurement error will be close to this average 'bias'. However, in a single small sample, the effect may differ appreciably from this average (Sorahan and Gilthorpe 1994). In these cases random error can sometimes even lead to an effect measure estimated from approximate exposures that is more extreme than that with the true exposure. It remains more likely, however, that if true exposure has an effect it is stronger than the estimate using the approximate measurement (Wacholder *et al.* 1995).

Prediction. It has been assumed in this chapter that it is the relationship between the true exposure and health outcome that is of interest. Sometimes this is not the case. If you wish to use the study to predict risks in subjects using the same approximate measure of exposure and drawn from the same population, then the naïve effect estimate (e.g. β_{Obs}) is appropriate.

Multiplicative error (proportional to the true exposure), with lognormal distribution of true exposures, is common in environmental and occupational epidemiology. Here measurement error changes the shape of the regression, for example, from a quadratic curve to a straight line (Doll and Peto 1978; Pierce *et al.* 1991).

Ecologic studies, which have groups as the unit of analysis, have some unexpected error effects. The exposure is proportion of individuals in the area with an attribute (e.g. proportion of smokers) and the individual measure is subject to misclassification, then the slope of the regression of outcome against proportion with the attribute will be greater than the true individual effect of the attribute on the outcome, that is, bias is away from the null (Greenland 1992). Where the group exposure measure is a good approximation to the mean true exposure across individuals in the group, then error is Berksonian, as discussed earlier, and little or no bias results.

Causality. The impact of random non-differential exposure measurement error on inference about the size of an effect is fairly clear once a causal relationship is assumed— the true effect of exposure is most likely to be greater than that estimated. The impact of measurement error on the evidence that such a study brings on whether a causal relationship exists is more problematic. The following points should be considered:

(1) One should usually be more cautious, if there is measurement error, in concluding from a 'negative' study that no causal association exists. The reduced power implies that it is more likely that a true underlying association has been missed.

(2) One should not use the (uncorrected) confidence interval for RR (or other measure of effect) to indicate the highest risk that is compatible with the data. For example, an uncorrected confidence interval for RR of (0.80, 1.25) suggests that relative risks in excess of 1.25 can be excluded. With exposure measurement error, however, the true uncertainty is greater, so that a higher RR is possible.

(3) Random non-differential measurement error should not lead us to discount an observed association of exposure with disease—observing a positive association is no more likely with measurement error. On the other hand, one cannot assume that a small non-significant or even significant estimated effect of exposure would be larger and more significant in the absence of exposure measurement error. Such small associations could be due to chance or to uncontrolled bias or confounding, in which case they would not be larger, on average, in the absence of measurement error.

Further reading

Most textbooks in epidemiology discuss the effect of misclassification of exposure on estimates of RR, and some give methods for calculating and correcting for bias due to measurement error. The book by Armstrong *et al.* (1992) (no relation!) on exposure measurement in epidemiology is the most accessible source for most of the results discussed in this chapter. There are several articles on this topic published recently in journals. A simple Medline search showed that articles published from 1981 to 2001 had the words 'measurement error' and 'epidemiology' in the title or abstract—most in the last 5 years. For statisticians, Carroll *et al.* (1995) is an excellent review monograph with a particular focus on logistic regression, and with most examples from epidemiology. Also, by Carrol (2000) is a briefer and updated review, somewhat more accessible to non-statisticians. Limited but more accessible reviews are given by Armstrong (1989) (especially useful for further discussion of and references on Berkson errors and errors in confounders), De Klerk *et al.* (1989) (especially useful for results on the impact of error on comparisons of risk in quantiles of the exposure distribution), and Armstrong (1996) (a precursor to this chapter!).

References

Armstrong, B. (1996). Optimizing power in allocating resources to exposure assessment in an epidemiologic study. *American Journal of Epidemiology*, **144**, 192–7.

Armstrong, B. G. (1989). The effects of measurement errors on relative risk regressions. *American Journal of Epidemiology*, **132**, 1176–84.

Armstrong, B. K., White, E., and Saracci, R. (1992). *Principles of exposure measurement in epidemiology*. Oxford University Press, Oxford.

Bland, J. M. and Altman, D. G. (1986). Statistical methods for assessing agreement between two methods of clinical measurement. *Lancet*, **I**, 307–10.

Breslow, N. E. and Day, N. E. (1987). *Statistical methods in cancer research. Vol. II. The design and analysis of cohort studies*. IARC Lyon.

Carroll, R. (2000). Measurement error in epidemiologic studies. In *Encyclopedia of epidemiologic method* (ed. M. H. Gail and J. Benichou), pp. 530–57. Wiley, New York.

Carroll, R. J., Ruppert, D., and Stefanski, L. A. (1995). *Measurement error in nonlinear models*. Chapman and Hall, New York.

De-Klerk, N. H., English, D. R., and Armstrong, B. K. (1989). A review of the effects of random measurement error on relative risk estimates in epidemiological studies. *International Journal of Epidemiology*, **18**, 705–12.

Doll, R. and Peto, R. (1978). Cigarette smoking and bronchial carcinoma: dose and time relationships among regular smokers and lifelong non-smokers. *Journal of Epidemiology and Community Health*, **32**, 303–13.

Greenland, S. (1988). Statistical uncertainty due to misclassification: implications for validation substudies. *Journal of Clinical Epidemiology*, **41**, 1167–74.

Greenland, S. (1992). Divergent biases in ecologic and individual-level studies. *Statistics in Medicine*, **11**, 1209–23.

Lagakos, S. W. (1988). Effects of mismodelling and mismeasuring explanatory variables on tests of their association with a response variable. *Statistics in Medicine*, **7**, 257–74.

Liu, K., Stamler, J., Dyer, A., *et al.* (1978). Statistical methods to assess and minimize the role of intra-individual variability in obscuring the relationship between dietary lipids and serum cholesterol. *Journal of Chronic Disease*, **31**, 399–418.

Pierce, D. A., Preston, D. L., *et al.* (1991). Allowing for dose-estimation errors for the A-bomb survivor data. *Journal of Radiation Research*, **32** (Suppl), 108–21.

Shoukri, M. M. (2000). Agreement, measurement of. *Encyclopedia of epidemiologic method* (ed. M. H. Gail and J. Benichou), pp. 35–48. Wiley, New York.

Sorahan, T. and Gilthorpe, M. S. (1994). Non-differential misclassification of exposure always leads to an underestimation of risk: an incorrect conclusion. *Occupational and Environmental Medicine*, **51**, 839–40.

Spiegelman, D. and Valanis, B. (1998). Correcting for bias in relative risk estimates due to exposure measurement error: a case study of occupational exposure to antineoplastics in pharmacists. *American Journal of Public Health*, **88**, 406–12.

Wacholder, S., Hartge, P., Lubin, J. H., and Dosemeci, M. (1995). Non-differential misclassification and bias towards the null: a clarification. *Occupational and Environmental Medicine*, **52**, 557–8.

Wacholder, S., Armstrong, B., *et al.* (1993). Validation studies using an alloyed gold standard. *American Journal of Epidemiology*, **137**, 1251–8.

Zeger, S. L., Thomas, D., *et al.* (2000). Exposure measurement error in time-series studies of air pollution: concepts and consequences. *Environmental Health Perspectives*, **108**, 419–26.

Zhao, L. P. and Lipsitz, S. (1992). Designs and analysis of two-stage studies. *Statistics in Medicine*, **11**, 769–82.

II Current topics

13. Allergen exposure and occupational respiratory allergy and asthma

Dick Heederik

13.1 Introduction

Occupational asthma is defined as a disease characterized by variable airway airflow limitation and/or airway hyper-responsiveness due to causes and conditions attributable to a particular environment and not to stimuli encountered outside the workplace (Bernstein *et al.* 1999). Usually, occupational asthma with and without a latency period is distinguished. Asthma with a latency period includes all forms of asthma for which an immunologic mechanism has been identified. In most cases an IgE mediated allergy is the underlying mechanism. Causes of immunologic asthma are low and high molecular weight (HMW) sensitisers of which more than 250 have been identified (Chan-Yeung and Malo 1994). Low molecular weight sensitizers are often chemicals such as iso-cyanates, acid anhydrides, metals and metal salts, and also plicatic acid from Western red cedar wood. Exposure to low molecular weight sensitizers occurs in a wide range of industries and especially the iso-cyanates are known as a major hazard in spray painters, foam rubber production workers, as well as in metal workers who make resin supported moulds. Many HMW sensitizers are naturally occurring water-soluble proteins in the 10–60 kDa molecular weight range that in a hydrophilic environment like the respiratory mucosa are released readily from, for example, skin scales, plant fibres, pollen grains, and other tissue matrices. Exposure has been associated with major outbreaks of Type I/IgE mediated allergies, like those described for occupational exposures in the detergent industry in the 1970s (Flindt 1996). The increased use of latex products, particularly in health care professions, has also resulted in an epidemic of latex associated respiratory and dermal allergies (Toraasen *et al.* 2000). These allergies are caused by proteins in the sap of the *Hevea brasiliensis* tree, which is used to produce latex.

Good quantitative epidemiological studies with state-of-the-art exposure assessment have been lacking for a long time for most allergens. An important explanation was the absence of methods to measure the exposure accurately, especially for HMW sensitizers. Exposure response studies for a number of these allergens have become available only recently. Exposure response modelling for sensitizing agents is also considered a complex issue. Asthma is a variable condition and when sensitized, an individual reacts to levels to which he or she did not react before becoming sensitized. This might complicate identification of levels that induced the condition. These issues are probably best illustrated by some quotes from a chapter on the epidemiology of occupational asthma by Becklake (1999):

...this level (provoking the onset of the condition) is likely to differ according to whether the mechanism triggering the hyper-responsiveness is allergic and IgE mediated, or irritative through stimulation of irritant receptors, or pharmacological as was originally postulated for conditions like byssinosis. Theoretically, therefore, the slope and intercept of the exposure–response relationship might differ between individuals in the same workplace, according to the mechanism of disease provocation (and therefore host factors). While it seems unlikely that exposure measurements including personal monitoring would ever be sufficiently detailed and accurate to permit between individual differences in exposure response relationships to be modelled or measured in epidemiological studies, they nevertheless need to borne in mind in any discussion of the distribution and determinants of asthma and asthma like conditions in workplaces.

Although very true, the issues mentioned do not necessarily make exposure response analyses impossible. In many other fields of (occupational) epidemiology differences between individuals in terms of the magnitude of the response (susceptibility) or the nature of the response (mechanism) play a role as well, and often cannot be measured and included in the study. In the field of allergy and asthma, one of the major effect modifiers, atopy, can actually be measured at the feno-typical level and taken care of in the analysis. Careful inclusion of these aspects in the design and especially the analysis of the data can lead to important and useful results. Temporal issues, such as a changed responsiveness after sensitization, can be taken into account in longitudinal designs. In addition, great progress has been made over the last decade with the development of more refined exposure assessment strategies that yield refined exposure estimates for use in epidemiological studies.

These issues, and several others, play a role in the evaluation of exposure to allergens and exposure response studies: instrumental issues, alternative exposure routes, and effective analysis of exposure response relationships, and all will be highlighted in this chapter.

13.2   Instrumental issues

13.2.1   Sampling

Low molecular weight sensitizers are usually gaseous or partially in gas and solid phase, and have to be measured using conventional equipment for gaseous or mixed phase (solid and gaseous) pollutants. Until recently, dust sampling has been the only tool for exposure assessment for HMW sensitizers. In the past, total dust levels have been measured as a crude surrogate of exposure, but because the definition of total dust is not similar in different areas of the world, leading to different results, the use of this approach has discontinued in the early 1990s. Nowadays, sampling equipment is based on particle size selective sampling using health-based definitions of particular size fractions such as respirable dust, thoracic dust, and inhalable dust (ISO 1992). Since sensitization and respiratory symptoms can occur along the upper and lower airways (rhinitis and asthma, respectively) inhalable dust, reflecting the dust particles that can penetrate the respiratory organ, is the dust fraction that is measured most commonly in modern epidemiological studies. A wide range of European personal samplers is available for this purpose, among which the British IOM sampler, the Dutch PAS6 sampler, the German GSP sampler, and extensive validation studies have been undertaken under varying conditions in wind tunnel and field experiments (Kenny *et al.* 1997). The development continues and has recently led to the development of personal samplers that measure size fractions. Most samplers can be used in combination with (immuno) chemical techniques to measure the allergen content of the dust. Information on up to date equipment can be found in occupational hygiene textbooks (Perkins 1997, 2003).

Recently, a nasal sampler has been developed and used for measurement of allergens in the air (O'Meara *et al.* 1998). This miniature slit sampler captures particulates by impaction on tape inside the sampler and is promoted as an alternative to conventional active air sampling that makes use of sampling heads and filtering techniques. The nasal sampler found some wider application for measurement of several domestic allergens and rat and latex allergen particulates in the work environment (O'Meara *et al.* 1998; Graham *et al.* 2000; Poulos *et al.* 2002; Renström *et al.* 2002). This sampler has been used in combination with immuno-staining techniques by which the allergen containing particles were identified and could be counted (see Section 13.2.2), in addition to conventional extraction and immuno-chemical analysis of the allergen content. Sampling times are usually short between 10–60 min, and the collection is driven by the subject's inhalation pattern. Although sampling of particles below $5 <$ is not efficient (Graham *et al.* 2000), correlations reported between results obtained by the nasal sampler and a conventional sampler are in the order of magnitude around 0.8 (Pearson R) (Poulos *et al.* 2002; Renström *et al.* 2002). However, an accurate comparison cannot always be made because the units differ (allergen/nostril for the nasal sampler vs. allergen level per cubic metre for a conventional dust sampler, or comparison based on the number of particulates per nostril or per cubic metre of air, respectively). Moreover, the comparison has focussed so far on the correlation between measurements, but the slopes of the regression lines, relating results from the conventional samplers with the nasal sampler, seem to differ depending on the type of dust and the (work) environment (Poulos *et al.* 2002; Renström *et al.* 2002). An issue not yet studied is the effect of mouth breathing on the sampling efficiency. These issues and the observation that certain particulates are not captured or captured with low efficiency in comparison with the inhalable dust convention curve, raises the concern that the nasal sampler does not have the potential to fulfill modern personal sampler design criteria. The experiences so far suggest that systematic differences could occur probably because these samplers do not measure according to inhalable dust criteria, and this certainly limits their use. The major argument in favour of the nasal sampler is the lower detection limit compared to conventional dust sampling. However, immuno-staining can also be combined with filtration techniques as developed for pollen exposure in the recent past (Holmquist and Vesterberg 1999, 2000) and the detection limit is than expected to be in the same order of magnitude and can be as low as a few particulates per cubic metre or in the low picogram per cubic metre range. A major application of the nasal sampler is in places where conventional sampling equipment cannot be used or is inconvenient to use, for example, measurement of tasks and activities of short duration. Renström *et al.* (2002)

used the nasal sampler, for instance, to evaluate the protective effect of face masks in laboratory animal facilities.

13.2.2   Measurement of allergen levels

Several studies have used conventional dust sampling techniques to characterize the exposure, and some have been successful in demonstrating differences in risk between high- and low-exposure categories for sensitization and respiratory symptoms or asthma. An important breakthrough took place when immuno-assays for measurement of HMW sensitizers became available in the early and mid-1980s. With these assays it was possible to measure individual allergens or allergen mixtures in environmental as well as personal dust samples. Immunochemical methods use antibodies specifically directed against antigen(s) that should be measured. These antibodies form measurable antigen–antibody complexes with the antigen(s) of interest present in dust samples. These complexes can be detected by using different labels, isotopes, enzymes, fluorescents, or luminescents. Most immunoassays for the measurement of allergens are either inhibition or sandwich assays. Both are solid phase assays in which antigen–antibody complex formation occurs at a surface coated with a known amount of well-characterized antibody or antigen. The binding of its specific counterpart from a fluid phase is quantified by subsequent binding of another, so-called detecting antibody. Enzyme labelled reagents (ELISA), with chromogenic substrates, are commonly used. In sandwich assays the allergen to be measured is captured between the antibody-coated surface and the detecting antibody, which is then directed to the allergen itself. In inhibition assays the concentration of allergen in, for example, a dust extract is quantitatively determined as the capability to inhibit the binding of anti-allergen antibodies to an allergen-coated surface. The activity of a small amount of allergen can be quantitatively detected, without interference by other non-specific agents present in the dust. Validation studies for each immunoassay are necessary and the outcome depends on sensitivity and particularly specificity of the antibodies used. Specificity of antibodies as well as the properties and purity of calibration standards or other reference preparations can be assessed by, for example, gel electrophoresis and immunoblotting, which have also been used to compare reagents used in analogous assay procedures of different laboratories. Sensitivity of inhibition assays depends mainly on the avidity and concentration of the inhibited antibodies in the assay. With high-avidity antibodies—Ka values of 10^9–10^{10} M^{-1}—a sensitivity of 10–20 ng ml^{-1} for protein allergen molecules of 10–20 kDa can be reached. Sandwich assays can be much more sensitive, depending on the quality of the reagents; if sufficiently specific, the detection system can be markedly amplified by using various secondary reagents, and in some assays sensitivities in the pg/ml range are possible.

Amplification techniques are being introduced that allow detection of allergens at considerably lower levels (Renström et al. 1997). This is especially relevant for domestic and public buildings where cat allergens are brought in through contaminated clothing in the absence of direct sources (cats). The levels in these premises are extremely low but still seem to be health relevant (Almqvist et al. 2001). Immuno-staining techniques, which make use of antibodies as well, can be used to detect allergenic particulates directly on a filter or on other media. Examples have been published for pollen allergens, *Fel d* 1 from cats, and *Hev b* 1, a major latex allergen (O'Meara *et al.* 1998; Holquist and Vesterberg 1999, 2000; Poulos *et al.* 2002).

Antibody sources

Antibodies used in immunoassays can be specific IgE antibodies from sensitized workers, polyclonal antibodies isolated from serum of animals (e.g. rabbits) immunized with an occupational allergen, or monoclonal antibodies produced by hybridomas made with spleen cells of immunized animals—usually mice or rats. Specific human IgE is theoretically the ideal antibody, since by definition it detects the allergen to be measured, but is available only in limited quantities. Absolute concentrations of specific IgE in serum are low, even in sensitized individuals. Alternatively, specific human IgG antibodies might be used, which are found in higher concentrations and are exposed in larger numbers. IgG4 class antibodies may be specifically recommended, since many IgE inducing allergen molecules induce IgG4 responses. Since reaction profiles of individual sera with a complex mixture of antigens may show marked differences, antigen measurements should be performed with pooled sera from at least 5–10 sensitized workers to prevent exclusive or preferential measurement of only one or a few relevant components. Use of antibody sources other than human IgE requires validation studies showing that the alternative antibodies have the same or very similar specificity as the IgE antibodies in sensitized workers. Fig. 13.1 gives an example for fungal α-amylase. The assay to measure fungal α-amylase in the air utilized rabbit IgG antibodies. Production of anti-sera may be time consuming but results, if successful, in large amounts of immune reagents with high titer. Monoclonal antibodies have the obvious additional advantage of being highly specific. For several major allergens, monoclonal antibodies are available commercially.

Allergen standards

When no purified allergen is available one has to identify an allergen extract as the working standard. In many cases, potentially more than one allergen is present in complex dust mixtures like latex dust. The allergen extracts should be prepared from

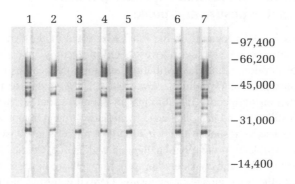

Fig. 13.1 Comparison of IgE responses sensitized in bakers and IgG response in rabbits.

industrial environment dusts, which are most likely to contain the allergen(s). The allergen concentration can be expressed in relative units (equivalents or EQ) or in mass units of the allergen extract or protein content of the allergen extract. However, results cannot be compared between studies when different standards have been used. Sometimes only one protein is involved, that is, when bakery workers are exposed to α-amylase, in which case the purified protein can be used as a working standard. This allows the allergen concentration to be expressed more easily in comparable mass units.

Validation and standardization

Few studies are available that evaluate the comparability of immuno-assays that have been used to measure aeroallergen levels (Gordon *et al.* 1992; Zock *et al.* 1996; Renström *et al.* 1997, 1999; Hollander *et al.* 1999; Lillienberg *et al.* 2000). The most detailed comparison has been made as part of a collaborative European project (see Table 13.1) (Hollander *et al.* 1999; Renström *et al.* 1999). Methods to measure rat and mouse urinary aeroallergens of three institutes were contrasted by comparing parallel ambient air inhalable dust samples from animal facilities. Median rat allergen levels obtained with a competitive inhibition radio immuno assay (RIA) method were considerably (by a factor of 3000 and 1700 times) higher compared to the levels measured by enzyme immuno assay (EIA)-sandwich methods. The difference between the two EIA-sandwich methods was considerably smaller (factor 2.2). Differences were smaller for the mouse allergen levels. Type of elution buffer and antibodies used were identified as the two major factors that caused the observed differences between sandwich assays. Variation in antibody specificity or variation in allergenic epitopes in the air samples may contribute as well as standards used (purified allergens, crude extract). Despite the systematic differences, correlation between allergen levels obtained with different assays was high. Validation and comparison of different assays by intra-laboratory comparisons is urgently needed. The optimal situation to analyse allergens immunochemically is reached when the allergen has been identified, and purified allergen and monoclonal or polyclonal antibodies against the allergen are available.

13.2.3   Exposure routes and exposure patterns: dermal exposure and peaks

Most studies so far have focused on the inhalation route of the exposure. Allergy to natural rubber latex has recently been investigated in mice by subcutaneous injection, percutaneous absorption, intranasal instillation, and intra-tracheal instillation with non-ammoniated latex proteins (Woolhiser *et al.* 2000). These studies demonstrated dose-dependent induction of specific IgE through all exposure routes. Mice sensitized by intra-tracheal instillation and later challenged with latex protein demonstrated a significant broncho-constrictive response compared to naïve mice, sham-sensitized mice, or to mice sensitized with latex protein but challenged with saline. Studies like this raise an important issue that has been considered in only very few studies, the issue of potential exposure routes other than inhalation exposure. Dermal exposure has been an issue in case of latex allergy where dermal exposure plays an important role and causes dermal effects as well. Poulos *et al.* (2002) describe results of an exploratory study in which

Table 13.1 Median and range of rat and mouse urinary allergen (RUA and MUA) levels ($ng\,m^{-3}$) found in ambient air dust samples taken in animal facilities of three participating laboratories

| | Filters taken in | | | | | | | | |
| | UK | | | The Netherlands | | | Sweden | | |
Method	N	Median ($ng\,m^{-3}$)	Range	N	Median ($ng\,m^{-3}$)	Range	N	Median ($ng\,m^{-3}$)	Range
RUA									
NHLI	13	11000	172–52900	35	3730	<10.9–47200	25	775	<10.9–21700
WU	13	0.37	<0.16–15.0	35	0.86	<0.16–31.9	25	<0.16	<0.16–3.6
NIWL	14	1.95	<0.11–11.8	35	2.0	<0.11–43.4	25	0.71	<0.11–11.6
MUA									
NHLI	10	9.92	0.89–162	21	11.0	0.8–4610	20	9.37	0.74–82.5
WU	13	<0.16	<0.16–32.6	34	1.1	<0.16–1560	25	<0.16	<0.16–3.0
NIWL	14	0.24	<0.11–71.5	35	2.8	0.13–446	25	0.36	<0.11–6.1

NHLI, National Heart and Lung Institute, United Kingdom; WU, Wageningen University, The Netherlands; NIWL, National Institute of Working Life, Sweden (Hollander et al. 1999).

latex allergens from gloves, on hands and work surfaces, were measured by use of adhesive tape. They were able to show that latex levels on the hands were considerably higher after removal of powdered latex gloves compared to vinyl gloves. Dermal exposure may be a secondary source of inhalation exposure after resuspension, but it might also play a role in the sensitization process. However, the importance of the dermal route for respiratory allergies has not been shown yet in convincing epidemiological studies. Recently, dermal exposure is hypothesized to play a role in specific respiratory sensitization to iso-cyanates. This hypothesis is based on its common use in experimental animal studies to induce respiratory sensitization by means of skin exposure. A study by Scheerens *et al.* (1999) describes this issue specifically. In a workshop held by the British Health and Safety Executive (HSE), the majority of experts believed that skin exposure could, at least in theory, induce the relevant immunological responses, (HSE 1999). However, dermal exposure has not been considered so far in human observational studies of iso-cyanate exposure.

It has been suggested that peak exposures play a crucial role in the development of allergy and asthma. This hypothesis is partly based on observations in which workers developed asthma after being exposed to incidental or accidental high concentration of chemicals such as di-isocyanates due to spills and splashes (Ott *et al.* 2000). Further, peak exposures are known to be relevant in the induction of RADS and have been described in di-isocyanate-exposed workers (Leroyer *et al.* 1998). This hypothesis has as yet not been supported by strong epidemiological evidence, but deserves more detailed analysis. Measurement of short-term exposure to soluble platinum salts in the air did not produce any supportive evidence that the peaks contributed significantly to the overall airborne exposure (Maynard *et al.* 1997). The authors also concluded that there were no indications for changes in work practices during the measurements, and that since they observed sensitization at exposure levels below the exposure standard it is not completely protective or that an alternate (dermal) route of exposure might play a role and explain the sensitization at low levels of airborne exposure. A study among bakery workers at least showed that peak exposures are very common and peak levels are orders of magnitude above the average shift exposure levels, but relationships with sensitization risk or asthma were not evaluated because of the strong correlation between peak and average shift exposure levels (Nieuwenhuijsen *et al.* 1995). Figure 13.2 shows part of a DataRam recording for a bakery worker. Analysis of this type of information shows that a typical bakery or dough maker is exposed to 200–600 exposure peaks per days (arbitrarily defined as a level above 0.5 $mg\,m^{-3}$). Background levels are extremely low, which indicates that the exposure over a working day is actually built up out of a series of short, long, low, and high peaks.

13.2.4   Exposure assessment in epidemiology

Exposure assessment in epidemiology has developed into a discipline on its own and covers issues such as categorizing the population into exposure categories, allocation of sampling effort over these categories in order to obtain accurate estimates of the average exposure, use of exposure modelling approaches to estimate the exposure, and evaluation of different exposure assessment strategies as part of the optimization process (Boleij *et al.* 1996). These issues have received little attention so far in the field of

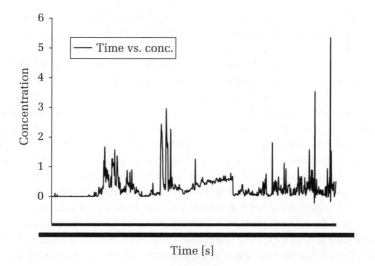

Fig. 13.2 Peak exposure pattern of a bakery worker.

allergen exposure since the emphasis has been on instrumental issues such as developing assays and monitoring techniques. Only few examples exist of application of these principles in epidemiological studies, however this area urgently needs more attention (Nieuwenhuijsen *et al.* 1995; Tielemans *et al.* 1998; van Tongeren *et al.* 1998).

13.2.5   The analysis of exposure–response relationships

A distinction has to be made between different types of exposure–effect or exposure–response variables. Challenge testing shows that the reactivity between individuals differs even between sensitized individuals. Theoretically, challenge testing allows evaluation of exposure–effect relationships on the individual level, for instance, between dose of the allergen and FEV_1 change. Peak expiratory flow (PEF) testing, and analysis of PEF changes in relation to workplace exposure is the real life parallel to challenge testing. Outcomes of individual PEF readings, such as amplitude or variability during working days in comparison to off workdays can be used to compare responsiveness between individuals, but can also be used as input for epidemiological analysis (Hollander *et al.* 1998). In epidemiological studies usually exposure–response relationships are being evaluated with the response defined as a dichotomous outcome, usually based on a measurement on a continuous scale (IgE titer) transformed to a dichotomous scale. The most evaluated exposure–response relationships in allergic respiratory disease are exposure–sensitization and exposure–symptom relationships. However, examples exist in which, for instance, time to sensitization also has been evaluated (Kruize *et al.* 1997).

The development of respiratory allergy is usually described as follows. Exposure leads to sensitization and development of an inflammatory response, which is accompanied by symptoms, bronchial hyper-responsiveness, airflow variability, etc. When exposure is continued, chronic changes and severe airflow impairment might occur. This process can develop rapidly and as a result it seems likely that workers may try to influence their exposure when they develop symptoms or leave the workforce (healthy worker effect). This process has not been studied directly but it is believed to play an important role. For each step risk modifying variables have been identified. There is clear evidence that the sensitization risk against HMW sensitizers is higher in atopic workers. Smoking and gender might modify the sensitization risk as well, but the evidence is weak and their roles depend on the type of sensitizing agent. In case of low molecular sensitizers such as platinum salts there are stronger indications that smokers are at higher risk and atopy seems no risk modifier. The consequence of these observations is that the exposure–response relationship is potentially modified by these factors, and that the slope of the relationship may differ for different subcategories of workers, and this has to be evaluated carefully in the epidemiological analysis. This has consistently been done in the more recent paper in which quantitative exposure–response relationships were explored for several HMW sensitizers such as wheat allergens, fungal α-amylase, and rat urinary proteins (Cullinan *et al.* 1994*a,b*; Houba *et al.* 1996*a,b*, 1998; Hollander *et al.* 1996, 1997; Heederik *et al.* 1999; Nieuwenhuijsen *et al.* 2002). In all cases it was clear that the slope of the exposure–response relationship was steeper for atopics compared to non-atopics. In some cases there was a suggestion that an elevated sensitization risk only occurred in the highly exposed non-atopic individuals; the exposure–response relationship was also shifted somewhat to the right.

When there is interest in the relationship between exposure to allergens and (work related) symptoms, all modifiers on the causal pathway between exposure and symptoms have to be considered. This makes sense because it is paramount that the risk for developing or having symptoms is higher for work-related sensitized individuals and may be higher for atopics without work-related sensitization. In addition, the symptom prevalence may be influenced by classical determinants such as smoking and age, and these have to be considered as well. Despite the fact that this problem has been recognized in the basic literature by Becklake (1999), it has not been translated into appropriate analytical strategies in the data analysis in most studies (see Section 13.2.6).

13.2.6   Exposure–sensitization relationships

Early studies in populations such as bakery and wood workers already gave some indications that exposure–response relationships could be observed in the exposure range encountered in some industries. Musk *et al.* (1989) showed that bakery workers with a 'high dust rank' were more often sensitized against one or more bakery allergens compared to workers with a low dust rank. The dust rank classification was validated with a series of total dust measurement. However, even more recent studies still use conventional dust sampling and are able to unravel exposure–response relationships for rhinitis and asthma in bakers (Brisman *et al.* 2000). However, this is probably explained by the observation that the wheat allergen levels in flour dust correlate reasonably with the dust level (Nieuwenhuijsen *et al.* 1995; Houba *et al.* 1996*a*), which is not often the case because the dust and allergen levels do not always share the same sources.

Most evidence on existence of exposure–response relationships is available for specific IgE mediated sensitization. Recent overviews of the available exposure–response studies (Baur *et al.* 1998; Heederik *et al.* 2002) show that several allergens like, for example, rat urinary proteins and fungal α-amylase, appear to be very potent and are already associated with increased sensitization rates at exposure levels in the nano or even picogram per cubic metre range for as little as a few hours per week (Houba *et al.* 1996*b*; Heederik *et al.* 1999; Nieuwenhuijsen *et al.* 1999). Other allergens like wheat proteins seem less potent and sensitization rates increase when exposure occurs in the low microgram per cubic metre range (Houba *et al.* 1998). One of the few longitudinal exposure–response studies in bakers seems to confirm cross-sectional studies on fungal α-amylase and wheat allergen exposure (Cullinan *et al.* 2001). Clear-cut exposure–response relationships in humans have as yet not been observed for latex proteins, since few epidemiological studies on latex sensitization have yet been conducted in which exposure was assessed with the use of latex-specific immunoassays.

Similar exposure–response relationships have been observed for common allergens from house dust and cats, but usually the allergen levels are measured in floor dust, the major reservoir, instead of airborne dust because of detection issues and the fact that most particles remain airborne for a very brief period because of the large particle size (Munir *et al.* 1997; Platt-Mills *et al.* 2001*a,b*). Exposure–sensitization relationships have been established for some low molecular weight sensitizers as well such as platinum salts (Merget *et al.* 2000).

As allergen exposure is accurately measured and sensitization has very specific end-points (one might argue that theoretically, apart from potential cross-sensitization, the relationship is mono-causal), relationships between allergen exposure and sensitization are usually very strong, with clear and relatively large increases in sensitization risk with increasing exposure. Sometimes statistical modelling might be complicated by the fact that sensitization does not occur in the controls or low-exposed individuals. This complicates the statistical analysis and makes evaluation of exposure–response relationships sometimes difficult. For instance, in the study by Hollander *et al.* (1997) in laboratory animal workers, only three sensitized individuals were observed in the internal reference group consisting of 86 individuals. The estimated relative sensitization risk for exposed workers then strongly depends on this baseline rate that is estimated with only poor precision. The situation becomes even more complex when deviations occur from simple linear relationships. The choice of a cut-point can have considerable impact on the outcome of the analysis. Novel approaches such as smoothing techniques might be helpful in this phase of the analysis to overcome these problems.

13.2.7   Exposure–symptom relationships

Several investigators have also evaluated exposure–symptoms relationships with mixed success, mainly because of the complex analysis and pitfalls. Several papers have been published in which the relationship between exposure and symptoms has been analysed in a simple straightforward way with the result that no clear relationship could be observed. Relationships between exposure and symptoms can only be studied in a meaningful way when the analysis is stratified for modifying variables along the causal pathway. This includes at least work-related sensitization and atopy in case of high-molecular sensitizers. Houba *et al.* (1998) analysed the relationship between wheat allergen exposure and upper- and lower-airway symptoms in a cross-sectional study among bakery workers. The relationship was more strong within sensitized individuals compared to non-sensitized workers, as expected. Similar observations were made by

Table 13.2	Relationship between aero-allergen levels of rat urinary proteins and respiratory symptoms after stratification for atopy and specific sensitization against rats (from Nieuwenhuijsen *et al.* 2003)

	SPT +ve				SPT −ve			
Symptoms by RUA categories	Cases (n/N)	Cumulative incidence (%)	RR	95% CI	Cases (n/N)	Cumulative incidence (%)	RR	95% CI
Any symptoms								
1-low	16/75	21.3	1		14/75	18.7	1	
2	3/13	23.1	1.7	0.5–6.2	18/68	26.5	1.8	0.9–3.7
3	6/15	40.0	9.1	2.6–31.9	21/88	23.9	1.8	0.9–3.7
4-high	2/7	28.6	3.0	0.6–14.4	30/71	42.3	2.1	1.1–3.9
Chest symptoms								
1-low	2/71	2.8	1		2/71	2.8	1	
2	2/13	15.4	2.9	0.5–17.8	5/70	7.1	2.8	0.5–14.4
3	8/16	50.0	11.1	2.7–45.9	5/87	5.7	2.5	0.5–12.9
4-high	5/10	50.0	9.9	2.2–44.9	5/74	6.8	2.3	0.5–12.1
Eyes/nose symptoms								
1-low	7/67	9.0	1		13/74	17.6	1	
2	4/15	26.7	4.6	1.3–16.2	13/69	18.8	1.3	0.6–2.8
3	10/17	58.8	12.9	4.4–37.7	11/82	13.4	1.1	0.5–2.5
4-high	3/9	33.3	8.8	3.1–24.9	12/76	15.8	0.8	0.3–1.8
Skin symptoms								
1-low	1/69	1.4	1		4/73	5.5	1	
2	2/12	16.7	9.2	1.3–67.1	8/69	11.6	2.2	0.5–9.4
3	7/16	43.8	19.9	3.8–105.0	7/84	8.3	2.3	0.6–9.4
4-high	7/11	63.6	43.6	7.5–254.4	12/76	15.8	3.8	1.0–13.5

RR, rate ratio; 95% CI, 95% confidence interval; the estimates are adjusted for smoking and atopic status (see text for RRs).

Nieuwenhuijsen *et al.* (2003) in a study among laboratory animal workers (see Table 13.2). Strong relationships between exposure and symptoms were observed within rat-sensitized workers, while among non-sensitized workers the relationship was considerably weaker. These results show that it is possible to observe relationships between exposure and symptoms as long as the proper analytical procedures are followed. This relationship can best be studied in a longitudinal design. De Zotti and Bovenzi (2000) showed that a history of allergic disease and the presence of skin sensitization to allergens from the work environment (wheat or fungal amylase) were strong predictors of development of symptoms in a small longitudinal study among apprentices. Although exposure was not considered in the analysis, especially this type of analysis based on longitudinal studies, it is useful to unravel the complex associations between exposure, sensitization, and symptoms. Similar observations have been made for low molecular weight sensitizers such as platinum salts (Calverly *et al.* 1995) and acid anhydrides (Barker *et al.* 1998).

13.2.8 New developments in the evaluation of exposure–response relationships

Recently more interest developed in the shape of the exposure–response relationship. This interest developed from two directions, from the perspective of risk assessment and from the perspective of disease aetiology. In risk assessment for occupational allergens it is relevant to know if exposure thresholds can be observed and with what model the shape of relationships can be described (Heederik *et al.* 2002). From the perspective of disease aetiology suggestions have been made that the exposure–response relationship flattens off at higher exposure levels as a result of development of tolerance possibly associated with a specific IgG4 response (Platt-Mills *et al.* 2001*a,b*).

Thus far, most studies do not allow inferences about the presence of exposure thresholds. The exposure has been characterized in a relatively crude way for a limited number of exposure categories, and the data analysis was not focused on this particular aspect. In one study among bakery workers with approximately 400 bakery workers and 546 allergen measurements it could be shown that when smoothing approaches were used to describe the exposure–response relationship for wheat sensitization, the sensitization risk increased rapidly from the low end of the exposure distribution, levelled off at intermediate levels, and dropped off again at higher exposures (see Fig. 13.3).

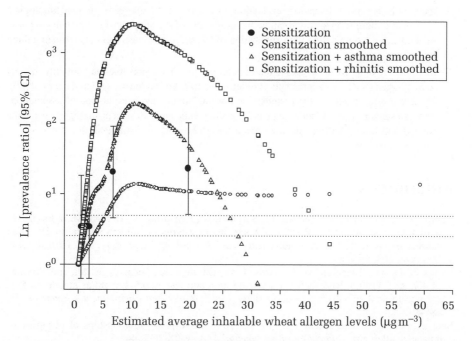

Fig. 13.3 Smoothed relationship between wheat allergen levels and wheat sensitization and work-related wheat allergy, defined as wheat sensitization and work-related rhinitis or asthma symptoms, respectively (from Heederik *et al.* 2001).

There were no indications of an exposure threshold or exposure level below which the sensitization risk was not increased. There is a need for more and new studies in which similar approaches in the analysis can be applied.

Evidence on the flattening off of the exposure–response relationship, possibly associated with specific IgG and IgG4 responses, has been published recently by Platts-Mills *et al.* (2001*a,b*). They found in a cross-sectional study among school children that strong IgG4 responses to the major cat allergen (Fel d1) were negatively associated with both atopic sensitization and symptomatic allergic disease. Since Fel d1-specific IgG4 titres were positively related to the estimated level of cat allergen exposure, it was suggested that these allergen-specific IgG4 responses may account for the unexpected negative associations between the presence of pets at home during early childhood and the risk of asthma and symptomatic allergy in children at later age and in young adults, as found in several recently reported population studies. Others have found that children from farmers and farmer apprentices with a farming background have a lower prevalence of asthma compared to urban populations (Douwes *et al.* 2002). Among many other explanations, endotoxin exposure on the farm has been suggested to play a role in the development of atopy. These examples illustrate that insight in the aetiology of allergy and asthma changes rapidly. The role of environmental exposures and interactions between agents such as allergens and endotoxins are at present an area of intensive research, and this will also have an impact on how exposure–response relationships will be evaluated in epidemiological studies. It is to be expected that:

(1) there will be more focus on evaluation of exposure to allergens in epidemiological studies in a more refined way to allow the evaluation of the shape of the exposure–response relationship in combination with application of advanced statistical tools such as smoothing techniques;

(2) there will be more focus on evaluation of exposure to other agents that may possibly interact with allergens such as disinfectants (Preller *et al.* 1996) or endotoxins (Gereda *et al.* 2000); because a requirement in these studies will be the simultaneous evaluation of associations between sensitization and more than one exposure, exposure assessment strategies need to be refined and have a sufficiently high resolution to be able to distinguish the effects of the different exposure variables.

References

Almqvist, C., Wickman, M., Perfetti, L., Berglind, N., Renstrom, A., Hedren, M., Larsson, K., Hedlin, G., and Malmberg, P. (2001). Worsening of asthma in children allergic to cats, after indirect exposure to cat at school. *American Journal of Respiratory and Critical Care Medicine*, **163**, 694–8.

Barker, R. D., van Tongeren, M. J., Harris, J. M., Gardiner, K., Venables, K. M., and Newman Taylor, A. J. (1998). Risk factors for sensitisation and respiratory symptoms among workers exposed to acid anhydrides: a cohort study. *Occupational and Environmental Medicine*, **55**, 684–91.

Baur, X., Chen, Z., and Liebers, V. (1998). Exposure–response relationships of occupational inhalative allergens. *Clinical and Experimental Allergy*, **28**, 537–44.

Bernstein, I. L., Chan-Yeung, M., Malo, J.-L., and Bernstein, D. I. (1999). Definition and Classification of Asthma. In *Asthma in the workplace* (ed. I. L. Bernstein, M. Chan-Yeung, J.-L. Malo, and D. I. Bernstein, 2nd edn). Marcel Dekker, New York.

Becklake, M. (1999). Epidemiological approaches in occupational asthma. In *Asthma in the workplace* (ed. I. L. Bernstein, M. Chan-Yeung, J.-L. Malo, and D. I. Bernstein, 2nd edn). Marcel Dekker, New York.

Boleij, J., Buringh, E., Heederik, D., Kromhout, H. (1995). Occupational hygiene of chemical and biological agents. Elsevier, Amsterdam.

Brisman, J., Jarvholm, B., and Lillienberg, L. (2000). Exposure–response relations for self reported asthma and rhinitis in bakers. *Occupational and Environmental Medicine*, **57**, 335–40.

Calverley, A. E., Rees, D., Dowdeswell, R. J., Linnett, P. J., and Kielkowski, D. (1995). Platinum salt sensitivity in refinery workers: incidence and effects of smoking and exposure. *Occupational and Environmental Medicine*, **52**, 661–6.

Chan-Yeung, M. and Malo, J.-L. (1994). Aetiological agents in occupational asthma. *European Respiratory Journal*, **7**, 346–71.

Chan-Yeung, M. and Malo, J.-L. (1999). Natural history of occupational asthma. In *Asthma in the workplace* (ed. I. L. Bernstein, M. Chan-Yeung, J.-L. Malo, and D. I. Bernstein, 2nd edn), Marcel Dekker, New York.

Cullinan, P., Lowson, D., Nieuwenhuijsen, M. J., Sandiford, C., Tee, R. D., Venables, K. M., McDonald, J. C., and Newman Taylor, A. J. (1994a). Work related symptoms, sensitisation, and estimated exposure in workers not previously exposed to flour. *Occupational and Environmental Medicine*, **51**, 579–83.

Cullinan, P., Lowson, D., Nieuwenhuijsen, M. J., Gordon, S., Tee, R. D., Venables, K. M., McDonald, J. C., and Newman-Taylor, A. J. (1994b). Work related symptoms, sensitisation, and estimated exposure in workers not previously exposed to laboratory rats. *Occupational and Environmental Medicine*, **51**, 589–92.

Cullinan, P., Cook, A., Nieuwenhuijsen, M. J., Sandiford, C., Tee, R. D., Venables, K. M., McDonald, J. C., Newman Taylor, A. J. (2001). Allergen and dust exposure as determinants of work-related symptoms and sensitization in a cohort of flour-exposed workers; a case-control analysis. *Ann Occup Hyg*, **45**, 97–103.

De Zotti, R. and Bovenzi, M. (2000). Prospective study of work related respiratory symptoms in trainee bakers. *Occupational and Environmental Medicine*, **57**, 58–61.

Douwes, J., Pearce, N., and Heederik, D. (2002). Does environmental endotoxin exposure prevent asthma? *Thorax*, **57**, 86–90.

Flindt, M. L. (1996). Biological miracles and misadventures: identification of sensitization and asthma in enzyme detergent workers. *American Journal of Industrial Medicine*, **29**, 99–110.

Gereda, J. E., Leung, D. Y., Thatayatikom, A., *et al.* (2000). Relation between house-dust endotoxin exposure, type 1 T-cell development, and allergen sensitisation in infants at high risk of asthma. *Lancet*, **355**, 1680–3.

Gordon, S., Tee, R. D., Lowson, D., and Newman Taylor, A. J. (1992). Comparison and optimization of filter elution methods for the measurement of airborne allergens. *Annals of Occupational Hygiene*, **36**, 575–87.

Graham, J. A., Pavlicek, P. K., Sercombe, J. K., Xavier, M. L., and Tovey, E. R. (2000). The nasal air sampler: a device for sampling inhaled aeroallergens. *Annals of Allergy, Asthma and Immunology*, **84**, 599–604.

Heederik, D., Venables, K., Malmberg, P., Hollander, A., Karlsson, A.-S., Renström, A., Doekes, G., and Nieuwenhuijsen, M. (1999). Exposure–response relationships for occupational respiratory sensitization in workers exposed to rat urinary allergens: results from an European study in laboratory animal workers. *Journal of Allergy and Clinical Immunology*, **103**, 678–84.

Hollander, A., Heederik, D., and Doekes, G. (1996). Rat allergy exposure–response relationships in laboratory animal workers. *American Journal of Respiratory and Critical Care Medicine*, **155**, 562–7.

Hollander, A., Heederik, D., and Brunekreef, B. (1998). Work related changes in peak expiratory flow among laboratory animal workers. *European Respiratory Journal*, **11**, 929–36.

Hollander, A., Renström, A., Gordon, S., Thissen, J., Doekes, G., Larsson, P., Venables, K., Malmberg, P., and Heederik, D. (1999). Comparison of methods to assess airborne rat and mouse allergen levels. I. Analysis of air samples. *Allergy*, **54**, 142–9.

Holmquist, L. and Vesterberg, O. (1999). Luminiscence immunoassay of pollen allergens on air sampling polytetrafluoroethylene filters. *Journal of Biochemical and Biophysical Methods*, **41**, 49–60.

Holmquist, L. and Vesterberg, O. (2000). Miniaturized direct on air sampling filter quantification of pollen allergens. *Journal of Biochemical and Biophysical Methods*, **42**, 111–14.

Houba, R., van Run, P., Heederik, D., and Doekes, G. (1996a). Wheat allergen exposure assessment for epidemiologic studies in bakeries using personal dust sampling and inhibition ELISA. *Clinical and Experimental Allergy*, **26**, 154–63.

Houba, R., Heederik, D., Doekes, G., and van Run, P. (1996b). Exposure-sensitization relationship for α-amylase allergens in the baking industry. *American Journal of Respiratory and Critical Care Medicine*, **154**, 130–6.

Houba, R., Heederik, D., and Doekes, G. (1998). Wheat sensitization and work related symptoms in the baking industry are preventable: an epidemiological study. *American Journal of Respiratory and Critical Care Medicine*, **158**, 1499–503.

HSE (1999a). *Does the skin react as a route for respiratory allergy?* Report from a HSE workshop held at the Radisson SAS Hotel. HSE (Health and Safety Executive); 18–19 November, Manchester, UK.

ISO (1992). *Air quality—particle size fraction definitions fro health related sampling*. ISO/CD 7708 International Standardization Organization, Geneva.

Kenny, L. C., Aitken, R., Chalmers, C., Fabries, J. F., Gonzalez-Fernandez, E., Kromhout, H., Liden, G., Mark, D., Riediger, G., and Prodi, V. (1997). A collaborative European study of personal inhalable aerosol sampler performance. *Annals of Occupational Hygiene*, **41**, 135–53.

Kruize, H., Post, W., Heederik, D., Martens, B., Hollander, A., and van der Beek, M. (1997). Respiratory allergy in laboratory animal workers: a retrospective cohort study using pre-employment screening data. *Occupational and Environmental Medicine*, **11**, 830–5.

Leroyer, C., Perfetti, L., Cartier, A., Malo, J. L. (1998). Can reactive airways dysfunction syndrome (RADS) transform into occupational asthma due to "sensitisation" to isocyanates? *Thorax* **5**, 723–3.

Lillienberg, L., Baur, X., Doekes, G., Belin, L., Raulf-Heimsoth, M., Sander, I., Stahl, A., Thissen, J., and Heederik, D. (2000). Comparison of four methods to assess fungal alpha-amylase in flour dust. *Annals of Occupational Hygiene*, **44**, 427–33.

Maynard, A. D., Northage, C., Hemingway, M., and Bradley, S. D. (1997). Measurement of short-term exposure to airborne soluble platinum in the platinum industry. *Annals of Occupational Hygiene*, **41**, 77–94.

Merget, R., Kulzer, R., Dierkes-Globisch, A., Breitstadt, R., Gebler, A., Kniffka, A., Artelt, S., Koenig, H. P., Alt, F., Vormberg, R., Baur, X., and Schultze-Werninghaus, G. (2000). Exposure-effect relationship of platinum salt allergy in a catalyst production plant: conclusions from a 5-year prospective cohort study. *Journal of Allergy and Clinical Immunology*, **105**, 364–70.

Munir, A. K., Kjellman, N. I., and Bjorksten, B. (1997). Exposure to indoor allergens in early infancy and sensitization. *Journal of Allergy and Clinical Immunology*, **100**, 177–81.

Musk, A. W., Venables, K. M., Crook, B., Nunn, A. J., Hawkins, R., Crook, G. D., Graneek, B. J., Tee, R. D., Farrer, N., Johnson, D. A., Gordon, D. J., Darbyshire, J. H., and Newman Taylor, A. J. (1989). Respiratory symptoms, lung function, and sensitisation to flour in a British bakery. *British Journal of Industrial Medicine*, **46**, 636–42.

Nieuwenhuijsen, M. J., Sandiford, C. P., Lowson, D., Tee, R. D., Venables, K. M., and Newman Taylor, A. J. (1995). Peak exposure concentrations of dust and flour aeroallergen in flour mills and bakeries. *Annals of Occupational Hygiene*, **39**, 193–201.

Nieuwenhuijsen, M. J., Lowson, D., Venables, K. M., and Newman Taylor, A. J. (1995). Correlation between different measures of exposure– in a cohort of bakery workers and flour millers. *Annals of Occupational Hygiene*, **39**, 291–8.

Nieuwenhuijsen, M. J., Heederik, D., Doekes, G., Venables, K. M., and Newman Taylor, A. J. (1999). Exposure–response relationships for α-amylase sensitization in British bakeries and flour mills. *Occupational and Environmental Medicine*, **56**, 197–201.

Nieuwenhuijsen, M. J., Putcha, V., Gordon, S., Heederik, D., Venables, K. M., Cullinan, P., and Newman-Taylor, A. J. (2003). Exposure–response relationships among laboratory anumal workers exposed to rats. *Occupational and Environmental Medicine*, **60**, 104–8.

O'Meara, T. J., De Lucca, S., Sporik, R., Graham, A., and Tovey, E. (1998). Detection of inhaled cat allergen. *The Lancet*, **351**, 1488–9.

Ott, M. G., Klees, J. E., and Poche, S. L. (2000). Respiratory health surveillance in a toluene di-isocyanate production unit, 1967–97: clinical observations and lung function analyses. *Occupational and Environmental Medicine*, **57**, 43–52.

Perkins, J. L. (ed.) (1997). *Modern industrial hygiene: Vol. I. Recognition, evaluation of chemical agents*. American Conference of Governmental Industrial Hygienists, Cincinnati, OH, USA, Van Nostrand Reinhold, New York, USA.

Perkins, J. L. (ed.) (2003). *Modern Industrial Hygiene: Vol. II. Biological aspects*. American Conference of Governmental Industrial Hygienists, Cincinnati, OH, USA, Van Nostrand Reinhold, New York, USA (in press).

Platts-Mills, T., Vaughan, J., Squillace, S., Woodfolk, J., and Sporik, R. (2001*a*). Sensitisation, asthma, and a modified Th2 response in children exposed to cat allergen: a population-based cross-sectional study. *Lancet*, **357**, 752–6.

Platts-Mills, T. A., Vaughan, J. W., Blumenthal, K., Pollart Squillace, S., and Sporik, R. B. (2001*b*). Serum IgG and IgG4 antibodies to Fel d 1 among children exposed to 20 microg Fel d 1 at home: relevance of a nonallergic modified Th2 response. *International Archives of Allergy and Immunology*, **124**, 126–9.

Poulos, L. M., O'Meara, T. J., Hamilton, R. G., and Tovey, E. R. (2002). Inhaled latex allergen (Hev b 1). *Journal of Allergy and Clinical Immunology*, **109**, 701–6.

Preller, L., Doekes, G., Heederik, D., Vermeulen, R., Vogelzang, P. F., and Boleij, J. S. M. (1996). Disinfectant use as a risk factor for atopic sensitization and symptoms consistent with asthma: an epidemiological study. *European Respiratory Journal*, **9**, 1407–13.

Renström, A., Gordon, S., Larsson, P. H., Tee, R. D., Newman Taylor, A. J., and Malmberg, P. (1997). Comparison of a radioallergosorbent (RAST) inhibition method and a monoclonal enzyme linked immunosorbent assay (ELISA) for aeroallergen measurement. *Clinical and Experimental Allergy*, **27**, 1314–1321.

Renstrom, A., Larsson, P. H., Malmberg, P., and Bayard, C. (1997). A new amplified monoclonal rat allergen assay used for evaluation of ventilation improvements in animal rooms. *Journal of Allergy and Clinical Immunology*, **100**, 649–55.

Renström, A., Hollander, A., Gordon, S., Thissen, J., Doekes, G., Larsson, P., Venables, K., Malmberg, P., and Heederik, D. (1999). Comparison of methods to assess airborne rat or mouse allergen levels: II Factors influencing antigen detection. *Allergy*, **54**, 150–7.

Renström, A., Karlsson, A.-S., and Tovey, E. (2002). Nasal sampling for the assessment of occupational allergen exposure and the efficacy of respiratory protection. Accepted for publication.

Scheerens, H., Buckley, T. L., Muis, T. L., Garssen, J., Dormans, J., Nijkamp, F. P., *et al.* (1999). Long-term topical exposure to toluene diisocyanate in mice leads to antibody production and *in vivo* airway hyperresponsiveness three hours after intranasal challenge. *American Journal of Respiratory and Critical Care Medicine*, **159**, 1074–80.

Tielemans, E., Kupper, L., Kromhout, H., Heederik, D., and Houba, R. (1998). Individual-based and group-based exposure assessment: some equations to evaluate different strategies. *Annals of Occupational Hygiene*, **42**, 115–119.

van Tongeren, M. J., Barker, R. D., Gardiner, K., Harris, J. M., Venables, K. M., Harrington, J. M., and Newman Taylor, A. J. (1998). Retrospective exposure assessment for a cohort study into respiratory effects of acid anhydrides. *Occupational and Environmental Medicine*, **55**, 692–6.

Toraasen, M., Sussman, G., Biagini, R., Meade, J., Beezhold, D., and Germolec, D. (2000). Latex allergy in the workplace. *Toxicological Sciences*, **58**, 5–14.

Woolhiser, M. R., Munson, A. E., and Meade, B. J. (2000). Immunological responses of mice following administration of natural rubber latex proteins by different routes of exposure. *Toxicological Sciences*, **55**, 343–51.

Zock, J.-P., Hollander, A., Doekes, G., and Heederik, D. (1996). The influence of different filter elution methods on the measurement of airborne potato antigens. *American Industrial Hygiene Association Journal*, **57**, 567–70.

14. Particulate matter

Helen H. Suh

14.1 Introduction

Exposure assessment plays a clear and important role in all aspects of environmental epidemiological studies. In its most obvious role, exposure assessment is used in epidemiological studies to assess exposures for their study population, either for individuals or for a population. Exposure assessment also plays a role in health assessment, helping to address issues of exposure error, confounding, and effect modification. As a result of its varied and wide roles, the utility and importance of exposure assessment are also varied. Exposure assessment can be used to help interpret results from epidemiological studies, design new epidemiological studies, and to generate hypotheses for future health effect studies.

Exposure assessment's role and importance in environmental epidemiological studies encompass all study types and pollutants. Perhaps the best illustration of its role and importance, however, is provided by particulate matter (PM), which has been the focus of considerable attention by scientists, regulators, and industry representatives over recent years. This attention has in large part resulted from the US EPA's recent revision of the National Ambient Air Quality Standard (NAAQS) for PM, which now also regulates particles with an aerodynamic diameter less than 2.5 μm ($PM_{2.5}$) and effectively lowers the allowable concentration of PM in the US. This revision was prompted primarily by results from epidemiological studies, which found associations between ambient particulate concentrations and a variety of adverse health indicators, including increased mortality, hospital admissions, blood inflammation markers, and reduced lung function (Pope 2000; US EPA 2002).

During the EPA revision process and the ensuing debate over the appropriate standard, numerous questions were raised about the validity of the epidemiological study findings and highlighted the need for research to address these outstanding questions. In a report by the National Research Council, the research questions were listed as ten research priorities (National Research Council 1998):

- outdoor measures vs. actual exposures,
- exposures of susceptible sub-populations to toxic PM, components,
- source–receptor measurement tools,
- application of methods and models,
- assessment of hazardous PM components,

- dosimetry,
- combined effects of PM and gaseous co-pollutants,
- susceptible subpopulations,
- mechanisms of injury,
- analysis and measurement.

Of these ten areas, six were related to exposure assessment, clearly demonstrating the importance of exposure assessment to our ability to understand particulate health effects and to develop effective regulatory policies. In response to these needs, numerous exposure assessment studies have been performed in recent years, with results from these studies having important implications for our understanding of particulate health effects. This chapter uses this PM exposure research to illustrate the importance of exposure-related research to health effect research and ultimately to public policy.

14.2   Exposure measurement

For air pollution epidemiological studies, exposures have historically been assessed using concentrations measured at centrally located stationary ambient monitoring (SAM) sites. However, more recent epidemiological studies have expanded their exposure measurements to include micro-environmental or personal exposure measurements as well. These additional exposure measurements have been made possible by the development of new methods to measure particulate exposures, which have improved dramatically over the past 10 years. This improvement has resulted from the development of new methods to measure particulate exposures (1) over shorter time periods, (2) in a variety of micro-environments, including personal micro environments, and (3) together with other air pollutants.

14.2.1   Integrated samplers

Among the latest integrated methods to measure personal and micro-environmental air pollutant concentrations is the multi-pollutant sampler, which was developed to allow personal particulate and gaseous exposures to be measured simultaneously over 24-h periods (Chang *et al.* 1999). The multi-pollutant sampler is essentially several individual samplers that have been joined to form a simple, compact, and relatively lightweight personal monitor. In its most complete form, the multi-pollutant sampler can be used to measure personal exposures and micro-environmental concentrations of PM_{10}, $PM_{2.5}$, the particle components elemental carbon (EC), organic carbon (OC), sulphate (SO_4^{2-}), nitrate (NO_3^-), and the elements, and the gases ozone (O_3), sulphur dioxide (SO_2), and nitrogen dioxide (NO_2) simultaneously.

For PM_{10} and $PM_{2.5}$, the multi-pollutant sampler includes small, low-flow inertial impactors, typically referred to as personal exposure monitors (PEMs), which operate at flow rates of approximately 2 LPM. These samplers use Teflon filters as the particle collection media and include drain disk rings to prevent metal contamination for possible elemental analysis by ICP-MS. The $PM_{2.5}$ and PM_{10} PEMs are attached to either side of the multi-pollutant monitor using a 10 cm long elutriator. Mini-samplers to measure SO_4^{2-}, NO_3^-, and/or EC and OC concentrations, which are based on traditional monitoring methods, are attached to the front of the elutriator using clips. Similarly, passive O_3 and SO_2/NO_2 badges are placed in the side of the elutriator, with their faces exposed to the sample air stream to allow for constant sampler collection rates. Sample air streams through the elutriator, PEMs, and mini-samplers are drawn using a personal pump operating at approximately 5.2 LPM. The fully configured multi-pollutant sampler plus pump and battery pack weighs approximately 7 lb.

This multi-pollutant sampler has been used in various configurations in several studies conducted throughout the US. In these studies, the performance of the multi-pollutant sampler has been shown to be excellent, with sufficient sensitivity to measure personal, indoor, and outdoor concentrations in most areas within the US. In a study conducted in Los Angeles, California, for example, the precision of $PM_{2.5}$ measurements was high, with values ranging from 6.5 to 9.7 per cent (Chang and Suh 2003). The accuracy of the PEM $PM_{2.5}$ was similarly high, with slopes of the regression of mini-PEM on the traditional HI measurements ranging from 1.2 to 1.3.

Consistent with these findings, mini-samplers have been shown to measure sulphate and nitrate concentrations with a high degree of accuracy. In field validation tests conducted in Boston, Massachusetts, and Southern California, respectively, sulphate and nitrate concentrations measured using mini-samplers were compared to those measured using reference Harvard Impactors (HI). Both mini-samplers were composed of an inlet-impaction section to remove particles larger than 2.5 μm. The sulphate mini-sampler included a Fluoropore filter to collect sulphate, while the nitrate mini-sampler included a coated honeycomb denuder to remove acidic gases, and a Na_2CO_3-coated glass fibre filter to collect nitrate. Results from these tests showed that the mini-samplers performed excellently. For sulphate, regression of the mini-PEM on HI concentrations resulted in slope and R^2 values close to 1 and an insignificant intercept. Similar results were found for nitrate, with an R^2 of 1.0, a slope of 1.04 (± 0.02), and a non-significant intercept when mini-PEM concentrations were regressed on HI concentrations.

The performance of the EC/OC mini-sampler was evaluated in Boston, Massachusetts. Twenty-four hour EC concentrations measured by the mini-sampler were compared to those measured using the reference ChemComb, which consists of a cartridge that contains a $PM_{2.5}$ inlet with impactor, two honeycomb denuders for the removal of selected gases, and a four-stage 47-mm diameter filter pack for the collection of particle-related components. Although the sample size was small ($n = 9$), results of the EC comparison tests showed that the mini-sampler performed well, with a slope of 1.08 (± 0.05), a non-significant intercept, and an R^2 of 0.62. The relatively low R^2 value may be attributed to the fact that samples were collected over a relatively narrow range in ambient EC levels.

14.2.2 Continuous methods

Continuous particulate instruments tend to be larger, more expensive, and more energy intensive than integrated methods. As a result of these size and expense considerations, many continuous instruments cannot be used in personal exposure studies, while others are not suitable or practical for wide-scale use in personal monitoring studies. Several recent exposure studies, however, have used personal nephelometers—a light-scattering technique—to measure short-term (<1 h) particulate mass exposures and to identify important particulate sources (Quintana *et al.* 2000; Chang *et al.* 2001; Howard-Reed *et al.* 2002). The performance of these nephelometers has been shown to be reasonable, particularly when used along with an integrated filter sampler. In a hourly exposure study conducted in Baltimore, Maryland (Chang *et al.* 2001), for example, $PM_{2.5}$ concentrations recorded by the personal nephelometer (Dustrak with an upstream Nafion diffusion dryer) were twice that measured by a 12-h $PM_{2.5}$ filter-based PEM. $PM_{2.5}$ concentrations measured by the nephelometer were, however, strongly associated with those measured using the PEM, with R^2 values of 0.87 and 0.81 in summer and winter, respectively. These results suggest that the nephelometer can be used as a qualitative indicator of $PM_{2.5}$ levels, and if used together with integrated measurements can provide a measure of the temporal and spatial variation in $PM_{2.5}$ exposures.

14.3   Exposure characterization and error

14.3.1   Correlation

As mentioned previously, air pollution epidemiological studies typically use SAM site measurements to assess exposures for their study populations. Since people do not spend all their time at these sites, these measurements clearly are a surrogate measure of exposure and are associated with some amount of error. The amount and direction of this exposure error has been the source of debate, as has its effect on the accuracy and precision of risk coefficients from these epidemiological studies.

Zeger *et al.* (2000) identified three major components of exposure error in time-series epidemiological studies. The first component is the difference between the exposures of the population and people within the population, which can be considered as a measure of the inter-individual variation in exposure. This error component has received little attention, since it is thought to introduce no bias in the effect estimate. However, results from recent exposure studies (as discussed below) have shown that systematic differences in individuals' exposures may exist, which suggests that the effect of this error component on risk estimates may be important to consider. The second error component is that related to spatial variability in ambient concentrations and is stated mathematically as the difference from the true and measured ambient concentrations. For PM, particularly $PM_{2.5}$, this component is thought to contribute little to overall exposure error, since ambient $PM_{2.5}$ concentrations are relatively uniform across large areas (Burton *et al.* 1996). However, for specific components of $PM_{2.5}$ the contribution of spatial variability to exposure error may be more substantial and may be important to consider. The final component is the difference between the average population exposure and the true ambient concentration, which as illustrated using data from the PTEAM study is thought to be the largest contributor to overall exposure error (Zeger *et al.* 2000), with the magnitude of its error varying by particulate component.

The impact of this third component on exposure error in time-series epidemiological studies has been examined in a series of exposure studies (Janssen *et al.* 1997, 2000; Ebelt *et al.* 2000; Evans *et al.* 2000; Rojas-Bracho *et al.* 2000, 2002; Sarnat *et al.* 2000; Williams *et al.* 2000). In these studies, some combination of 12- or 24-h personal, indoor, and outdoor concentrations were measured repeatedly for a cohort of sensitive individuals. The most recent of these studies have focused on $PM_{2.5}$, since it is thought to be the particulate component posing the greatest health hazard (Schwartz *et al.* 1997). Data from these studies were used to examine the individual-specific associations between ambient particulate concentrations and personal exposures, with study findings generally discussed relative to the median, individual-specific personal–ambient correlation coefficient for the study cohort. Results from these studies have consistently showed that the associations between personal exposures and ambient $PM_{2.5}$ concentrations are strong over time. Results from the Janssen *et al.* (2000) study of senior citizens, for example, showed mean personal, indoor, and outdoor concentrations in the Netherlands to equal 24.3, 28.6, and 20.6 $\mu g\,m^{-3}$, respectively. Higher personal and indoor concentrations were attributed to environmental tobacco smoke. Since ETS exposure was limited to few homes, however, its ability to affect the association between personal and outdoor concentrations was limited, as the personal–ambient correlation over time remained high (median $r = 0.79$).

As shown on Table 14.1, the ability of ambient concentrations to act as a surrogate of personal exposures over time is strong in many areas, as similarly strong personal–ambient associations have been shown for studies conducted in the Eastern US (Rojas-Bracho *et al.* 2000; Sarnat *et al.* 2000; Williams *et al.* 2000), and Santiago, Chile (Janssen *et al.* 1997, 2000; Rojas-Bracho *et al.* 2002). More limited data from the Western US (Evans *et al.* 2000; Chang and Suh 2003) and Western Canada (Ebelt *et al.* 2000) indicate that personal–ambient associations are weaker in Western versus Eastern

Table 14.1 Median subject-specific correlation coefficients for the comparison of personal vs. ambient $PM_{2.5}$ levels: by study cohort and location

Cohort	No. of subjects	Days/ Subject	*r* value Median	Range
Children				
The Netherlands[1]	13	6	0.86	−0.11–0.09
Santiago, Chile[2]	20	5	0.80	
Elderly				
Fresno, CA[3]	16	24	0.84	
Baltimore, MD[4]	15	12	0.76	−0.21–0.95
Baltimore, MD[5]	21	5–22	0.80	0.38–0.98
COPD				
Vancouver, BC[6]	16	7	0.48	−0.68–0.83
Boston, MA[7]	18	12–18	0.61	0.10–0.93
Elderly w/CVD				
The Netherlands[8]	36	22	0.79	−0.41–0.98
Helsinki, Finland[8]	46	27	0.76	−0.12–0.97

[1]Janssen *et al.* (1997). [2]Rojas-Bracho *et al.* (2002) pooled *r* value. [3]Evans *et al.* (2000). [4]Sarnat *et al.* (2000). [5]Williams *et al.* (2000). [6]Ebelt *et al.* (2000). [7]Rojas-Bracho *et al.* (2000). [8]Janssen *et al.* (2000).

cities, suggesting that regional or particle compositional differences may impact on the observed personal–ambient.

For PM_{10}, a pollutant with more indoor sources and greater spatial variability, the results are less consistent. In Mexico City, where PM_{10} levels are much higher, the correlation between personal and ambient PM_{10} levels was low with a value of only 0.26 (pooled r value) (Santos-Burgoa *et al.* 1998), while in Japan in a study with minimal indoor sources, an r value close to one was found (Tamura *et al.* 1996). These findings suggest that the presence of local particulate sources, either indoors or outdoors, may reduce the ability of ambient concentrations to act as exposure surrogates.

For potentially sensitive subgroups, such as children, the elderly, or those with pre-existing disease, it is possible that the relationship between personal and ambient exposures over time may differ from those of the general population. These differences may reflect the influence of activity patterns, where children, for example, may spend more time outdoors than adults. Conversely, senior citizens, especially those with pre-existing disease, may be less active as compared to the general population and as a result, may participate in fewer activities that generate particles, such as cooking, cleaning, or tobacco smoking, and may spend less time outdoors. Numerous studies intended to characterize particulate exposures for sensitive subgroups have recently been conducted, with many underway. From the results published to date, the association between personal exposures and ambient concentrations, as reflected by the median personal–ambient correlation coefficient, tends to be comparable across sensitive subgroups (Table 14.1), with perhaps the exception of individuals with chronic obstructive pulmonary disease (COPD), for which the median correlation coefficients are somewhat lower.

For each subgroup, including that for individuals with COPD, however, the personal–ambient association exhibited substantial interpersonal variability, as evidenced by the range in observed correlation coefficients. Results indicate that personal exposures are strongly associated with corresponding outdoor concentrations for some, but not all individuals. This inter-individual variability in the personal–ambient association suggests that although ambient $PM_{2.5}$ may be an appropriate surrogate for population exposures, it may be less able to reflect the exposures of individuals adequately.

14.3.2   Effect modification

Interpersonal variability in the personal–ambient association has been attributed to a number of factors, including residential locations, indoor sources, and housing characteristics. Through their effect on the personal–ambient association, these factors may also account for some of the observed variability in the risks posed by air pollution, both on the individual and population level.

Traffic

Exposure studies, for example, have shown that traffic may have significant impacts on particulate exposures, as studies that use tracers of motor vehicle emissions to reflect traffic-related particulate emissions demonstrate strong gradients in motor vehicle pollution. In a recent report by Salmon *et al.* (1997), 1995 annual average particulate mass concentrations were higher at urban as compared to rural sites in the Northeastern US. Observed differences between urban and rural particulate levels were attributed to corresponding differences in their concentrations of elemental carbon (EC), a tracer of motor vehicle and diesel exhaust, as urban EC levels were considerably higher than corresponding rural levels while urban and rural sulphate concentrations were comparable.

Within a city, both ambient EC concentrations and filter blackness—an indicator of EC—may also vary substantially in relation to local traffic (Nitta *et al.* 1993; Brunekreef *et al.* 1997). In a Harlem, New York City, study, Kinney *et al.* (2000) measured 8-h ambient $PM_{2.5}$ and EC concentrations on four geographically distinct sidewalks and collected corresponding diesel truck, bus, car, and pedestrian count data for each of these sites. Although mean $PM_{2.5}$ concentrations at the four sites varied only slightly, EC concentrations varied widely, with a 4-fold difference observed between the sites. This difference was associated with bus and truck counts on adjacent streets. In inner city Boston, Massachusetts, Levy *et al.* (2001) examined personal exposure to $PM_{2.5}$ in subjects living near a major bus depot. There was considerable variation in exposure to traffic particles, which was related to proximity to the bus depot and diesel traffic. Roorda-Knape *et al.* (1998) have reported strong variations in traffic particles within a city in Europe. Similarly, Belander *et al.* (2001) reported an 11-fold range of variation in estimated exposure to NO_2, a pollutant that originates outdoors predominantly from traffic, across 11,000 residential addresses in Stockholm. Together, these results suggest that exposures to traffic-related pollution will vary spatially, with the highest levels found in areas with a greater density of bus and truck depots, diesel and car traffic, and roads. The magnitude and extent of these exposure gradients are not currently well understood. However, it is likely that the magnitude of these gradients will depend on factors that govern how people are exposed to traffic-related particles and to other particles of outdoor origin.

Further research in this area is needed, as gradients in exposures to traffic-related pollutants may be associated with poorer health. In a recent study of children at risk of asthma, Kramer *et al.* (2000) examined 317 children in three German communities. NO_2 measurements were made outside the homes of each of the children, and personal NO_2 exposures were measured for each child. Outdoor NO_2 concentrations at the homes were shown to vary with traffic density, with the highest levels found at homes with the highest traffic density. The outdoor NO_2 measurements, but not the personal exposures (which reflect indoor generated NO_2 as well), were significant predictors of hay fever, symptoms of allergic rhinitis, wheezing, and sensitization against pollen, house dust mites, or cats. Since outdoor NO_2 is predominantly from traffic, this indicates that traffic pollution, but probably not the NO_2 from traffic, is associated with atopy and wheezing. If NO_2 per se is not the relevant exposure, than diesel particles, or some component of those particles, such as elemental carbon or polycyclic aromatic hydrocarbons (PAHs), may be the most important aetiologic component. In a related study, Lin *et al.* (2002) geo-coded the residential addresses of children admitted to the hospital in Erie County, New York (excluding Buffalo), for asthma and for age-matched controls admitted for non-respiratory conditions. Residential addresses were subsequently linked to Department of Transportation data on vehicle miles traveled on their street. Results from this study showed that (1) the odds of asthma (adjusted for poverty level) for living within 200 m of a street with the highest tertile of traffic density was 1.93 (95% CI 1.13, 3.29) and (2) the asthmatic children were more likely to have truck traffic on their street.

Ventilation

Ventilation conditions may be the most important modifier of exposures to particles of outdoor origin, as ventilation can influence the effective penetration efficiency of particles. In a study by Sarnat *et al.* (2000), personal particulate and gaseous exposures were measured repeatedly for a cohort of senior citizens living in Baltimore, Maryland. In addition to these exposure measurements, participants kept detailed diaries in which they documented information about their activities, including the nature and location of each activity. For activities located indoors, participants were asked to record whether the windows were open. Measured personal particulate and gaseous exposures were subsequently compared to ambient concentrations measured at federal and state SAM sites to examine the influence of various factors on the personal–ambient relationship. Results from this study showed that ventilation, expressed as the fraction of time spent in indoor environments with open windows (f_v), was a significant predictor of the association between ambient and personal $PM_{2.5}$, with the association strongest for individuals spending most of their time in well-ventilated environments (Fig. 14.1(a)) and weakest for individuals spending their time in poorly ventilated environments (Fig. 14.1(b)). Weaker associations for individuals in the poor ventilation category were attributed to lower effective penetration efficiency of $PM_{2.5}$ and to increased influence of indoor particle sources.

The relative importance of these factors was investigated further using the corresponding ambient–personal relationship for sulphate (SO_4^{2-}), a pollutant that has few indoor sources (Koutrakis *et al.* 1992; Tolocka *et al.* 2001) and can therefore be considered a tracer of fine particles of outdoor origin. Unlike $PM_{2.5}$, the strength of the personal–ambient associations for SO_4^{2-} were comparable across ventilation categories (Fig. 14.2(a) and (b)), suggesting that ambient concentrations are strong exposure surrogates of $PM_{2.5}$ of ambient origin. However, the effective penetration efficiency of SO_4^{2-}, as shown by the slope of the personal on ambient regression lines, did vary with ventilation, with the lowest effective penetration efficiencies observed for individuals spending time in poorly ventilated environments. These results suggest that the $PM_{2.5}$ exposures of ambient origin will increase by a smaller amount for people spending time in poorly ventilated as compared to well-ventilated homes for the same increase in outdoor $PM_{2.5}$ concentrations.

These differences may have important implications for epidemiological studies of ambient air pollution. In a recent analysis of data from the National Morbidity, Mortality, and Air Pollution Study (NMAPS), Janssen *et al.* (2002) found differences in ventilation to explain some of the observed variation in the city-specific risk coefficients for hospital admissions and ambient PM_{10} from 14 US cities. In their analyses, risk coefficients from each of the 14 cities were regressed against a population indicator of ventilation— the percentage of air conditioners used in each of these cities—to examine whether ventilation conditions modify the risk posed by outdoor particles. Cities were stratified by whether their PM_{10} levels peaked in the winter or non-winter months.

For both winter and non-winter peaking cities, the risk coefficients were found to decrease with increasing prevalence of air conditioners (Fig. 14.3). This finding is consistent with exposure studies that have shown air conditioner use to be associated with lower air exchange rates, which are in turn associated with lower effective penetration

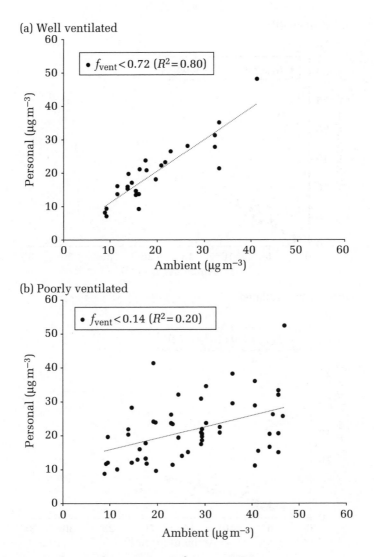

Fig. 14.1 Personal vs. ambient PM$_{2.5}$: Baltimore, MD*.

Source: Adapted from Sarnat *et al.* (2000).

efficiencies for fine particles. As a result, for the same outdoor concentration, exposures will be lower in cities in which air conditioner use is more prevalent as compared to other cities, thus resulting in lower observed risk coefficients for ambient particles. Correspondingly, cities with winter-peaking PM$_{10}$ concentrations were found to have lower risks as compared to other cities. Again, these lower risks may be attributed to home ventilation, where for a given increase in outdoor levels, exposures are lower during the winter months when homes are more tightly sealed.

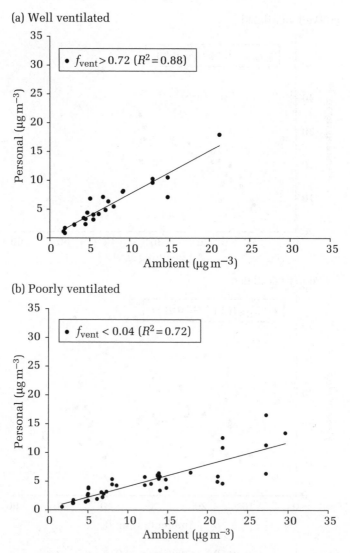

Fig. 14.2   Personal vs. ambient SO$_4^{2-}$: Baltimore, MD*.

Source: Adapted from Sarnat *et al.* (2000).

Particle composition and sources

Particle composition may vary substantially by location. In the Eastern United States, for example, sulphate is the major component of $PM_{2.5}$, accounting for approximately 38 per cent of fine particulate mass (USEPA 2002). By contrast, sulphate constitutes on average only 11 per cent of $PM_{2.5}$ in Western US (USEPA 2002). Similar differences in composition can be found for other $PM_{2.5}$ components, such as crustal materials and elemental carbon. Both components contribute approximately 4 and 15 per cent to

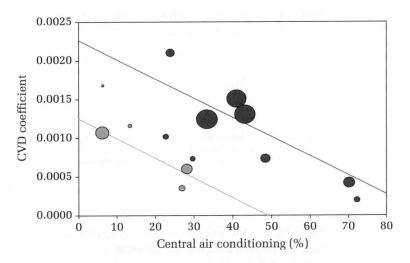

Fig. 14.3 Percentage of homes with AC vs. Regression Coefficients for CVD-related hospital admissions. Dark circles represent cities with non-winter peaking PM_{10} concentrations; light shaded circles represent cities with winter-peaking PM_{10} concentrations. Circle area is proportional to the inverse of the variance of the effect estimate. Lines represent inverse variance weighted regression equations (fixed effect model) (adapted from Janssen *et al.* 2002).

$PM_{2.5}$ in the Eastern and Western US, respectively (USEPA 2002). Results from exposure studies have shown that these differences in particle composition may also modify the impact of particle exposures on health and have provided information that better define the roles of particles as potential causative factors of respiratory and cardiovascular disease.

The impact of particle composition on health has been examined using a variety of techniques, including the use of specific particle components as source tracers, particle emission inventories to examine the impact of particle sources on health, and source apportionment and other statistical methods to quantify source contributions. Using source apportionment methods, for example, Laden *et al.* (2000) showed that traffic particles were associated with daily deaths, independent of particles from coal or residual oil burning, and that their effect was triple that of the coal-derived particles (Table 14.2). Janssen *et al.* (2002) used particle emission inventories from the US Environmental Protection Agency (EPA) to examine the contribution of particle sources to variability in the cardiovascular health risks in their 14-city reanalysis of NMAPS data (Table 14.3). Results from this reanalysis showed that the city-specific effect size for heart disease admissions (adjusted for the proportion of homes with central air conditioning) increased with the fraction of PM_{10} emissions from traffic and oil combustion. PM_{10} hospital admission coefficients increased by 55 per cent (standard error 10%) and 38 per cent (standard error 9%) for traffic and oil combustion emissions, respectively, for an inter-quartile range increase in the proportion of PM_{10} emissions from traffic.

Table 14.2. Percentage increase in daily deaths by specific $PM_{2.5}$ sources: six cities study (1979–88)*

Source factor	% Increase	95% CI
Crustal (Si)	−2.3	−5.8–1.2
Motor vehicles (Pb)	3.4	1.7–5.2
Coal (Se)	1.1	0.3–2.0

*Percentage increase in daily deaths associated with 10 $\mu g\,m^{-3}$ increase in mass concentration from source. Cities: Boston, MA, St. Louis, MO, Knoxville, TN, Madison, WI, Steubenville, OH, Topeka, KS. Adapted from Laden *et al.* (2000).

Table 14.3. Percentage change in ambient PM_{10} on CVD-hospital admissions coefficients by source type*

	β CVD, Lag 0/1	
Source parameter	% change	s.e. (%)
% PM_{10} from		
Highway vehicles	55.3**	9.9
Highway diesels	52.8**	9.4
Coal combustion	0.6	2.6
Oil combustion	37.5**	9.3
Wood burning	2.7	3.2
Metal processing	29.0**	13.0
Fugitive dust	−49.4**	16.5

*Percentage change for inter-quartile increase in source parameter, adjusted for central AC.
**$p<0.05$.
Source: Adapted from Janssen *et al.* (2001).

14.3.3 Confounding

Exposure assessment research has been able to address directly whether confounding by gaseous pollutants is possible in epidemiological studies of PM. Traditionally, the issue of confounding has been examined in epidemiological studies indirectly using multi-pollutant statistical models and by examining correlations among ambient $PM_{2.5}$ and ambient co-pollutant concentrations. The recent development of the multi-pollutant monitor, however, has allowed the relationship between personal $PM_{2.5}$ exposures and personal gaseous pollutant exposures to be assessed for the first time.

Over the past 5 years, several studies have been conducted that measure personal particulate and gaseous exposures simultaneously; however, results from most of these studies have not yet been finalized. In one of the earliest of these studies (Sarnat *et al.* 2000), associations among personal exposures to $PM_{2.5}$, coarse particles, ozone, sulphur dioxide, and nitrogen dioxide were examined for a cohort of senior citizens living in Baltimore, Maryland. Their exposures were compared to those among the ambient concentrations and to those between the ambient concentrations and personal exposures for the individual pollutants (Sarnat *et al.* 2001).

As shown in Table 14.4, results from this study showed that ambient $PM_{2.5}$ concentrations were strongly associated with corresponding ambient concentrations of several gaseous co-pollutants, including ozone, although the strength and direction of these associations differed by season. For example, ambient ozone was positively associated with ambient $PM_{2.5}$ in the summer and negatively associated with ambient $PM_{2.5}$ in the winter. Based on ambient results alone, then, it is reasonable to assume that confounding by gaseous co-pollutants may impact observed associations between ambient $PM_{2.5}$ and health. With the exception of $PM_{2.5}$, however, ambient pollutant concentrations were weak indicators of their respective personal exposures. Similarly, the associations among the personal $PM_{2.5}$ and gaseous pollutant exposures were also weak. These weak associations among personal $PM_{2.5}$, ozone, nitrogen dioxide, and sulphur dioxide, together with the strong personal–ambient associations for $PM_{2.5}$, provide evidence that the observed $PM_{2.5}$-associated health effects are not due to confounding by the gaseous pollutants, at least for individuals with similar exposure profiles and living in similar urban locations. While exposures to the gaseous co-pollutants are unlikely to be potential confounders of $PM_{2.5}$ for this study population, ambient co-pollutant concentrations were found to be surrogates of personal $PM_{2.5}$. Ambient ozone was significantly correlated with personal $PM_{2.5}$, with the same seasonal pattern observed as in the associations between their ambient levels.

The generalizability of the Baltimore study findings to other cities and to other cohorts is not yet known, but should become clearer as results from more multi-pollutant exposures studies become available. Despite this, results from the Baltimore study have

Table 14.4 Relationship between ambient concentrations and personal exposures to $PM_{2.5}$ and ozone

Comparison	Total $PM_{2.5}$			$PM_{2.5}$ of ambient origin		
	n^*	Slope	*t*-value	n	Slope	*t*-value
Ambient $PM_{2.5}$ vs. ambient O_3						
Summer	48	0.84	5.98			
Winter	37	−0.67	−5.56			
Personal $PM_{2.5}$ vs. personal O_3						
Summer	24/193	0.21	1.31	15/130	0.22	1.56
Winter	45/434	−0.05	−0.20	30/282	−0.18	−1.66
Personal $PM_{2.5}$ vs. ambient O_3						
Summer	24/225	0.28	4.00	15/150	0.37	6.23
Winter	45/487	−0.29	−4.86	30/301	−0.36	−14.04

*For personal exposure comparisons, n indicates the number of subjects and the total number of person days.
Source: Adapted from Sarnat *et al.* (2001).

already helped explain results from epidemiological air pollution studies, as illustrated by Sarnat *et al.* (2001) using ozone mortality results from the NMAPS. In the NMAPS, data from 90 cities were compiled to assess the percentage change in mortality associated with changes in ambient air pollutant concentrations. Among other findings, ozone was found to be positively associated with mortality in the summer but to have a seemingly protective effect in the winter months. This wintertime protective relationship was 'puzzling and (may) reflect some unmeasured confounding factor'. The Baltimore study findings suggest that the wintertime ozone finding may be due to ambient ozone acting as a surrogate for $PM_{2.5}$ exposures, where the observed negative wintertime associations between ambient ozone and mortality reflect a corresponding negative association between ambient ozone and personal $PM_{2.5}$ exposures.

14.4 Summary

Particulate matter provides just one example of how exposure assessment research is a critical and necessary component of health effect studies. Similar examples of the importance of exposure assessment research can also be found using other pollutants as case studies, including gaseous air pollutants, such as ozone and nitrogen dioxide, as well as other single- or multi-media pollutants, such as lead and polychlorinated biphenyls.

Exposure assessment has multiple roles. It is a tool to measure and characterize exposures for study populations. It also plays an important role in the quantification of exposure error, in the identification of factors that may modify exposure–disease relationships, and in the examination of the potential for confounding by other ambient pollutants. Moreover, together with epidemiological and toxicological studies, results from future exposure studies will help to answer current questions about particle health effects regarding sensitive populations, biological mechanisms, and chemical composition. The benefits provided by these advances will likely be far-reaching, as they will ultimately be used to develop sound and cost-effective regulatory policies to protect public health.

References

Belander, T., Berglind, N., Gustavsson, P., Jonson, T., Nyberg, F., Pershagen, G., and Jarup, L. (2001). Using geographic information systems to assess individual historical exposure to air pollution from traffic and house heating in Stockholm. *Environmental Health Perspectives*, **109**, 633–9.

Brunekreef, B., Janssen, N. A. H., deHartog, J., Hassema, H., Knape, M., and vanVliet, P. (1997). Air pollution from truck traffic and lung function in children living near motorways. *Epidemiology*, **8**, 298–303.

Burton, R. M., Suh, H. H., and Koutrakis, P. (1996). Characterization of outdoor particle concentrations within metropolitan Philadelphia. *Environmental Science and Technology*, **30**, 400–7.

Chang, L.-T., Sarnat, J., Wolfson, J. M., Rojas-Bracho, L., Suh, H. H., and Koutrakis, P. (1999). Development of a personal multi-pollutant exposure sampler for particulate matter and criteria Gases. *Pollution Atmosphérique*, **10**, 31–9.

Chang, L. T., Suh, H. H., Wolfson, J. M., Misra, K., Allen, G. A., Catalano, P., and Koutrakis, P. (2001). Laboratory and field evaluation of measurement methods for one-hour exposures to O_3, $PM_{2.5}$, and CO. *Journal of the Air and Waste Management Association*, **51**, 1414–22.

Chang, L. T. and Suh, H. H. (2003). *Characterization of the Composition of Personal, Indoor, and Outdoor Particulate Exposures*. Report to the California Air Resources Board. Contract No. 98-330.

Ebelt, S. T., Petkau, A. J., Vedal, S., Fisher, T. V., and Brauer, M. (2000). Exposure of chronic obstructive pulmonary disease patients to particulate matter: relationships between personal and ambient air concentrations. *Journal of the Air and Waste Management Association*, **50**, 1081–94.

Evans, G. F., Highsmith, R. V., Sheldon, L. S., Suggs, J. C., Williams, W. R., Zweidinger, R. B., Creason, J. P., Walsh, D., Rhodes, C. E., and Lawless, P. A. (2000). The 1999 Fresno particulate matter exposure studies: comparison of community, outdoor, and residential PM mass measurements. *Journal of the Air and Waste Management Association*, **50**, 1700–3.

Howard-Reed, C., Rea, A. W., Zufall, M. J., Burke, J. M., Williams, R. W., Suggs, J. C., Sheldon, L. S., Walsh, D., and Kwock, R. (2002). Use of a continuous nephelometer to measure personal exposure to particles during the U. S. Environmental Protection Agency Baltimore and Fresno panel studies. *Journal of the Air and Waste Management Association*, **50**, 1125–32.

Janssen, N. A. H., Hoek, G., Harssema, J., and Brunekreef, B. (1997). Childhood exposure to PM_{10}: Relation between personal, classroom, and outdoor concentrations. *Occupational and Environmental Medicine*, **54**, 888–94.

Janssen, N. A. H., De Hartog, J. J., Hoek, G., Brunekreef, B., Lanki, T., Timonen, K. L., and Pekkanen, J. (2000). Personal exposure to fine particulate matter in elderly subjects: relation between personal, indoor, and outdoor concentrations. *Journal of the Air and Waste Management Association*, **50**, 1133–43.

Janssen, N. A. H., Schwartz, J., Zanobetti, A., and Suh, H. H. (2002). Air conditioning and source-specific particles as modifiers of the effect of PM_{10} on hospital admissions for heart and lung disease. *Environmental Health Perspectives*, **110**, 43–9.

Kinney, P. L., Aggarwal, M., Northridge, M. E., Janssen, N. A. H., and Shepard, P. (2000). *Environmental Health Perspectives*, **108**, 213–18.

Koutrakis, P., Briggs, S. L. K., and Leaderer, B. P. (1992). Source apportionment of indoor aerosols in Suffolk and Onondaga Counties, New York. *Environmental Science and Technology*, **26**, 521–7.

Kramer, U., Koch, T., Ranft, U., Ring, J., and Behrendt, H. (2000). Traffic related air pollution is associated with atopy in children living in urban areas. *Epidemiology*, **11**, 64–70.

Laden, F., Neas, L. M., Dockery, D. W., and Schwartz, J. (2000). Association of fine particulate matter from different sources with daily mortality in six US cities. *Environmental Health Perspectives*, **108**, 941–7.

Levy, J. I., Houseman, E. A., Spengler, J. D., Loh, P., and Ryan, L. (2001). Fine particulate matter and polycyclic aromatic hydrocarbon concentration patterns in Roxbury, Massachusetts: a community-based GIS analysis. *Environmental Health Perspectives*, **109**, 341–7.

Lin, S., Munsie, J. P., Hwang, S. A., Fitzgerald, E., and Cayo, M. R. (2002). Childhood asthma hospitalization and residential exposure to state route traffic. *Environmental Research*, **88**, 73–81.

National Research Council (1998). *Research priorities for airborne particulate matter. 1. Immediate priorities and a long-range research portfolio*. National Academy Press, Washington, DC.

Nitta, H., Sato, T., Nakai, S., Maeda, K., Aoki, S., and Ono, M. (1993). Respiratory health associated with exposure to automobile exhaust. I: Results of cross-sectional studies in 1979, 1982, and 1983. *Archives of Environmental Health*, **48**, 53–8.

Pope, C. A. (2000). Review: epidemiological basis for particulate air pollution health standards. *Aerosol Science and Technology*, **32**, 4–14.

Quintana, P. J. E., Samimi, B. S., Kleinman, M. T., Liu, L. J., Soto, K., Warner, G. Y., Bufalino, C., Valencia, J., Francis, D., Hovell, M. H., and Delfino, R. J. (2000). Evaluation of a real-time passive personal particle monitor in fixed site residential indoor and ambient measurements. *Journal of Exposure Analysis and Environmental Epidemiology*, **10**, 437–45.

Rojas-Bracho, L., Suh, H., and Koutrakis, P. (2000). Relationship among personal, indoor, and outdoor fine and coarse particulate concentrations for individuals with COPD. *Journal of Exposure Analysis and Environmental Epidemiology*, **10**, 294–306.

Rojas-Bracho, L., Suh, H. H., Oyola, P., and Koutrakis, P. (2002). Measurements of children's exposures to particles and nitrogen dioxide in Santiago, Chile. *Science of the Total Environment*, **287**, 249–64.

Roorda-Knape, M. C., Janssen, N. A., de Hartog, J., Van Vliet, P. H., Harssema, H., and Brunekreef, B. (1998). Air pollution from traffic in city districts near motorways. *Atmospheric Environment*, **32**, 1921–30.

Salmon, L. G., Cass, G. R., Pederen, D. U., Durant, J. L., Gibb, R., Lunts, A., and Utell, M. (1997). *Determination of fine particle concentration and chemical composition in the Northeastern United States*, 1995. Report to NESCAUM.

Samet, J. M., Dominici, F., Curriero, F. C., Coursac, I., and Zeger, S. L. (2000). Fine particulate air pollution and mortality in 20 U. S. cities, 1987–1994. *New England Journal of Medicine*, **343**, 1742–9.

Santos-Burgoa, C., Rojas-Bracho, L., Rosas-Perez, I., Ramierez-Sanchez, A., Sanchez-Rico, G., and Mejia-Hernandez, S. (1998). Particle exposure modeling in the general population and risk or respiratory disease. *Gaceta Médica de México*, **134**, 407–17.

Sarnat, J., Koutrakis, P., and Suh, H. H. (2000). Assessing the relationship between personal particulate and gaseous exposures of senior citizens living in Baltimore, MD. *Journal of the Air and Waste Management Association*, **50**, 1184–98.

Sarnat, J. A., Schwartz, J., Catalano, P. J., and Suh, H. H. (2001). Gaseous pollutants in particulate matter epidemiology: confounders or surrogates? *Environmental Health Perspectives*, **109**, 1053–61.

Schwartz, J., Dockery, D. W., and Neas, L. M. (1997). Is daily mortality associated specifically with fine particles? *Journal of the Air and Waste Management Association*, **46**, 927–39.

Tamura, J. K., Ando, M., Sagai, M., and Matsumoto, Y. (1996). Estimation of levels of personal exposures to suspended particulate matter and nitrogen dioxide in Tokyo. *Environmental Science (Japan)*, **4**, 37–51.

Tolocka, M. P., Solomon, P. A., Mitchell, W., Norris, G. A., Gemmill, D. B., Wiener, R. W., Vanderpool, R. W., Homolya, J. B., and Rice, J. (2001). East versus West in the US: chemical characteristics of $PM_{2.5}$ during the Winter of 1999. *Aerosol Science and Technology*, **34**, 88–96.

US Environmental Protection Agency (2002). *Third external review draft of air quality criteria for particulate matter*. Office of Research and Development, Washington, DC.

Williams, R., Creason, J., Zweidinger, R., Watts, R., Sheldon, L., and Shy, C. (2000). Indoor, outdoor, and personal exposure monitoring of particulate air pollution: the Baltimore elderly epidemiology-exposure pilot study. *Atmospheric Environment*, **34**, 4193–204.

Zeger, S. L., Thomas, D., Dominici, F., Samet, J. M., Schwartz, J., Dockery, D., and Cohen, A. (2000). Exposure measurement error in time-series studies of air pollution: concepts and consequences. *Environmental Health Perspectives*, **108**, 419–26.

15. Exposure assessment in studies of chlorination disinfection by-products and birth outcomes

Mark J. Nieuwenhuijsen

15.1 Introduction

15.1.1 Chlorination disinfection by-products

Chlorination has been the major disinfectant process for drinking water and swimming pools in many countries for many years. The added chlorine reacts with naturally occurring organic matter such as humic and fulvic acids, to form a wide range of halogenated organic compounds, which were first reported just over 25 years ago (Rook 1974). These compounds are referred to as chlorination disinfection by-products (DBPs). They include trihalomethanes (THMs), haloacetonitriles (HANs), haloketones (HKs), chloropicrin (CP), and haloacetic acids (HAAs) (Krasner *et al.* 1989) (Table 15.1). Epidemiological research of adverse birth outcomes has mainly focussed on the THMs, a volatile group of compounds, which consists of chloroform, bromodichloromethane (BDCM), chlorodibromomethane (CDBM), and bromoform, as these occur in the highest quantities and are routinely measured throughout water supplies. They are used as a marker for other DBPs, which may or may not always be appropriate. The major difficulty in studying such epidemiological associations lies in the exposure assessment (Reif *et al.* 1996; Swan and Waller 1998; Nieuwenhuijsen *et al.* 2000*a,b*; Arbuckle *et al.* 2002). This chapter discusses the issues in the exposure assessment, the approaches that have been used, and the way ahead.

15.1.2 Variation in DBPs

There is temporal and spatial variation in DBP levels. Chloroform is usually the most prevalent by-product compound formed, although brominated THMs can occur at high levels when waters with high bromide levels are chlorinated. The formation of the by-products is a function of disinfection processes and chemicals, water source, pH, temperature, concentration of chlorine residual, residence time, reaction time, total or organic carbon (TOC), and bromide content. DBP levels are generally much lower in ground water compared to surface water (Arora *et al.* 1997). Residence time in the distribution system affects the concentration of various DBPs; THMs increase with increasing residence time, whilst mean concentrations of HANs, HKs, CP, and HAAs

Table 15.1   Disinfection by-products and highest quarterly averages as measured by Krasner *et al.* (1989) in the US

Disinfection by-product	Highest quarterly average (μg l^{-1})
Trihalomethanes	44
Chloroform	
Bromodichloromethane	
Chlorodibromomethane	
Bromoform	
Haloacids	21
Monochloroacetic acid	
Dichloroacetic acid	
Trichloroacetic acid	
Monobroacetic acid	
Dibromoacetic acid	
Aldehydes	6.9
Formaldehyde	
Acetaldehyde	
Haloacetonitriles	4.0
Trichloroacetonitrile	
Dichloroacetonitrile	
Bromochloroacetonitrile	
Dibromoacetronitrile	
Haloketones	1.8
1,1-Dichloropropanone	
1,1,1-Trichloropropanone	
Miscellaneous	
Chloropicrin	
Chloral hydrate	
Cyanogen chloride	
2,4,6-Trichlorophenol	

decrease (Krasner *et al.* 1989; Stevens *et al.* 1989; Chen and Weisel 1998; Krasner 1999). Higher temperatures in the warm season and possibly differences in the type and quantity of organic matter present in the source water may increase the production of TTHMs, dichloroacetonitrile, bromochloroacetonitrile, 1,1,1-trichloropropanone, and chloropicrin in the water as compared with the cold season (Chen and Weisel 1998), although this pattern may not always be so consistent (Whitaker *et al.* 2003a). Higher pHs have been associated with higher TTHMs levels but with lower levels of some HAAs (Stevens *et al.* 1989; Krasner 1999), while higher levels of both bromide and TOC have been associated with higher THM levels (Krasner *et al.* 1994; Arora *et al.* 1997). The TCAA/THM ratio was higher in humic acid-rich waters compared with fulvic acid rich waters resulting in a good correlation between specific UV absorbance, which is higher for the humic acid and Trichloroacetic acid- (TCAA)/THM ratio (Reckhow *et al.* 1990).

15.1.3 Correlation between DBPs

Krasner *et al.* (1989) found a high correlation between the sum of all the disinfection by-products levels and TTHM levels ($r = 0.96$), and a good correlation between the sum of non-THM disinfection by-products and TTHM levels ($r = 0.76$). The correlation between TTHMs and HANs was also high ($r = 0.9$), as was the correlation between dibromoacetic acid (DBAA) and CDBM ($r = 0.91$), but the correlation between TTHMs and HKs was low ($r = 0.06$). Keegan *et al.* (2001) reported a high correlation between TTHMs and chloroform ($r = 0.97$), but less so for TTHMs and BDCM ($r = 0.65$) and TTHM and both CDBM and bromoform ($r < 0.2$).

15.1.4 Exposure pathways and routes

Exposure to DBPs may occur via several exposure pathways and routes and the relative importance of these may be different for different DBPs. For non-volatile compounds, such as the HAAs, ingestion appears to be the major route of exposure (Weisel *et al.* 1999; Kim *et al.* 1999). However, exposure to volatile compounds present in tap water, such as the THMs, occurs not only via ingestion, but also via inhalation, and dermal absorption, for example, during showering, bathing, swimming, boiling water, and dish washing (see Chapter 1, Fig. 1.2). Chloroform uptake due to inhalation and dermal absorption can be considerably greater than through ingestion (Levesque *et al.* 1994; Weisel and Jo 1996; Gordon *et al.* 1998; Whitaker *et al.* 2003c). Temperature can affect the uptake of chloroform, for example, dermal absorption during bathing was calculated to be 30 times higher in water at 40°C than in water at 30°C (Gordon *et al.* 1998). Little work has been done on DBPs other than THMs and HAAs.

15.1.5 Biomonitoring

Total uptake of DBPs can be estimated by modelling the DBP uptake, for example, by combining information on the ingestion rate and levels of DBPs in water and/or combining the frequency and duration of exposure of various DBP-related activities (e.g. showering and swimming), inhalation and skin absorption rate and levels of DBPs in water in case of, for example, the volatile THMs. Alternatively total uptake can be estimated by biomonitoring, which provides an integrated measure of the uptake (see Chapter 11). DBPs can be measured in, for example, human exhaled breath, serum, or urine. To estimate chloroform and other THM uptake exhaled breath sampling techniques can be used (Levesque *et al.* 1994; Aggazotti *et al.* 1995; Weisel and Jo 1996; Gordon *et al.* 1998; Weisel *et al.* 1999) and/or serum measurements can be obtained (Levesque *et al.* 1994; Aggazotti *et al.* 1995; Backer *et al.* 2000; Lynberg *et al.* 2001). As the concentration of a volatile compound in exhaled breath is related to its concentration in the bloodstream, it can be used as a proxy to determine changes in body burden with time. Simple linear regression analyses between alveolar chloroform and plasma chloroform showed a good correlation ($r = 0.91$) (Levesque *et al.* 1994). Measurement of the concentration of chloroform in alveolar air is at times preferred over serum chloroform because air sampling is more practical and less invasive, although its use is limited because it is not as sensitive as serum measurements. The main drawback of biomonitoring is the fairly short biological half-life of chloroform (approximately 30 min). It is therefore important to account for time since last exposure. Ashley and Prah (1997) have suggested that the decay is a complex three-order process and possibly four. The complex decay allows a very short half-life after acute exposure, but also bioaccumulation with repeated exposure, followed by slow release.

TCAA and Dichloroacetic acid (DCAA) uptake has been estimated recently using urine monitoring (Kim and Weisel 1998; Kim *et al.* 1999; Weisel *et al.* 1999). TCAA appeared to have a longer biological half-life (70–120 h) than DCAA (<2 h) and showed a fairly good correlation with ingestion exposure (Kim *et al.* 1999). Weisel *et al.* (1999) found a strong correlation between estimated ingested exposure and TCAA in urine ($r = 0.81$), but not for estimated ingested exposure and DCAA ($r = -0.1$) for a group of people who did not work outside the home.

15.1.6   PBPK modelling

Physiologically based pharmacokinetic (PBPK) models have been used, based often on parameters obtained by Corley *et al.* (1990) to model the relative uptake from various exposure routes and the distribution of chloroform in the body but the main target organs were generally the kidney and liver, and they have not been used in epidemiological studies (Nieuwenhuijsen *et al.* 2000*b*). PBPK modelling offers great opportunities to refine exposure assessment (see Chapter 10).

15.2   Exposure indices used in epidemiological studies of DBPs and reproductive outcomes

The epidemiological studies of birth outcomes that have been carried out so far can be categorized into three approaches according to the exposure indices they have used: (a) water source and/or treatment, (b) modelled or measured routinely collected THMs in the water zone or region, and (c) modelled or measured routinely collected THMs in the water zone or region combined with some form of personal exposure estimate such as ingested amount or duration while showering or swimming they are summarised in Table 15.2. A more detailed discussion of the interpretation of the epidemiological studies can be found elsewhere (Nieuwenhuijsen *et al.* 2000*a*; Gravecker Graves *et al.* 2001).

15.3   Discussion of the various approaches

The different approaches have their strengths and limitations and none are perfect. Design issues such as sample size and data sources in the epidemiological studies play an important role in the choice of exposure assessment. Many studies have used routinely collected health data (registry data) and in this case only limited exposure-related information could be obtained from the subjects in the study, for example, address but

Table 15.2   Exposure indices used in reproductive epidemiological studies

Study	Exposure indices
Water source and water treatment	
Aschengrau *et al.* (1989)	Based on maternal residential address to ascertain type of water supply; surface vs. ground water, chlorination vs. chloraminated water for surface water
Aschengrau *et al.* (1993)	Based on maternal residential address to ascertain type of water supply, chlorination vs. chloramination, and ground/mixed water vs. surface water.
Kanitz *et al.* (1996)	Based on maternal residential address to ascertain type of water source, chlorine dioxide and/or hypochlorite vs. not treated.
Magnus *et al.* (1999) Jaakkola *et al.* (2001)	Based on maternal residential address to ascertain type of water supply; chlorination yes vs. no, colour high vs. low
Kallen *et al.* (2000)	Based on maternal residential address to ascertain type of water supply; no vs. sodium hypochlorite, no vs. chlorine dioxide
Yang *et al.* (2000*a*) Yang *et al.* (2000*b*)	Based on maternal residential address to ascertain type of water supply; chlorinated (>95% pop. served chlorin. water) vs. non-chlorinated (<5% pop. served chlorin. water)
Routinely collected THM water measurements (including some modelling	
Kramer *et al.* (1992)	Based on maternal residential address and one municipal water survey to estimate individual THM levels in water (2 or 3 exposure categories).
Bove *et al.* (1995)	Based on maternal residential address and municipal water surveys to estimate monthly TTHM levels (5 or 6 exposure categories)
Gallagher *et al.* (1998)	Based on maternal residential address and municipal water surveys. Estimate of household TTHM level during last trimester based on hydraulic modelling (4 exposure categories)
Dodds *et al.* (1999) King *et al.* (2000) Dodds and King (2001)	Based on maternal residential address and TTHM levels for public water facilities (3 sampling locations) modelled using linear regression on the basis of observations by year, month, and facility (4 exposure categories)
Routinely or specially collected THM and other DBP water measurements combined with information on personal exposure	
Savitz *et al.* (1995)	Based on maternal residential address and quarterly municipal water surveys to estimate average TTHM levels. Analysis of: (a) surface vs. ground water source (b) TTHM levels (3 exposure categories) (c) consumption during pregnancy (d) water source × amount (e) TTHM dose (level × amount)
Waller *et al.* (1998)	Based on maternal residential address and quarterly municipal water surveys to estimate average TTHM and individual THM levels. Analysis based on: (a) THM levels (3 or 10 exposure categories) (b) consumption during first trimester from interview (2 exposure categories)
Klotz and Pyrch (1999)	Based on residential address and public water facility TTHM data, and tap-water sampling for TTHMs, HANs, and HAAs (3–5 exposure categories)

not personal information on DBP-related characteristics. Also, for studies with a large study population it is difficult to carry out an individual exposure assessment taking into account, for example, personal characteristics, because of the time and effort involved and financial restraints. In both cases routinely collected THM data have been used as the basis for an exposure index. One of the main problems is that the putative agent is unknown, if there is any at all. THM data have generally been used as a marker for the total DBP load, but often there may not be a good relation between THMs and other by-products, in which case exposure misclassification may occur. The largest proportion of TTHM is often chloroform, and TTHM levels show only moderate correlation with the other THMs. This suggests that when studies have used TTHM as an exposure index, they were most likely examining the effects of chloroform or other substances strongly correlated with TTHMs or chloroform. While various studies used TTHM exposure levels as the exposure index, several others have used individual THMs and showed independent effect(s), particularly for bromodichloromethane (Kramer *et al.* 1992; Waller *et al.* 1998; King *et al.* 2000; Dodds and King 2001).

None of the epidemiological studies have included all the exposure pathways and routes for an integrated measure, for example, for THMs. For the major non-volatile disinfection by-products, the HAAs, ingestion appears to be the major route of uptake, but only one study so far has examined HAAs (Klotz and Pyrch 1999). Differences in routes of uptake may explain differences in epidemiological findings and potentially allows inferences about putative agents. The California study suggested that the major exposure route for a putative agent of spontaneous abortion would be ingestion and that it would be a brominated compound, or a substance correlated with it (Swan *et al.* 1998; Waller *et al.* 1998; Waller *et al.* 1999).

A limitation of all the epidemiological studies to date has been that only THM exposures at home were taken into account and not those outside the home, for example, at work, where THM levels might be different. This may lead to exposure misclassification. Water consumption outside the home can be considerable (Hopkins and Ellis 1980; Shimokura *et al.* 1998). Waller *et al.* (1998) carried out separate analyses for women employed outside the home, and found that risk estimates for those employed outside the home were considerably lower compared with those at home, suggesting either attenuation of risk estimates as a result of misclassification of exposure or a confounding factor associated with the home. Also, given that an American study found that over 20 per cent of pregnant women moved residence between the time of conception and delivery (Shaw and Halinka 1991), the possibility of confounding or risk attenuation from residential mobility during pregnancy cannot be ruled out for the various studies.

15.4   Personal or water zone estimates

Epidemiological studies require accurate, precise, and biologically relevant exposure estimates, preferably with a large range, which, as can be seen from this review, makes the exposure assessment fairly challenging. Inaccurate and imprecise exposure estimates may lead to loss of power and precision and attenuation in health-risk estimates, depending on the type of error model (see Chapter 12). Researchers generally have to perform some cost–benefit analysis when it comes to choosing an exposure estimate for an epidemiological study. Improving the accuracy of the exposure estimate will improve study power and the accuracy and/or precision of the effects of the exposure, but it is likely to come at a financial cost. For example, personal exposure assessment such as questionnaire data on water-related activities combined with subjects' tap water DBP levels or biomonitoring of exhaled breath or urine may provide a much more accurate exposure estimate for each study subject than a group estimate such as a water zone mean estimate, at least when a sufficient number of samples are taken. However it may come at a financial cost that is also considerably higher, and may be well out of reach of the study. Relative large sample sizes may be needed for epidemiological studies of birth outcomes, for example, for prospective cohort studies, given that many of the outcomes of interest are rare. Case–control studies may require fewer subjects, but the biomonitoring has to take place after the relevant exposure period and is therefore likely to be less informative than in other study designs with a retrospective exposure assessment. Questionnaire data are also likely to be less accurate than in a prospective design.

In epidemiological studies using personal (i.e. individual) estimates, the variability in these personal activities may lead to measurement error, and therefore attenuation of health-risk estimates, under the classical error model (see Chapter 12). Attenuation is less likely to occur when a group estimate is used as an exposure index, such as the mean estimates of water zones, because the Berkson error model may apply. In linear, and often in log-linear models, Berkson error is generally unlikely to lead to attenuation in health-risk estimates, only to less precise ones, which may reduce study power. The efficiency in this case is equal to the proportion of variance of personal uptake explained by water zone means, that is, the square of the correlation between personal uptake and water zone mean.

There is little information on variation in individual exposure estimates in epidemiological studies, partly because the estimates are only obtained once, rather than repeatedly, in which case it is difficult to estimate the extent of attenuation. There is information on the relation between DBP levels in water and actual uptake as discussed previously, including how personal estimates can be improved. For example, Weisel *et al.* (1999) found a strong relation between concentrations of chloroform in water and exhaled breath shortly after showering, suggesting the former is an important determinant of the latter, but there is no relation between TCAA in water and urine. However, they found a fairly good relation between TCAA in water and urine when they included water ingestion patterns, suggesting that ingestion patterns are an important determinant, which is essential information for the design of epidemiological studies including power calculations. Answers to questionnaires could also be a source of variability, which may lead to attenuation in risk estimates in individual epidemiological studies, therefore validation of the questionnaire is important. Shimokura *et al.* (1998) compared a tap water questionnaire with a three-day diary (the 'gold standard') and found a good correlation ($r = 0.78$) for drinking water intake, but estimates obtained by questionnaire were almost twice as high as those obtained by the diary (0.75 vs. 0.40 $1 day^{-1}$). However, analysis of the daily water consumption questionnaires showed that the largest proportion in the variation in consumption is explained by differences between individuals (ICC $= 0.61$), which is good for an epidemiological study, although there were differences between full-time (ICC $= 0.42$) and part-time or less-employed (ICC $= 0.81$) women.

But when using ecological exposure estimates such as water zone estimates, what is the relationship between the water zone estimates and the actual uptake of DBPs? Lynberg *et al.* (2001) and Backer *et al.* (2000) carried out a number of studies in which they measured the THM concentrations in water and in serum, as background levels and after showering. When plotting the average values for the three regions, the plots show that there is a good relationship between water and serum chloroform levels for both background and after showering concentrations, suggesting that chloroform levels in

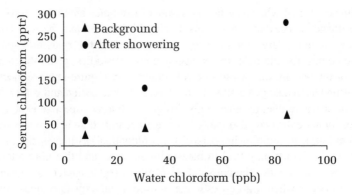

Fig. 15.1   Chloroform in serum vs. chloroform in water before and after showering.

water may be a good indicator for uptake of chloroform (Fig. 15.1). The serum background levels suggest that some bioaccumulation and slow release of chloroform has
taken place (Ashley and Prah 1997; Lynberg *et al.* 2001). The data also suggests that
uptake during showering is large and increases the serum chloroform levels well
beyond the background levels. Furthermore, there was a lot of variability in the chloroform levels within the three regions, which may be explained by differences in personal
behaviour and suggests that the relationship is not as smooth as the figure suggests
(Backer *et al.* 2000; Lynberg *et al.* 2001).

Whitaker *et al.* (2003*c*) simulated the relationship between chloroform levels in the
water (average of tap-water samples in a water zone) and predicted uptake of chloroform in pregnant women to assess the potential extent of exposure misclassification and
measurement error in epidemiological studies. They used available data from the literature to assign statistical distributions to the frequency and duration of swimming,
showering, and bathing, average daily tap-water intake, and swimming pool chloroform
concentrations. They used results of studies that measured blood chloroform concentrations after swimming, showering, bathing, and ingesting tap water to estimate the
average chloroform uptake per minute per microgram per litre chloroform in the water
spent on showering, bathing, and swimming and chloroform uptake (μg) for every litre
of ingested tap water per microgram per litre chloroform in the water (Fig. 15.2).
Chloroform concentrations were obtained from their epidemiological study region in
the north of England. An average daily chloroform uptake (μg) over a 90-day period
was simulated for 300,000 mothers. They found a moderate correlation between the
chloroform levels in water and the actual chloroform uptake for the whole population
($r = 0.6$) and good correlation when swimming was excluded ($r = 0.87$), suggesting that
chloroform levels in water may be a reasonable indicator for actual uptake of chloroform, but that there may be a considerable loss of power (assuming a Berkson error
model). It also showed that uptake of chloroform during swimming dominated the total
uptake of chloroform. The relationship may be better when fewer exposure pathways
and routes play a role, for example, for HAAs. The simulation exercise was fairly crude
and focussed only on the main exposure pathways, but at least it provided some
indication of how to interpret epidemiological study results.

Chloroform concentration	Chloroform levels in tap water (μg/l) ×	Chloroform levels in tap water (μg/l) ×	Chloroform levels in tap water (μg/l) ×	Chloroform levels in pool water (μg/l) ×
Activity level	Ingested amount of tap water (L) ×	Frequency and duration (min) of showering ×	Frequency and duration (min) of bathing ×	Frequency and duration (min) of swimming ×
Rate of uptake	Uptake of chloroform (μg) per μg/l tap water for ingestion	Uptake of chloroform (μg/min) per μg/l tap water for showering	Uptake of chloroform (μg/min) per μg/l tap water for bathing	Uptake of chloroform (μg/min) per μg/l pool water for swimming
	↓	↓	↓	↓
Uptake	Chloroform + uptake (μg) through ingestion	Chloroform + uptake (μg) through showering	Chloroform + uptake (μg) through bathing	Chloroform = uptake (μg) through swimming	Total chloroform uptake (μg)

Fig. 15.2 A schematic overview of the simulation of chloroform uptake.

As mentioned above, issues that are cause for concern when using the water zone estimates, are the mobility of the cohort members between water zones (or any exposure index used), the accuracy and precision of the water zone mean estimate, and any variation in the composition of the TTHM estimate, which includes the issue of the use of TTHM or individual THM as a marker for other disinfection by-products, for example, HAAs. The first two are likely to lead to attenuation in health-risk estimates, while the last one will improve the interpretation. Mobility from zone to zone, which could, for example, be caused by the home and workplace being in different water zones, should therefore be estimated and adjusted for in the epidemiological analysis. The accuracy and precision of the water zone estimates are likely to be low when based on only a few measurements, for example, four per water zone year in the UK, and this may affect the risk estimates as was illustrated, for example, by Waller *et al.* (2001). In particular, when exposure is estimated for a pregnancy trimester this may be a problem because of the temporal variability in DBP levels. Exposure estimates can be improved by modelling techniques, including, for example, regression modelling (Dodds *et al.* 1999; King *et al.* 2000; Dodds and King 2001) and Bayesian mixture modelling (Whitaker *et al.* 2003b), and water supply or hydraulic modelling taking into account determinants of DBP levels and composition (Gallagher *et al.* 1998). Further works need to be done on the development and validation of models.

The composition of disinfection by-products (e.g. ratio of THMs/HAAs and brominated/non-brominated) can differ depending on, for example, the total organic compound

(TOC) and bromide levels, pH, temperature, fulvic or humic acid content, and residual time. Krasner (1999) hypothesized that the different findings in recent studies in California (Waller *et al.* 1998), North Carolina (Savitz *et al.* 1995), and Canada (Dodds *et al.* 1999) may be a result of the different composition of the DBPs in water, with California having a relatively high level of brominated DBPs, Canada a relatively low level, and North Carolina in between. Relatively little information is generally available on the composition of DBPs by geographical area. This information is needed when routinely collected THMs are used as markers for the total THM load, and studies should be carried out to determine the composition.

Classical and Berkson error models represent two extremes of a continuum, and may not be as clear-cut as presented here. Most exposure errors combine elements of each. Water zone estimates have been combined with personal exposure information, which may sometimes make it more difficult to interpret health risk estimates, if a clear understanding is not achieved as to the effect of the various exposure errors. It may even be more difficult when exposure categories are formed from continuous measurements, since this may in certain cases lead to a reversal of the true direction of an exposure–response relationship (Flegal *et al.* 1991; Brenner and Loomis 1994).

15.5   Future work

A recent international workshop on the exposure assessment of DBPs for epidemiological studies brought together experts from several disciplines (e.g. chemistry, engineering, toxicology, biostatistics, epidemiology) and they made many recommendations for further work in the various areas (Arbuckle *et al.* 2002).

Table 15.3 indicates some specific areas for further research that would help the interpretation of epidemiological studies. As indicated earlier, when personal estimates of exposure are used in epidemiological studies, measurement error and attenuation in health-risk estimates are likely, particularly when there is substantial within-subject variability and a limited number of measurements is obtained. Repeated measurements could be obtained, at least in a subset of the population, to improve the exposure estimate, or to estimate the within- and between-subject variance, which will enable the estimation of attenuation in health-risk estimates.

Accurately and precisely estimated mean THM water zone estimates may be a valid and useful index of exposure for epidemiological studies of reproductive health outcomes. They are most likely to be the cheapest option in financial terms, particularly since they are commonly available. However uncertainties remain in the interpretation of the health-risk estimates unless further work is carried out for validating the assumptions that have to be made, and the relationship between personal uptake and water zone mean estimates. This can be done in smaller-scale exposure assessment studies.

If we want to use personal exposure estimates, it is unlikely that we will ever be able to measure the DBP uptake of every subject in an epidemiological study, given the time and cost involved, although some crude indicator (approximate) may well be within reach of most studies. Study power can be optimized by balancing sample size and

Table 15.3 Specific areas for further DBP research

When using water zone means as exposure index
Within- and between-variance in DBPs in tap-water sampling points within water zones to
  determine the validity of water zone means as marker for tap concentrations in the water zone
The validity of TTHM as marker of total DBP load, including
(a) the composition of DBPs in previous and current epidemiological study areas
(b) the determinants of the level and composition
(c) the correlation between various DBPs
Refinement of the hydraulic kinetic model that can predict DPB concentrations at tap
Improved statistical techniques to estimate water zone means and variability using a limited
  number of samples per water zone
The correlation between water zone mean and personal uptake of DBPs
Estimating mobility between water zones

When using personal exposure estimates as an exposure index
Development and validation of water consumption and activities (e.g. showering, bathing,
  swimming) questionnaires
Validation of existing biomarkers, particularly for TCAA (including effect of other
  substances) and development and validation of new biomarkers, particularly for those that
  have none and for new techniques such as adducts
Estimation of within- and between-subject variance in DBP exposure and uptake, including
  the variation in exposure route, biomarkers, and questionnaire data
Determinants of DBP exposure and uptake, in particular to identify the main ones that can be
  used in epidemiological studies
Correlation between DBP exposure and uptake
Estimating the effect of adding water consumption and activities information on the relation
  between DBP exposure and uptake
Correlation between DBP uptake and potential confounders
Development and validation of a PBPK model specifically for reproductive outcomes

General
Possible gene–environment interactions

Source: After Nieuwenhuijsen *et al.* (2000*b*).

exposure approximation or accuracy. It is likely to be more efficient to develop models
of uptake in a subset of the population, using routinely collected data, questionnaires,
biomarkers, and PBPK modelling, and use these to model the uptake in the wider population under study (see Chapter 6). Major determinants of uptake should be identified
in the models, keeping in mind that they need to be used for assessment in the wider
population, and be fed back into the model to obtain an estimate for each subject in
the study.

Although the available epidemiological evidence suggests that the risks, if any, are
small, the large number of people exposed to chlorinated water supplies implies that the
population attributable risk is potentially high. To estimate this risk, a detailed and
refined exposure assessment is essential.

References

Aggazotti, G., Fantuzzi, G., Righi, E., and Predieri, G. (1995). Environmental and biological monitoring of chloroform in indoor swimming pools. *Journal of Chromatography A*, **710**, 181–90.

Arbuckle, T. E., Hrudey, S. E., Krasner, S. W., *et al.* (2002). Assessing exposure in epidemiologic studies to disinfection by-products in drinking water: report from an international workshop. *Environmental Health Perspective*, **110**, 53–60.

Arora, H., LeChevallier, M. W., and Dixon, K. L. (1997). DBP occurrence survery. *Journal of the American Water Works Association*, **89**, 60–8.

Aschengrau, A., Zierler, S., and Cohen, A. (1989). Quality of community drinking water and the occurrence of spontaneous abortion. *Archives of Environmental Health*, **44**, 283–9.

Aschengrau, A., Zierler, S., and Cohen, A. (1993). Quantity of community drinking water and the occurrence of late adverse pregnancy outcomes. *Archives of Environmental Health*, **48**, 105–13.

Ashley, D. L. and Prah, J. D. (1997). Time dependence of blood chloroform concentrations during and after exposure to a mixture of volatile organic compounds. *Archives of Environmental Health*, **52**, 25–33.

Backer, L. C., Ashley, D. L., Bonin, M. A., Cardinalli, F. L., Kieszak, S. M., and Wooten. J. V. (2002). Household exposures to drinking water disinfection by-products: whole blood tri-halomethane levels. *Journal of Exposure Analysis and Environmental Epidemiology*, **10**, 321–6.

Bove, F. J., Fulcomer, M. C., Klotz, J. B., Esmart, J., Dufficy, E. M., and Savrin, J. E. (1995). Public drinking water contamination and birth outcomes. *American Journal Epidemiology*, **141**, 850–62.

Brenner, H. and Loomis, D. (1994). Varied forms of bias due to non differential error in measuring exposure. *Epidemiology*, **5**, 510–17.

Chen, W. and Weisel, C. (1998). Halogenated DBP concentrations in a distribution system. *Journal of the American Water Works Association*, **90**, 151–63.

Corley, R. A., Mendrala, A. L., Smith, F. A., Staats, D. A., Gargas, M. L., Conolly, R. B., Andersen, M. E., and Reitz, R. H. (1990). Development of a physiologically based pharmaco-kinetic model for chloroform. *Toxicological and Applied Pharmacology*, **103**, 512–27.

Dodds, L., King, W., Woolcott, C., and Pole, J. (1999). Trihalomethanes in public water supplies and adverse birth outcomes. *Epidemiology*, **3**, 233–7.

Dodds, L. and King, W. D. (2001). Relation between trihalomethane compounds and birth defects. *Occupational and Environmental Medicine*, **58**, 443–6.

Flegal, K. M., Keyl, P. M., and Nieto, F. J. (1991). Differential misclassification arising from non-differential errors in exposure measurement. *American Journal Epidemiology*, **134**, 1233–44.

Gallagher, M. D., Nuckols, J. R., Stallones, L., and Savitz, D. A. (1998). Exposure to tri-halomethanes and adverse pregnancy outcomes. *Epidemiology*, **9**, 484–9.

Gordon, S. M., Wallace, L., Callaghan, P., Kenny, D., and Brinkman, M. (1998). Effect of water temperature on dermal exposure to chloroform. *Environmental Health Perspectives*, **106**, 337–45.

Gravecker Graves, C., Matanoski, G. M., and Tradiff, R. (2001). Weight of evidence for an association between adverse reproductive and developmental effects and exposure to disinfection by-products: a critical review. *Regulatory Toxicology and Pharmacology*, **34**, 103–24.

Hopkins, S. M. and Ellis, J. C. (1980). *Drinking water consumption in Great Britain*. Water Research Centre (TR 137) 1980.

Jaakkola, J. J. K., Magnus, P., Skrondal, A., Hwang, B.-F., Becher, G., and Dybing, E. (2001). Foetal growth and duration of gestation relative to water chlorination. *Occupational and Environmental Medicine*, **58**, 437–42.

Kanitz, S., Franco, Y., Patrone, V., Caltabellotta, M., Raffo, E., Riggi, C., Timitilli, D., and Ravera, G. (1996). Association between drinking water disinfection and somatic parameters at birth. *Environmental Health Perspectives*, **104**, 516–20.

Keegan, T., Whitaker, H., Nieuwenhuijsen, M. J., Elliott, P., Toledano, M., and Morris, S. (2001). The use of routinely collected data for epidemiological purposes. *Occupational and Environmental Medicine*, **58**, 447–52.

Kim, H. and Weisel, C. P. (1998). Dermal absorption of dichloro- and trichloro acids from chlorinated water. *Journal of Exposure Analysis and Environmental Epidemiology*, **8**, 555–75.

Kim, H., Haltmeier, P., Klotz, J. B., and Weisel, C. P. (1999). Evaluation of biomarkers of environmental exposures: urinary haloacetic acids accociated with ingestion of chlorinated drinking water. *Environmental Research*, **80**, 185–95.

King, W. D., Dodds, L., and Allen, A. C. (2000). Relation between stillbirth and specific chlorination by-products in public water supplies. *Environmental Health Perspectives*, **108**, 883–6.

Klotz, J. B. and Pyrch, L. A. (1999). Neural tube defects and drinking water disinfection by-products. *Epidemiology*, **10**, 383–90.

Kramer, M. D., Lynch, C. F., Isacson, P., and Hanson, J. W. (1992). The association of waterborne chloroform with intrauterine growth retardation. *Epidemiology*, **3**, 407–13.

Krasner, S. W., Sclimenti, M. J., and Means, E. G. (1994). Quality degradation: implications for DBP formation. *Journal of the American Water Works Association*, **86**, 34–47.

Krasner, S. W., McGuire, M. J., Jacaugelo, J. G., Patania, N. L., Reagen, K. M., and Aieta, E. M. (1989). The occurrence of disinfection by-products in U.S. drinking water. *Journal of the American Water Works Association*, **81**, 41–53.

Krasner, S. W. (1999). *Chemistry and occurrence of disinfection by-products*. Abstract and presentation at ILSI Second International Conference on 'The Safety of water disinfection: balancing chemical and microbial risks' Miami Beach, US.

Levesque, B., Ayotte, P., LeBlanc, A., Dewailly, E., Prud Homme, D., Lavoie, R., Allaire, S., and Levallois, P. (1994). Evaluation of dermal and respiratory chloroform exposure in humans. *Environmental Health Perspectives*, **102**, 1082–7.

Lynberg, M., Nuckols, J. R., Lanlois, P., Ashley, D., Singer, P., Mendola, P., Wilkes, C., Krapfl, H., Miles, E., Speight, V., Lin, B., Small, L., Miles, A., Bonin, M., Zeitz, P., Tadkod, A., Henry, J., and Forrester, M. B. (2001). Assessing exposure to disinfection by-products in women of reproductive age living in Corpus Christ, Texas, and Cobb County, Georgia: descriptive results and methods. *Environmental Health Perspectives*, **109**, 597–604.

Magnus, P., Jaakkola, J. J. K., Skrondal, A., Alexander, J., Becher, G., Krogh, T., and Dybing, E. (1999). Water chlorination and birth defects. *Epidemiology*, **10**, 513–17.

Nieuwenhuijsen, M. J., Toledano, M. B., Eaton, N. E., Elliott, P., and Fawell, J. (2000*a*). Chlorination disinfection by-products in water and their association with adverse reproductive outcomes: a review. *Occupational and Environmental Medicine*, **57**, 73–85.

Nieuwenhuijsen, M. J., Toledano, M. B., and Elliott, P. (2000*b*). Uptake of chlorination disinfection by-products; a review and a discussion of its implications for epidemiological studies. *Journal of Exposure Analysis and Environmental Epidemiology*, **10**, 586–99.

Reckhow, D. A., Singer, P. C., and Malcolm, R. L. (1990). Chlorination of humic materials: by-product formation and chemical interpretations. *Environmental Science and Technology*, **24**, 1655–64.

Reif, J. S., Hatch, M. C., Bracken, M., Holmes, L. B., Schwetz, B. A., and Singer, P. C. (1996). Reproductive and developmental effects of disinfection by-products in drinking water. *Environmental Health Perspectives*, **104**, 1056–61.

Rook, J. J. (1974). Formation of haloforms during chlorination of natural waters. *Journal of the Society for Water Treatment and Examination*, **23**, 234–43.

Savitz, D. A., Andrews, K. W., and Pastore, L. M. (1995). Drinking water and pregnancy outcome in Central North Carolina: Source, amount and trihalomethane levels. *Environmental Health Perspectives*, **103**, 592–6.

Shaw, G. M. and Halinka, L. H. (1991). Residential mobility during pregnancy for mothers of infants with or without congenital cardiac anomolies. *Archives of Environmental Health*, **46**, 310–12.

Shimokura, G. H., Savitz, D. A., and Symanski, E. (1998). Assessment of water use for estimating exposure to tap water contaminants. *Environmental Health Perspectives*, **106**, 55–9.

Stevens, A. A., Moore, L. A., and Miltner, R. J. (1989). Formation and control of non-trihalomethane disinfection by-products. *Journal of the American Water Works Association*, **81**, 54–60.

Swan, S. H. and Waller, K. (1998). Disinfection by-products and adverse pregnancy outcomes: what is the agent and how should it be measured? *Epidemiology*, **9**, 479–81.

Waller, K., Swan, S. H., DeLorenze, G., and Hopkins, B. (1998). Trihalomethanes in drinking water and spontaneous abortion. *Epidemiology*, **9**, 134–40.

Waller, K. and Swan, A. H. (1999). Drinking water and spontaneous abortion; The authors reply. *Epidemiology*, **10**, 204.

Waller, K., Swan, S. H., Windham, G. C., and Fenster, L. (2001). Influence of exposure assessment methods on risk estimates in an epidemiologic study of trihalomethane exposuree and spontaneous abortion. *Journal of Exposure Analysis and Environmental Epidemiology*, **11**, 522–31.

Weisel, C. P. and Jo, W. K. (1996). Ingestion, inhalation and dermal exposure to chloroform and trichloroethane from tap water. *Environmental Health Perspectives*, **104**, 48–51.

Weisel, C. P., Kim, H., Haltmeier, P., and Klotz, J. B. (1999). Exposure estimates to disinfection by-products of chlorinated drinking water. *Environmental Health Perspectives*, **107**, 103–10.

Whitaker, H., Nieuwenhuijsen, M. J., Best, N., Fawell, J., Gowers, A., and Elliott, P. (2003*a*). Description of Trihalomethane Levels in Three UK Water Companies. *Journal of Exposure Analysis and Environmental Epidemiology*, **13**, 17–23.

Whitaker, H., Best, N., Nieuwenhuijsen, M. J., Wakefield, J., and Elliott, P. (2003*b*). Hierarchical modelling of trihalomethane levels in drinking water (in prep).

Whitaker, H., Nieuwenhuijsen, M. J., and Best, N. (2003*c*). The relationship between water chloroform levels and uptake of chloroform: a simulation study. *Environmental Health Perspectives* (in print).

Yang, C.-Y., Cheng, B.-H., Tsai, S.-S., Wu, T.-N., Lin, M.-C., and Lin, K.-C. (2000*a*). Association between chlorination of drinking water and adverse pregnancy outcome in Taiwan. *Environmental Health Perspectives*, **108**, 765–8.

Yang, C.-Y., Cheng, B.-H., Tsai, S.-S., Wu, T.-N., Hsu, T.-Y., and Lin, K.-C. (2000*b*). Chlorination of drinking water and sex ratio at birth in Taiwan. *Journal of Toxicology and Environmental Health*, **60**, 471–6.

16. Exposure assessment of pesticides in cancer epidemiology

Mustafa Dosemeci

16.1 Introduction

Pesticides are defined as 'substances or mixture of substances intended for destroying, preventing, repelling or mitigating any pest, including chemicals intended for use as plant regulators, defoliants or dessicant' (CFR 1986). The purpose is to control insects, animal vectors, and plants in human disease and to increase agricultural productivity. The generic term 'pesticides' includes insecticides, herbicides, fungicides, rodenticides, fumigants, growth regulators, and repellents.

In many epidemiological studies dealing with pesticides and cancer, assessment of exposure to agricultural pesticides has been limited to the use of surrogates of exposure such as type of farm operation, years of application, number of acres or animals treated, crop type, or frequency of pesticides use (Zahm *et al.* 1997). A limited number of studies have obtained information on years of use, days of application per year, and use of protective equipment while handling specific pesticides (Blair and Zahm 1995). Previous epidemiological studies have considered pesticides as a group without further characterization of chemical-specific exposures. Some epidemiological studies have evaluated risk of cancers by chemical-specific exposures, and frequency or duration (Baris *et al.* 1998; Blair *et al.* 1998), but intensity of exposure to individual pesticides has been largely ignored. This chapter briefly reviews procedures used to evaluate pesticide exposures in epidemiological studies of cancer, particularly in the agricultural setting and provides suggestions for more accurate assessment methods.

16.2 Methods for assessing exposure to pesticides in epidemiological studies of cancer

Accurate assessment of exposure to occupational and environmental risk factors is needed to assure that epidemiological studies meet their objectives in investigating the exposure–disease relationship. The basic principle of exposure assessment for epidemiological studies is to identify the determinants of exposure variability within the study population and to classify study subjects accurately with respect to their level of exposure to the risk factor of interest.

Exposure to pesticides may occur while transporting, mixing, loading, or applying chemicals, through cleaning or repairing equipment, or from re-entering treated fields. Factors affecting the level of exposure include type of activity (e.g. application, mixing, loading, or harvesting), method of application (e.g. air blast, backpack, aerial spray, hand spray, or ground boom application), pesticide formulation (e.g. dilute spray, aerosol, or dust), application rate (e.g. lbs. active-ingredient/acre), use of personal protective equipment [PPE] (e.g. gloves, respirators, face shield, boots, or overalls); and personal work habits and hygiene (e.g. changing into clean clothes/washing hands or taking bath/shower after the use of pesticide; frequency of health care visits). The challenge is to incorporate these exposure modifiers into an estimation of intensity of pesticide exposure (Dosemeci *et al.* 2002). The procedures for assessing exposures to pesticides depend on the availability of exposure information. The availability of pesticide exposure information in epidemiological studies can range from a simple job title (Blair *et al.* 1993) to subject-specific interview (Dosemeci *et al.* 2002) or biological monitoring data (Aronson *et al.* 2000). The following procedures have been used for assessing exposure to pesticides in epidemiological studies of cancer.

16.2.1   Assessing exposure using farmers and agricultural settings as surrogate

In early occupational epidemiological studies on cancer, job or industry titles have been used as surrogates of exposure to occupational risk factors, assuming that every study subject with the same job or industry title have the same level of exposure to all the risk factors in that occupation or industry. Epidemiological analyses usually have been carried out by evaluating the risk of cancer either among farming occupations (e.g. Dosemeci *et al.* 1994*a*; Settimi *et al.* 2001), pesticide applicators (Torchio *et al.* 1994; Fleming *et al.* 1999), or in various agricultural settings (Nanni *et al.* 1998; Rautiainen *et al.* 2002). Recently, several meta-analyses have been conducted to investigate cancer risk with farming, using agricultural settings as surrogates for pesticide exposures. These meta-analyses in agricultural settings evaluated risks of leukemia (Keller-Byrne *et al.* 1995), multiple myeloma (Khuder and Mutgi 1997), prostate cancer (Keller-Byrne 1997*a*), non-Hodgkin's lymphoma (Keller-Byrne *et al.* 1997*b*), and brain cancer (Khuder *et al.* 1998). Investigating cancer risk by occupation or industry may not be an appropriate approach to evaluate dose–response relationship between specific pesticide and cancer risk, but is a very useful tool for screening or for hypothesis generating studies.

16.2.2   Assessing pesticide exposure by job exposure matrices

Job-exposure matrices (JEMs) are designed to assign *a priori* exposure levels for study subjects based on their job and industry titles obtained from their work histories in case–control and surveillance studies (see Chapter 8).

In earlier applications of JEMs, exposure levels have been usually assigned directly on job title/industry combinations and they were limited to the specific study and not applicable for other studies (Acheson 1983). However, in later JEM applications (Dosemeci *et al.* 1994*b*), assignments of exposure levels have been carried out separately for job titles and industries and then integrated to specific occupation/ industry combinations using an algorithm (Dosemeci *et al.* 1989) to be applicable to any dataset having work histories with the same coding scheme. These JEMs are generic, can be applied to any occupational study, and have assignments of exposure levels (i.e. level of intensity), exposure probabilities (i.e. likelihood of occurrence of exposure), confidence on the assignments (i.e. accuracy of the estimates), and source indicators (i.e. whether the origin of exposure is based on the occupation or the industry). Although they provide us with semi-quantitative evaluations, assessing exposure by JEMs is a very practical approach in the evaluation of dose–response relationships. For example, the development of a JEM for pesticides have been described in detail (Wood *et al.* 2002) and several JEMs for pesticides have been applied in various case–control studies, including pancreatic cancer (Ji *et al.* 2001), reproductive disorders (Tielemans *et al.* 1999), and neurotoxicity (London and Myers 1998).

JEMs are very useful tools for investigations of an occupational or environmental agent and cancer risk. They provide us with an opportunity to group several occupations and industries by common pesticide exposures. However, they have some limitations compared to the workplace- or subject-specific exposure evaluation. Even though JEMs consider the exposure variability for a given job title in various agricultural settings, they do not provide us with available information between different farms or pesticide-used workplaces. For example, they still assume that the level of pesticide exposure for farmers is the same regardless of the variability between different farms. JEMs also has a potential for mis-classification by ignoring the variability of exposure between farmers working in the same farm or pesticide applicators working in the same workplaces. If a higher level of quan-tification was needed, as in some risk-assessment studies, then subject-specific exposure assessment approaches would be necessary to ensure the accuracy of the estimates.

16.2.3 Subject- and pesticide-specific exposure assessment using determinants of pesticide exposure

Because of the large exposure variability between individuals within the same pesticide-exposed jobs, such as farmers or pesticide applicators, subject-specific exposure information can play a significant role in reducing the potential exposure misclassification by considering the between-individual variability. One of the efficient ways of collecting subject-specific exposure information is the administration of the interview to study subjects. Questions related to the determinants of subject-specific exposures provide us with a great opportunity to calculate the overall exposure level for each study subject.

In the large prospective cohort of Agricultural Health Study (AHS) (Alavanja *et al.* 1996), a quantitative method was developed to estimate pesticide exposures of over 58,000 pesticide applicators in North Carolina and Iowa (Dosemeci *et al.* 2002). Self-reported exposure information on pesticide use from questionnaires as well as pesticide monitoring data from the literature, the Pesticide Handlers Exposure Database (PHED), and results of EPA pilot AHS pesticide monitoring surveys were utilized to estimate the levels of exposure to pesticides.

Questionnaire information

At enrollment into the study, approximately 58,000 pesticide applicators completed a questionnaire with time- and intensity-related pesticide exposure questions. The time-related information consisted of the duration (i.e. number of exposed years) and frequency (i.e. average annual number of days used) of handling (i.e. mixing, application for 22 pesticides: 10 herbicides, nine insecticides, one fumigant, and two fungicides). Intensity-related information included frequency of mixing pesticides, method of application, repairing application equipment, and use of PPE.

All applicators who completed the enrollment questionnaire were also given a self-administered take-home questionnaire to obtain additional information. Information includes pesticide handling, use of an enclosed mixing system, type of tractor (open cab or enclosed cab with or without a charcoal air filtration system), procedures used to clean pesticide application equipment, personal hygiene (e.g. timing of changing into clean clothes/washing hands, or taking bath/shower after application), the practice of changing clothes after a spill, and frequency of replacing old gloves, as well as information on lifestyle factors. In this questionnaire time- and intensity-related information was obtained for an additional 28 chemicals (i.e. eight herbicides, thirteen insecticides, three fumigants, and four fungicides).

Pesticide monitoring data

The pesticide monitoring data were extracted from more than 200 available published articles that had numerous measurements of pesticide exposures in relation to mixing, application, or work practices in agricultural settings. These articles provided extensive monitoring data on applicators' dermal, inhalation, and internal exposures.

Methods for determining dermal exposure include washing or wiping of the skin (Van Hemmen 1992), the use of pseudo-skin (e.g. pads or patches, special clothing, coveralls, caps, and gloves) (Nigg and Stamper 1985), and fluorescent tracer technique (Fenske 1988, see Chapter 9). In the assignment of exposure weights, the researchers relied on the results obtained by pseudo-skin and fluorescent tracer techniques, since the data from comparison studies suggested that washing or wiping may yield lower levels of exposure than sampling by means of pads and gloves (Fenske *et al.* 1989). Respirators were used to trap the inhaled particles and vapour to measure inhalation exposure in the early monitoring (Nigg and Stamper 1985). Later on, personal air sampling has been used to monitor the level of breathing zone pesticide exposure of applicators (Brouwer *et al.* 1992). Internal doses of pesticides are usually monitored by the measurements of the parent compound or its metabolites in urine, blood, faeces, adipose tissue, exhaled air, or sweat. The details of biological monitoring of internal doses of pesticides have been reported recently in two review articles (Maroni *et al.* 2000; Aprea *et al.* 2002).

The second source of information on monitoring data is the PHED (1992). The US Environmental Protection Agency (EPA), in conjunction with Health and Welfare Canada and the American Crop Protection Association, developed the PHED, a non-chemical specific summary database for investigating pesticide exposure to hands and to other dermal surfaces of the body, and inhalation while engaged in mixing, loading, and application activities.

The PHED consists of data collected from about 100 studies submitted primarily by companies that wish to register a specific pesticide. Even though this database contains many more records than any published study, there is some concern about its relevance to actual exposure situations because of the controlled, almost experimental, conditions under which the application occurs.

The other source of information used to assign exposure scores for the algorithms was the results of a pilot exposure monitoring survey conducted by the US EPA at six AHS farms in Iowa and North Carolina. For example, this monitoring survey showed that hand-spray applications resulted in approximately three times more exposure to the applicator than the ground-boom applications, which is consistent with the literature (Rutz and Krieger 1992; Brouwer *et al.* 1994).

Development of algorithms intensity levels

The questionnaire responses were used to develop chemical-specific exposure scenarios. Quantitative intensity levels for a given exposure scenario were calculated using two algorithms based on the reported information from the enrollment and take-home questionnaires. The first algorithm had fewer exposure variables than the detailed second algorithm, which is based on the information both from the more detailed self-administered take-home questionnaire and the enrollment questionnaire.

The enrollment algorithm and weights for the variables from the enrollment questionnaire are as follows:

Intensity = (Mix + Appl + Repair) × PPE

where: **Mix** = mixing status: score

- Never $= 0$
- <50% of time $= 3$
- 50% + of time $= 9$

Appl = application method:

- Aerial-aircraft $= 1$
- Distribute tablets $= 1$
- In furrow/banded $= 2$
- Boom on tractor $= 3$
- Backpack $= 8$
- Hand spray $= 9$
- Seed treatment $= 1$
- Air blast $= 9$
- Mist blower/fogger $= 9$
- Ear tags $= 1$
- Inject anima $= 2$
- Dip animal $= 5$
- Spray animal $= 6$
- Pour on animal $= 7$
- Powder duster $= 9$
- Gas canister $= 2$
- Row fumigation $= 4$
- Pour fumigant $= 9$

Repair = repair status

- Does not repair   = 0
- Repair   = 2

PPE = personal protective equipment use:

- Never used PPE   = 1.0
- Face shields/goggles = 0.8
- Fabric/leather gloves = 0.8
- Boots   = 0.8
- Cartridge respirator = 0.7
- Disposable clothing = 0.7
- Rubber gloves   = 0.6

In the take-home questionnaire, more pesticide-specific exposure information was used than that from the enrollment questionnaire. For example, intensity variables, such as mixing conditions, application type, and PPE used were collected by group of chemicals (i.e. herbicides, crop insecticides, livestock insecticides, fungicides, and fumigants). In addition, detailed questions were asked about work practices such as washing pesticide equipment after application, frequency of replacing old gloves, personal hygiene behaviour on changing into clean clothes and washing hands or taking bath/shower after application, and changing clothes after a spill.

For the information obtained from the take-home questionnaire, the following algorithm was used to calculate the intensity level for each exposure scenario:

$$\text{Intensity} = [(\text{Mix} \times \text{Enclosed}) + (\text{Appl} \times \text{Cab}) + \text{Repair} + \text{Wash}] \times \text{PPE} \times \text{Repl} \times \text{Hyg} \times \text{Spill}$$

where:

Enclosed = using enclosed mixing system

- Yes   = 0.5
- No   = 1.0

Cab = tractor with enclosed cab and/or charcoal filter

- Both cab and filter = 0.1
- Cab, but not filter = 0.5
- No cab, and no filter = 1.0

Wash = status of washing pesticide equipment after application

- Don't wash   = 0.0
- Hose down sprayer = 0.5
- Hose down tractor = 0.5
- Clean nozzle   = 3.0
- Rinse tank   = 1.0

Repl = replacing old gloves

- Change after each use = 1.0
- Change once a month   = 1.1
- Change when worn out   = 1.2

Hyg = personal hygiene: changing clean clothes and washing hands or taking bath/shower

- Change clothing right away   = 0.2
- Change clothing at the end of the day   = 0.4
- Change clothing at the end of the next day = 1.0
- Always use disposable clothing   = 0.2
- Hands/arms washed right away   = 0.2
- Bath/shower right away   = 0.2
- Bath/shower at lunch   = 0.4
- Bath/shower at the end of the day   = 0.6
- Hand/arms only at the end of the day   = 0.6

Spill = changing clothes after a spill

- Right away   = 1.0
- Always use disposable clothing   = 1.0
- At lunch   = 1.1
- At the end of the day   = 1.2
- At the end of the next day   = 1.4
- Later in the week   = 1.8

In both algorithms, an additive model was used for mixing, application, repair, and washing activities, because they are independent contributing factors for the overall body exposure, while a multiplicative model was used for the PPE and other potential protective factors, such as variables for 'Enclosed', 'Cab', 'Repl', 'Hyg', and 'Spill', because they are dependent to the basic exposure determinants.

To generate weights for the variables in the algorithms, the results of various monitoring data between individual exposure variables (e.g. mixing vs. applying) as well as within a selected variable (e.g. for 'Appl' variable: ground boom vs. backpack; for 'Cab' variable: open cab vs. closed cab) were compared using the results presented in these articles. The ratio between exposure levels of mixing and application depends on the method of application. For example, mixer/loaders have approximately 9-fold higher exposures than aerial applicators (Chester *et al.* 1987), hence the score '9', and have 3-fold higher exposure than ground-boom applicators (Rutz and Krieger 1992; Brouwer *et al.* 1994), which were assigned a score of '3'. The level of exposure for mixing/loaders was almost the same as the exposure level for hand-spray applicator (Rutz and Krieger 1992), which were assigned a score of '8'. The comparison between two application types, hand spray and ground boom, showed approximately 3-fold intensity differences (i.e. on the average, hand-spray application has three times more exposure than ground-boom application) using various monitoring results summarized in two review articles (Rutz and Krieger 1992; Van Hemmen 1992). In another study, both air-blast and hand-spray applications generated approximately three times higher intensity in levels of exposure than ground-boom applications (Nigg *et al.* 1990). The intensity levels of exposure were reviewed in their association with the use of various type of protective equipment. Rubber gloves provided approximately 50 per cent protection among fruit growers (De Cock *et al.* 1995). Similarly, closed cabs on tractors provided approximately 50 per cent protection, and closed cabs with air filter provided almost 90 per cent protection compared to tractors without cabs (Carman *et al.* 1982). To estimate intensity scores for PPEs, articles providing data on exposures by parts of the body were also used, by calculating proportion of the particular body part, which can be protected using PPE, in the overall body exposure (Davies *et al.* 1983; Marchado *et al.* 1992). There was almost no published data on measurements of human exposure from application of pesticides to animals. An NCI study in Iowa provided some data for estimating scores for the application techniques of hand spraying, pour on animal, and backpack, but not for other application methods (Stewart *et al.* 1999).

Relative comparisons between different application methods and various types of protective equipment in the PHED provided additional exposure information to refine the scoring system. For example, in the PHED, gloves provided about 40–50 per cent protection of the overall body exposure, regardless of application method, which is similar to the magnitude of protection reported in the peer-reviewed scientific literature (De Cock *et al.* 1995).

The AHS (Alavanja *et al.* 1996) was designed to capture chemical-specific intensity and duration-related pesticide exposure information. The enrollment and take-home questionnaires provided detailed information on mixing status, application techniques, types of PPE used, work practices, and personal hygiene, which are the known major determinants of exposure to pesticide in agricultural settings. These exposure data allowed us to develop quantitative exposure scores, including daily intensity or lifetime cumulative exposure to a specific pesticide, for use in analyses of disease risk and pesticide exposure.

To develop a weighting factor for each of the exposure variables, the study relied mostly on the results of the different exposure measurements from monitoring studies that used different individual pesticides for the same variables. Pesticide monitoring surveys suggest that the intensity of exposure variables, such as mixing status, application technique, or PPE type, is largely independent of the pesticide used (Stamper *et al.* 1988; Krieger *et al.* 1990). For example, studies indicated that the ratio of exposure levels between two application techniques or between mixing and a particular application technique was similar for different pesticides. These findings provided some additional confidence that the use of the non-chemical specific PHED to estimate relative-intensity weight factors might be a reasonable approximation of actual chemical-specific weight factors.

The exposure assessment approach proposed here represents a step forward in the estimation of pesticide exposure in an epidemiological cohort. The approach utilizes a mixture of professional judgement and the existing literature data to quantify potential pesticide exposure in a more detailed manner than has been attempted before. The intensity scores derived in these algorithms require further validation. The literature suggests that there is a substantial inter-applicator variability of exposure even for the same type application procedure (Van Hemmen 1992). Even with the many complexities in estimating exposures, a recent study has suggested that pesticide experts, industrial hygienists, and crop growing experts can identify the most important determinants of external exposures (De Cock *et al.* 1996).

16.2.4 Suggestions for future exposure assessment procedures

The main goal of the exposure assessment for epidemiological studies is to identify the variability of an exposure in the study population and then classify study subjects accurately with respect to their variability of exposure. In traditional exposure assessment approaches, we usually limit ourselves to dealing with the variability of external risk factors either in their concentrations in the ambient air or their intake into the body without considering the variability of host factors that determine the amount of internal dose from the external exposure. Because our main goal is to reduce the exposure misclassification in the evaluation of dose–response relationships between occupational/ environmental exposures and cancer risks, there is also a need to consider the variability of genetic susceptibility factors that eventually determine the internal dose, biologically effective dose, or in the case of evaluating cancer risk, cancer-causing dose of the external risk factors.

The evaluation of gene–environment interactions has power limitations when the prevalence of environmental risk factors and/or genetic susceptibility markers are low in the study population and multiple genetic markers interact with the exposure of interest. Recently, a method for estimating the biologically effective dose has been developed by integrating levels of external exposure with the protective ability of genetic susceptibility markers. In this process, the level of external occupational or environmental exposure may either be reduced or increased depending on the capacity of Phase I (activation), Phase II (detoxification), and DNA-repair enzymes. In this approach, genetic susceptibility markers (e.g. CYP1A1, CYP2E1, NAT1, NAT2, GSTM1, GSTT1, or DNA repair capacity) are used as if they were internal PPE. For example, low capacity of activation enzymes (e.g. CYP1A1) and high capacity of detoxification (e.g. NAT2) and DNA repair enzymes would have higher protective functions than high capacity of activation enzymes and low capacity of detoxification and DNA repair enzymes that may result in reducing cancer-causing doses of xenobiotics. This approach allows us to evaluate relationships between an unlimited number of genetic susceptibility markers and the exposure under investigation, without losing power. The challenge is to find appropriate biological markers that interact with pesticides in the carcinogenesis process. To find the appropriate markers, the starting point is to evaluate the gene–pesticide interactions on cancer risk estimates, and identify biomarkers related to pesticides and cancer site. Then protective factors of each pesticide-related biomarkers can be used as an internal protective factor to estimate the biologically effective dose.

Another way of reducing potential exposure misclassification caused by the retrospective nature of exposure assessment is to design prospective exposure assessment procedures based on biological monitoring data. The accuracy of the biological monitoring data depends on the time windows that represent the internal dose. If the chemical is a persistent one and the measured value represents the time window of the exposure period, such as the case for DDT or PCBs, then the biological monitoring would be a good index for the exposure assessment procedures. However, if the half-life of the chemical is short, such as for a couple of days as in 2,4-D or MCPA, then the current monitoring level would not be representative for the biological effective level of exposure needs to be used in epidemiological studies. If this were the case, then the only solution would be a prospective study design with frequent monitoring programs to cover the biologically effective dose. Depending on the half-life of the pesticide of interest, a prospective exposure assessment with estimated biologically effective dose would be the best approach for future epidemiological studies of pesticide and cancer.

16.3   Selection of the optimal index of pesticide exposure in occupational cancer epidemiology

A wide variety of exposure indices, ranging from very simple ones (e.g. ever/never exposed or duration of exposure) to complex ones (e.g. time-weighted cumulative exposure or biologically effective dose), have been developed and used in occupational epidemiological analyses. They can be classified into three major categories based on their associations with disease outcomes. The first group is the time-dependent exposure indices, such as duration of exposure, frequency of exposure, latency of exposure, and recentness of exposure. The second category is the intensity-dependent exposure indices, such as average intensity, highest intensity, longest intensity, and peak exposure. The last category is the combination of the first and the second, the time- and intensity-dependent indices, such as cumulative exposure, time-weighted cumulative exposure, intensity by duration, intensity by latency, intensity by recentness, cumulative exposure by latency, cumulative exposure by recentness, internal dose, or biologically effective dose. The selection of the optimum exposure index is based on the mechanism of the exposure–disease relationship. An exposure index may be optimum for certain relationships, acceptable for others, or may be totally inappropriate for some other relationships. Before deciding which index would be optimal, it is important to know about the characteristics of the metabolism of the agent of interest, such as the level of metabolic saturation, half-life in the body, and activity of metabolic enzymes.

The other important clue may come from epidemiological observations. For example, a cross-tabulation disease risk by a time-dependent exposure, such as duration of exposure, and by an intensity-dependent exposure index, such as average intensity, could give useful information for the selection of an optimum exposure index. If both the duration of exposure at various intensity levels and the intensity of exposure at various duration levels do not show associations with the disease risk, then it is unlikely that cumulative exposure would be an optimum index for that association. Because the role of exposure in disease process is the key factor for the selection of the optimum exposure index, and because the biologically effective dose requires understanding of the mechanism, it is recommended that the use of either of these indices be considered as a potential optimal index of exposure in the evaluation of an exposure– disease relationship.

References

Acheson, E. D. (1983). What are Job Exposure Matrices? in Acheson, E. D. (ed.) Job-exposure matrices: Proceedings of a conference held in April 1982 at the University of Southampton. Southampton, U.K.

Alavanja, M. C., Sandler, D. P., McMaster, S. B., Zahm, S. H., McDonnell, C. J., Lynch, C. F., Pennybacker, M., Rothman, N., Dosemeci, M., Bond, A. E., and Blair, A. (1996). The agriculture health study. *Environ Health Perspect*, **104**, 362–9.

Aprea, C., Colosio, C., Mammone, T., Minoia, C., and Maroni, M. (2002). Biological monitoring of pesticide exposure: a review of analytical methods. *Journal of Chromatography Analytical Technological and Biomedical Life Science*, **769**, 191–219.

Aronson, K. J., Miller, A. B., Woolcott, C. G., Sterns, E. E., McCready, D. R., Lickley, L. A., Fish, E. B., Hiraki, G. Y., Holloway, C., Ross, T., Hanna, W. M., SenGupta, S. K., and Weber, J. P.

(2000). Breast adipose tissue concentrations of polychlorinated biphenyls and other organo-chlorines and breast cancer risk. *Cancer Epidemiology, Biomarkers and Prevention*, **9**, 55–63.

Baris, D., Zahm, S., Cantor, K. P., and Blair, A. (1998). Agricultural use of DDT and risk of non-Hodgkin's lymphoma: pooled analysis of three case-control studies in the United States. *Occup Environ Med*, **55**, 522–27.

Blair, A., Dosemeci, M., and Heineman, E. F. (1993). Cancer and other causes of death among male and female farmers from twenty-three states. *American Journal of Industrial Medicine*, **23**, 729–42.

Blair, A. and Zahm, S. H. (1995). Agricultural exposures and cancer. *Environmental Health Perspectives*, **103**, 205–8.

Blair, A., Cantor, K., and Zahm, S. H. (1998). Non-Hodgkin's lymphoma and agricultural use of the insecticide Lindane. *American Journal of Industrial Medicine*, **33**, 82–7.

Brouwer, D. H., Brouwer, E. J., and Van Hemmen, J. J. (1992). Assessment of dermal and inhalation exposure to Zineb/Maneb in the cultivation of flower bulbs. *Annals of Occupational Hygiene*, **36**, 373–84.

Brouwer, D. H., Brouwer, E. J., and van Hemmen, J. J. (1994). Estimation of long-term exposure to pesticides, *American Journal of Industrial Medicine*, **25**, 573–88.

Carman, G. E., Iwata, Y., Pappas, J. L., O'Neal, J. R., and Gunther, F. A. (1982). Pesticide applicator exposure to insecticides during treatment of citrus trees with oscillating boom and air-blast units. *Archives of Environmental Contamination and Toxicology*, **11**, 651–9.

CFR (1986). Protection of Environment. *Office of Federal Register, National Archives and Records Administration*. 40-162.3. US Government Printing Office, Washington, DC.

Chester, G., Hatfield, L. D., Hart, T. B., Leppert, B. C., Swaine, H., and Tummon, O. J. (1987). Worker exposure to, and absorption of, cypermethrin during aerial application of an 'ultra low volume' formulation to cotton. *Archives of Environmental Contamination and Toxicology*, **16**, 69–78.

Davies, J. E., Dedhia, H. V., Morgade, C., Barquet, A., Maibach, H. I. (1983). Lindane poisonings. *Arch Dermatol*, **119**, 142–4.

De Cock, J., Heederik, D., Hoek, F., Boleij, J., and Kromhout, H. (1995). Urinary excretion of THPI in fruit growers with dermal exposure to captan. *American Journal of Industrial Medicine*, **28**, 245–56.

Dosemeci, M., Stewart, P. A., and Blair, A. (1989). Evaluating occupation and industry separately to assess exposure in case-control studies. *Applied Industrial Hygiene*, **4**, 256–9.

Dosemeci, M., Hoover, R. N., Figgs, L., Devesa, S., Grauman, D., Blair, A., and Fraumeni, J. F. Jr. (1994*a*). Farming and prostate cancer among African Americans in the southeastern United States. *Journal of National Cancer Institute*, **86**, 1718–19.

Dosemeci, M., Cocco, P., Gomez, M., Stewart, P. A., and Heineman, E. F. (1994*b*). Effects of three features of a job-exposure matrix on risk estimates. *Epidemiology*, **5**, 124–7.

Dosemeci, M. and Stewart, P. A. (1996). Recommendation to occupational hygienists to minimize the effects of exposure misclassification on risk estimates. *Occupational Hygiene*, **3**, 169–76.

Dosemeci, M., Alavanja, M. C. R., Rowland, A., Mage, D., Zahm, S. H., Rothman, N., Lubin, J., Sandler, D. P., and Blair, A. (2002). A quantitative approach for estimating exposure to pesticides in the agricultural health study. *Annals of Occupational Hygiene*, **46**, 245–60.

Fenske, R. A. (1988). Correlation of fluorescent tracer measurements of dermal exposure and urinary metabolite excretion during occupational exposure to malathion. *American Industrial Hygiene Association Journal*, **49**, 438–44.

Fenske, R. A., Birnbaum, S. G., Methner, M., and Soto, R. (1989). Methods for assessing field worker hand exposure to pesticides during peach harvesting. *Bulletin of Environmental Contamination and Toxicology*, **43**, 805–13.

Fleming, L. E., Bean, J. A., Rudolph, M., and Hamilton, K. (1999). Mortality in a cohort of licensed pesticide applicators in Florida. *Occupational and Environmental Medicine*, **56**, 14–21.

Ji, B. T., Silverman, D. T., Stewart, P. A., Blair, A., Swanson, G. M., Baris, D., Greenberg, R. S., Hayes, R. B., Brown, L. M., Lillemoe, K. D., Schoenberg, J. B., Pottern, L. M., Schwartz, A. G., and Hoover, R. N. (2001). Occupational exposure to pesticides and pancreatic cancer. *American Journal of Industrial Medicine*, **39**, 92–9.

Keller-Byrne, J. E., Khuder, S. A., and Schaub, E. A. (1995). Meta-analysis of leukemia and farming. *Environmental Research*, **71**, 1–10.

Keller-Byrne, J. E., Khuder, S. A., and Schaub, E. A. (1997a). Meta-analyses of prostate cancer and farming. *American Journal of Industrial Medicine*, **31**, 580–6.

Keller-Byrne, J. E., Khuder, S. A., Schaub, E. A., and McAfee, O. (1997b). A meta-analysis of non-Hodgkin's lymphoma among farmers in the central United States. *American Journal of Industrial Medicine*, **31**, 442–4.

Khuder, S. A. and Mutgi, A. B. (1997). Meta-analyses of multiple myeloma and farming. *American Journal of Industrial Medicine*, **32**, 510–16.

Khuder, S. A., Mutgi, A. B., and Schaub, E. A. (1998). Meta-analyses of brain cancer and farming. *American Journal of Industrial Medicine*, **34**, 252–60.

Krieger, R., Blewett, C., Edmiston, S., Fong, H., Gibbons, D., Meinders, D., O'Connell, L., Ross, J., Schneider, F., and Spencer, J. (1990). Gauging pesticide exposure of handlers (miner/load-ers/applicators) and harvesters in California agriculture. *La Medicina del Lavoro*, **81**, 474–9.

London, L. and Myers, J. E. (1998). Use of a crop and job specific exposure matrix for retrospective assessment of long-term exposure in studies of chronic neurotoxic effects of agrichemicals. *Occupational and Environmental Medicine*, **55**, 194–201.

Maroni, M., Colosio, C., Ferioli, A., and Fait, A. (2000). Biological monitoring of pesticide exposure: a review. Introduction. *Toxicology*, **143**, 1–118.

Marchado, J. G., Matuo, T., and Matuo, Y. K. (1992). Dermal exposure of pesticide applicators in staked tomato crops: efficiency of a safety measure in the application equipment. *Bulletin of Environmental Contamination and Toxicology*, **49**, 529–34.

Nanni, O., Falcini, F., Buiatti, E., Bucchi, L., Naldoni, M., Serra, P., Scarpi, E., Saragoni, L., and Amadori, D. (1998). Multiple myeloma and work in agriculture: results of a case–control study in Forli, Italy. *Cancer Causes and Control*, **9**, 277–83.

Nigg, H. N. and Stamper, J. H. (1985). Field studies: methods overview in dermal exposure related to pesticides use. *ACS Symposium Series*, **273**, 95–108.

Nigg, H. N., Stamper, J. H., and Mahon, W. D. (1990). Handgun applicator exposure to ethion in Florida citrus. *Bulletin of Environmental Contamination and Toxicology*, **45**, 463–8.

PHED, Pesticide Handlers Exposure Database (1992). US EPA, Health and Welfare Canada and the American Crop Protection Association. *Versar Publications*, Version 1.0. Springfield.

Rautiainen, R. H. and Reynolds, S. J. (2002). Mortality and morbidity in agriculture in the United States. *Journal of Agricultural Safety and Health*, **8**, 259–76.

Rutz, R. and Krieger, R. I. (1992). Exposure to pesticide mixer/loaders and applicators in California. *Review of Environmental Contamination and Toxicology*, **129**, 121–39.

Settimi, L., Comba, P., Bosia, S., Ciapini, C., Desideri, E., Fedi, A., Perazzo, P. L., Axelson, O. (2001). Cancer risk among male farmers: a multi-site case–control study. *International Journal of Occupational Medicine and Environmental Health*, **14**, 339–47.

Stamper, J. H., Nigg, H. N., Mahon, W. D., Nielsen, A. P., and Royer, M. D. (1989). Pesticide exposure to greenhouse handgunners. *Archives of Environmental Contamination and Toxicology*, **18**, 515–29.

Stewart, P. A., Fears, T., Kross, B., Ogilvie, L., and Blair, A. (1999). Exposure of farmers to phosmet, a swine insecticide. *Scandinavian Journal of Work and Environmental Health*, **25**, 33–8.

Tielemans, E., Burdorf, A., te Velde, E. R., Weber, R. F., van Kooij, R. J., Veulemans, H., and Heederik D. J. (1999). Occupationally related exposures and reduced semen quality: a case–control study. *Fertility and Sterility*, **71**, 690–6.

Torchio, P., Lepore, A. R., Corrao, G., Comba, P., Settimi, L., Belli, S., Magnani, C., and di Orio, F. (1994). Mortality study on a cohort of Italian licensed pesticide users. *Science of Total Environment*, **149**, 183–91.

Van Hemmen, J. J. (1992). Agricultural Pesticide exposure databases for risk assessment. *Review of Environmental Contamination and Toxicology*, **126**, 1–85.

Wacholder, S., Dosemeci, M., and Lubin, J. H. (1991). Blind assignment of exposure does not always prevent differential misclassification. *American Journal of Epidemiology*, **134**, 433–7.

Wood, D., Astrakianakis, G., Lang, B., Le, N., and Bert, J. (2002). Development of an agricultural job-exposure matrix for British Columbia, Canada. *Journal of Occupational Environmental Medicine*, **44**, 865–73.

Zahm, S. H., Blair, A., and Ward, M. H. (1997). Pesticides and cancer. *Occupational Medicine: State of the Art Review*, **12**, 269–89.

17. Radiofrequency exposure and cancer

Martie van Tongeren and Philip Chadwick

17.1 Introduction

The twentieth century witnessed a number of important developments in technology, one of which was the introduction of methods for telecommunication using radiofrequency electromagnetic radiation. Any electrical charge generates an electric field, whilst an electrical current generates a magnetic field. When the electrical charge and current oscillate, waves of electric and magnetic fields are created that travel with the speed of light. The frequency of the electromagnetic wave is determined by the frequency of oscillation of the electrical charge and current. Hence, electromagnetic fields (EMFs) from electrical wires in homes and from power lines have a frequency of 50 Hz in the UK. The term radiofrequency has generally been used to describe the frequencies that can be employed practically for wireless communications by the transmission of modulated electromagnetic waves, with frequencies between 3 kHz and 300 GHz.

The improved understanding and application of radiofrequency radiation has had a tremendous influence on modern society. During the Second World War, radar was developed to detect ships and planes, with the first radio services being introduced in the UK in the 1940s. Since then numerous applications have been developed for communications and broadcasting; industrial uses such as heating and sealing of plastics; medical uses such as hyperthermia for cancer therapy and diathermy for treating muscular injuries; and consumer uses such as cooking, security systems, and the use of mobile phones. The use of mobile phones has grown very rapidly in the late 1990s and the early years of the twenty-first century, and currently the majority of the UK population owns a mobile phone. Exposure to radiofrequency is now ubiquitous, and terms such as 'electro-smog' have been used by some scientists to describe this continuous, low-level background exposure.

17.2 Physiological effects and dosimetry

Radiofrequency radiation does not posses sufficient energy to directly remove electrons from atoms or molecules, and hence is classified as non-ionizing radiation. Therefore, in contrast to ionizing radiation, such as X-rays and γ-radiation, radiofrequency radiation is not genotoxic and does not damage DNA molecules. The established adverse

Table 17.1   Reference levels for occupational
exposure to radio frequency (10 MHz to 300 GHz)

Frequency range	E-field $(V m^{-1})$	H-field $(A m^{-1})$	Power density $(W m^{-2})$
10–400 MHz	61	0.16	10
400–2000 MHz	$3\sqrt{f}$	$0.008\sqrt{f}$	$f/40$
2–300 GHz	137	0.36	50

f is the frequency in MHz.

effects of exposure to radiofrequency fields and radiation are a result of heating of biological matter due to energy absorption by body tissues and currents induced in the body. The capacity of radiofrequency radiation to produce a measurable temperature rise in biological tissues and the susceptibility of certain tissues to thermal injury (such as skin, testes, and lens of the eye) has been the basis for protection guidelines in the UK and elsewhere.

The International Commission on Non-Ionizing Radiation Protection (ICNIRP) has formulated basic restrictions expressed in dosimetric quantities, such as the specific energy absorption rate (SAR) or current density in the central nervous system (ICNIRP, 1998). SAR is a measure of the power absorbed in the body per unit mass of tissue and is expressed in watts per kilogram $(W kg^{-1})$. Between 100 kHz and 10 GHz, the basic restriction for the whole body, expressed as SAR, is $0.4 W kg^{-1}$ for occupational and $0.08 W kg^{-1}$ for general public exposure, respectively. Basic restrictions are also given for localized exposure, such as for the head, which are (averaged over 10 g of tissue) $10 W kg^{-1}$ for occupational and $2 W kg^{-1}$ for exposure to the general public, respectively.

As the measurement of SAR is extremely difficult, reference levels of external electric strength (E-fields expressed as volts per metre), magnetic field strength (H-field expressed as ampere per metre), and power density (expressed as watts per metre) have been issued by ICNIRP (1998). These reference levels are frequency dependent and are shown in Table 17.1 for occupational exposures. Simple dosimetric models are used to relate the external electric and magnetic field exposure levels to the dosimetric quantities of SAR and current density inside the body. These models are conservative, in that compliance with the reference levels is intended to ensure that the basic restrictions will be met under all circumstances.

At a sufficiently large distance from the source (far-field region), the electric and magnetic fields are in general highly correlated, and it is often sufficient to measure one or the other. Closer to the source (near-field) the relationships between the electric and magnetic fields are much more complex and separate evaluation of the electric and magnetic fields need to be carried out (Bergqvist 2001).

17.3   Health effects

Comparatively little attention was paid to possible links between exposure to electro and magnetic fields and neoplastic diseases until, in 1979, Wertheimer and Leeper (1979) published results of a residential study indicating increased incidence of leukaemias and some other neoplasms in children, which they hypothesized as being due to EMFs. Milham (1982) first reported an increased mortality from leukaemia among electrical workers. Subsequently a large number of epidemiological studies have investigated the possible association between EMFs and cancer, with varying results. Initially, most studies investigated the potential health effects from exposure to extremely low frequency (ELF) EMFs. In a recent review by the International Agency for Research on Cancer (IARC) ELF-EMFs were evaluated as possibly carcinogenic to humans (Group 2B), based on the statistical association of higher level residential ELF magnetic fields and increased risk for childhood leukaemia (IARC 2001). There is no consistent evidence that residential or occupational exposures are related to excess risks of adult cancer (IARC 2001; NRPB 2001).

Fuelled by the enormous growth in use of mobile phone technology, attention has shifted somewhat on effects of exposure to higher (radio) frequencies emitted by mobile phone base stations and mobile phones. Subsequently, a number of reviews have appeared in recent years that have reviewed the scientific evidence for an association between radiofrequency exposure and possible health effects (Royal Society of Canada 1999; IEGMP 2000; Zmirou 2001). These reviews were specifically carried out to establish if there was a link between use of mobile phones and health effects and included evidence from toxicological, human volunteer, and epidemiological studies (both general population and occupational).

In the UK, the Independent Export Group on Mobile Phones (IEGMP) concluded that the current evidence does not suggest that exposures to radiofrequency radiation below ICNIRP guidelines cause adverse health effects. However, there was some evidence suggesting that there may be some biological effects occurring at exposures below these guidelines (IEGMP 2000). Examples of such effects were a decrease in reaction time (Preece *et al.* 1999; Koivisto *et al.* 2000), influences on sleep (Mann and Roschke 1996; Borbely *et al.* 1999), and event-related EEG changes during performance of cognitive tasks (Krause *et al.* 2000).

In addition, some *in vivo* studies show some effect from radiofrequency radiation, while others did not (Lai and Singh 1995, 1996; Malyapa *et al.* 1997*a,b*, 1998; Repacholi *et al.* 1997; Utteridge *et al.* 2002).

17.4 Epidemiology

Epidemiological studies on possible health effects of radiofrequency exposure can be categorized into three groups:

(1) studies of occupational radiofrequency exposures, including the armed forces and those exposed through hobbies, such as radio amateurs;
(2) studies of the general population living near radio transmitters; and
(3) studies of people using mobile phones or other telecommunication systems.

The following sections will briefly summarizes the epidemiological cancer and mortality studies in these three areas.

17.4.1   Occupational/military/hobbies

A number of studies have investigated the link between occupational radiofrequency exposure and cancer incidence and mortality. The exposure indices were generally broad exposure groups such as working in the industry or job title. These studies were carried out amongst military personnel (Robinette *et al.* 1980; Grayson *et al.* 1996; Szmigielski 1996; Groves *et al.* 2002), in professional or amateur radio operators (Milham 1988; Tynes *et al.* 1996), in other occupations (Davis and Mostofi 1993; Lagorio *et al.* 1997; Morgan *et al.* 2000), and in the general population (Thomas *et al.* 1987; Hayes *et al.* 1990; Demers *et al.* 1991; Tynes *et al.* 1992; Cantor *et al.* 1995). Most studies investigated links between radiofrequency exposure and morbidity or mortality due to cancer of the central nervous system or brain, breast (male and female), testis, and lymphatic/haematopoietic system.

Robinette *et al.* (1980) found no evidence of increased mortality amongst a cohort of Korean war veterans, whilst a follow-up study of the same population by Groves *et al.* (2002) found a relative risk for leukaemias of 1.5 (95% confidence interval (CI) 1.0–2.2). Szmigielski *et al.* (1996) found increased morbidity of malignancies of the haematopoietic system and lymphatic organs and nervous system amongst Polish military personnel exposed to radiofrequency compared to unexposed personnel. Grayson (1996) found an increased risk of brain tumours (OR 1.4, 95% CI 1.01–1.90) in members of the US Air Force exposed to radiofrequency or microwave radiation, although there was no exposure–response relationship with a cumulative exposure index.

Amongst female professional radio operators Tynes *et al.* (1996) found an increased risk of female breast cancers, but not for brain cancer and cancer of the lymphatic organs or haematopoietic system. Similarly, Milham (1988) did not find an increased risk of leukaemia and brain cancers amongst male amateur radio operators. A study by Morgan *et al.* (2000) amongst Motorola personnel in the US, showed no difference in mortality due to brain cancer or lymphatic/haematopoietic cancer in personnel exposed to relatively high intensity of radiofrequency compared to low-exposed personnel.

A number of general population case–control studies investigated links between brain cancers (Thomas *et al.* 1987), male and female breast cancers (Demers *et al.* 1991; Cantor *et al.* 1995), and testicular cancer (Hayes *et al.* 1990) and occupational radiofrequency exposure. Thomas *et al.* (1987) observed a relationship between radiofrequency exposure and primary brain cancer, but only in those who were also exposed to ELF and solvents. No effect was observed for those who were only exposed to radiofrequency and not to ELF and solvents. Demers *et al.* (1991) found an increased risk of male breast cancer in radio and communication workers (OR 2.9), but this relationship was not statistically significant and no relationship was found with duration of exposure. In a study of testicular cancer, Hayes *et al.* (1990) found an association between self-reported radiofrequency exposure (OR 3.1, 95% CI 1.4–6.9), but not for exposure to radar (OR 1.1, 95% CI 0.7–1.9). No association was found when expert exposure assessments based on job titles were used. Finally, Cantor *et al.* (1995) found an increased risk of breast cancer in white and black females, although this study looked at a large number of exposures, and therefore this could have been a chance finding.

Little is known about exposure levels in these industries and none of the forementioned studies attempted to quantify the personal exposure to radiofrequency radiation.

Tynes *et al.* (1996) provided some results from spot measurements from three representative Norwegian ships to describe radiofrequency fields in the radio rooms of such ships. Similarly, Robinette *et al.* (1980) used measurements made by the US Navy on ships carrying radar equipment to categorize different occupations as potentially of low or high exposure. Szmigielski (1996) reported that the exposure intensity for 80–85 per cent of the service posts where radiofrequency emitting equipment was used did not exceed $2\,\mathrm{W\,m^{-2}}$, whilst levels exceeding $6\,\mathrm{W\,m^{-2}}$ only occurred incidentally. Grayson (1996) utilized a central register that contained information on all incidents of high exposure ($>100\,\mathrm{W\,m^{-2}}$) to develop a job-exposure matrix, which provided an assessment of the probability of exposure, not the intensity.

In terms of intensity and duration of exposure, highest occupational exposure levels are likely to be found for operators of high-frequency (HF) heaters such as those used for plastic welding (Mantiply *et al.* 1997; Jokela and Puranen 1999). Allen *et al.* (1994) reported maximum electric field levels at the operator position near dielectric heaters (16–53 MHz) of 5–$330\,\mathrm{V\,m^{-1}}$. Mantiply *et al.* (1997) summarized the results of 12 studies of radiofrequency exposure levels near dielectric heaters (6.5–65 MHz). Electric field strengths varied from 20 to $1700\,\mathrm{V\,m^{-1}}$, with magnetic field varying from 0.04 to $14\,\mathrm{A\,m^{-1}}$, with typical values of $250\,\mathrm{V\,m^{-1}}$ and $0.75\,\mathrm{A\,m^{-1}}$. However, as these dielectric heaters operated with a duty cycle of 0.1–0.5, personal exposures will be less than these. Few studies have investigated possible links between radiofrequency exposures and cancer in this industry. Lagorio *et al.* (1997) investigated mortality in 481 female plasticware workers who were employed between 1962 and 1992. They found a slightly higher mortality due to all cancers, however it was not statistically significant; this study was limited due to its small size and confounding exposures.

17.4.2 Radio transmitters

A small number of studies have investigated health effects in residents living near radio and television transmitters (Hocking *et al.* 1996; Dolk *et al.* 1997*a,b*; McKenzie *et al.* 1998; Michellozzi *et al.* 2002). The exposure indices used were generally at a distance from the source, that is, transmitter. Dolk *et al.* (1997*a*) first investigated the cancer incidence between 1974 and 1986 in a small area near the Sutton Coldfield (UK) high-power radio and television transmitter. The study found an increased risk in leukaemia for adults living near the transmitter (<2 km) and there was a significant declining trend with increasing distance from the transmitter. Field strength measurements were made in the vicinity of the transmitter, which confirmed that average field strength or power density decreased with distance from the transmitter. When the study was expanded to all high-powered television and radio transmitters in the UK, no increased incidence of leukaemia was found for those living within 2 km of the masts, although there was a significant decline in leukaemia with distance from the masts (Dolk *et al.* 1997*b*). Hocking *et al.* (1996) found an increased incidence of childhood leukaemia (RR 1.6, 95% CI 1.1–2.3) in residential areas near a number of high-powered television and radio transmitters in Sydney. However, McKenzie *et al.* (1998) showed that this increase in childhood leukaemia only occurred in one municipality and not for all populations near the masts, indicating that the increased risk may have been a chance finding or caused by other factors. Michelozzi *et al.* (2002) found an excess risk of adult and childhood leukaemia within 2 km of the Vatican's radio transmitter with a declining risk with distance from the site. However, the study was based on a small number of cases (adult leukaemia, $n = 40$; childhood leukaemia, $n = 8$), and the excess mortality from leukaemia was found only amongst men, whereas no significant increase was observed amongst women. Finally, Hallberg and Johansson (2002) argued that there was a link between the increased melanoma incidence in four countries (Denmark, Norway, Sweden, and US) and the expanding FM broadcasting network. No studies have been reported on cancer incidence or mortality in relation to radiofrequency exposure from mobile phone base stations.

Although most of the forementioned studies provide some evidence that radiofrequency levels near the transmitter masts are higher than further away, it is unclear how this relates to personal exposure. Generally, radiofrequency exposure levels in urban areas are very low. Dahme (1999) reported electric fields of 0.1–$0.4\,\mathrm{V\,m^{-1}}$ at a distance of 1.5 km from radio and television broadcasting masts. However, much higher levels were found at 200 m distance from HF, LF, and MF broadcasting masts (43–$130\,\mathrm{V\,m^{-1}}$) (Dahme 1999). Schuz and Mann (2000) carried out spot measurement in nine locations in Mainz (Germany) near mobile phone base stations with results for electric field levels ranging from 0.012 to $0.343\,\mathrm{V\,m^{-1}}$ (equivalent to 0.4×10^{-6}–$3.1 \times 10^{-4}\,\mathrm{W\,m^{-2}}$). Mann *et al.* (2000) reported that the geometric mean of total radiofrequency exposure at 73 accessible locations near 17 mobile phone base stations was 18 millionth of the ICNIRP public reference level. Unfortunately, Schuz and Mann (2000) showed that distance from mobile phone base station transmitter is generally a poor indicator of exposure due to shielding effects and multiple reflections from house walls and other buildings. In addition, these reported levels are from spot measurements outside the homes, and it is unclear how these results are related to personal radiofrequency exposure.

17.4.3   Mobile phones

The first study reporting on a possible link between use of mobile phones and mortality was published in 1996 (Rothman *et al.* 1996). This study found no effect of the use of hand-held mobile phones on mortality due to brain cancers, amongst 250,000 phone users who were followed up for one year. Subsequently, a number of other studies have been published (Dreyer *et al.* 1999; Hardell *et al.* 1999, 2002; Muscat *et al.* 2000, 2002; Inskip *et al.* 2001; Johansen *et al.* 2001; Auvinen *et al.* 2002). Apart from one study by Hardell *et al.* (2002), in which an increased risk of brain tumours was observed amongst users of analogue mobile phones, the results of these studies were generally negative, with no evidence of any exposure–response relationship. However, as mobile phone use has become widespread only in recent years, it is possible that any increase in cancer may only be manifested after many more years of exposure.

Apart from the studies by Rothman *et al.* (1996) and Dreyer *et al.* (1999), all the forementioned studies were case–control studies, in which information on exposure (frequency, intensity, and duration of use, side of the head, etc.) was obtained by questionnaire or interview. The cohort studies by Rothman *et al.* (1996) and Dreyer *et al.* (1999) compared mortality amongst users of hand-held phones with users of other phones. None of the studies attempted to obtain quantitative information on exposure.

A large international case–control study coordinated by IARC is currently underway, with results not expected before 2004 (Cardis and Kilkenny 1999). Information on exposure is collected using computer-assisted personal interviews and validation studies are being carried out using software-modified phones to determine the validity of the information collected by the interview. In addition, the study will attempt to determine SAR levels at the tumour site using dosimetric models.

17.5 Exposure assessment

Ideally, exposure measurements for epidemiological studies on the effect of radiofrequencies would characterize the frequency and intensity of the radiofrequency exposure, the temporal variation in the exposure of each individual being investigated within the study, and possibly include an assessment of any modulation. Preferably, intensity would be measured not just in terms of external field strength, but also as anatomical site-specific SAR (Swerdlow 1999). Spatial and temporal variation in SAR can be determined: for example, it is possible to estimate maximum SAR in a small volume of brain, or as average SAR in the whole brain or even the whole body.

Few tools are available that will allow the assessment of SAR across a working day. However, it may be possible to measure body currents, for example, in plastic welders who are relatively stationary, or by measuring external electric and magnetic fields. In some situations, for example, close to high-power, medium-frequency radio transmitters, SAR can be estimated through measuring body currents by using transformer clamps around the wrist, ankle, or neck. Measurement of current flowing between the feet and the ground can be carried out using two parallel conducting plates, separated by a slab of dielectric material, and short circuited via a small resistance. Measurement of body currents is probably of only limited practicable use for epidemiological surveys, as currently there are no devices available that enable the measurements and storage of these indices over a full work shift.

Personal monitors for radiofrequency exposure are only just becoming available and are still in the early stages of development. In a recent study by the University of Birmingham and the National Radiological Protection Board, personal monitors were used to measure electric and magnetic field exposure in workers in the broadcasting and telecommunications industry (http://www.bham.ac.uk/ioh/mvtrfstudy/rf_page.htm). Personal monitors integrate the electric and/or magnetic fields over a certain frequency spectrum and the output is presented as a percentage of some *a priori* established limit (e.g. ICNIRP reference levels). Reporting of the electric or magnetic field intensity is not useful without information on the frequency of the signal as the absorption of energy by the body is dependent on frequency. In the study by the University of Birmingham and the NRPB exposure records were obtained from workers operating in different environments such as inside transmission buildings, outdoors at ground level, on rooftops, and on masts and towers with high-powered radio and television transmitters. The results showed that exposure levels when working on mobile phone base stations were generally below the noise level of the dosimeter unless other sources of radiofrequency were present, such as paging antennas. Highest levels were found whilst working on or near high-powered radio and television equipment.

One problem is that exposure cannot be measured at the port of entry in the body such as for airborne contaminants. Exposure levels when measured with a personal dosimeter worn on the lapel may not be relevant when investigating the relationship between radiofrequency exposure and brain tumours. For example, exposure to radiofrequency from the use of mobile phones is generally very localized whilst riggers climbing towers with high-powered broadcast antennas will have a whole-body exposure, possibly for sustained periods of time.

Generally, personal monitors that are currently commercially available lack sensitivity for personal assessment of exposure in general population studies, because the background levels of radiofrequency in homes are low, even close to transmitters. Therefore, these monitors can currently be used only to obtain detailed assessments of personal exposure for certain occupations, for example, where workers are in close proximity to live antennas of relatively high power. However, for studies in communities near television or radio broadcasting towers or mobile phone base stations other strategies need to be applied to obtain information on personal exposure. Schuz and Mann (2000) showed that distance from a base station is a very poor proxy for radiofrequency levels indoors. Therefore, assessment of radiofrequency exposure in general population studies will require detailed spot measurement surveys using very sensitive equipment such as spectrum analysers, combined with surveys of activity patterns of the relevant population.

Radiofrequency exposure from mobile phones is determined by a large number of factors related to the type of phone, such as type and geometry of antenna, operating power, and the way the phone is used (Balzano 1999). There are methods to assess SAR from mobile communication devices (e.g. mobile phones) using physical or computational models of the head and body. However, these are not of direct relevance to epidemiological studies, but are used to certify that mobile phones meet exposure guidelines. Using these physical or computational models it has been shown that when using a mobile phone the energy absorption is highest in the parts of the brain nearest to the antenna of the mobile phone, with a marked attenuation through the head. Dimbylow and Mann (1999) found that the maximum SAR in the ear region on the side of the head holding the phone is approximately 150–500 times greater than on the opposite ear, depending on the frequency.

SAR assessments are now routinely carried out in test laboratories throughout the world and the measurement procedures and protocols are well established. There are international standards for SAR assessments (CENELEC 2001) and test laboratories are accredited specifically for SAR testing. Simple homogeneous physical models of the head are used, filled with liquids whose electrical properties are similar to those of the brain. The shapes of the model heads and the properties of the liquids are specified so that measured SARs will always be greater than SARs encountered by mobile phone users.

SAR is assessed inside the model heads using a probe that measures the internal electric field strength inside the head. The probe is mounted on a robot arm that is controlled by a computer. The head is scanned by the robot and the highest SAR region identified. The system then performs a 'fine scan' of the SAR distribution around the position of highest SAR and records the SAR averaged over a specific volume— usually 1 or 10 g.

It is also possible to assess SAR using computational dosimetry, and this has the advantage that a more realistic head model, containing multiple tissue types and specific organs, can be used. Because of this, computational dosimetry may be a valuable adjunct to epidemiological studies. However, computational dosimetry is very much a research tool rather than a fully established dosimetric approach and is not at present specified in mobile phone assessment standards.

An important dosimetric variable that also must be taken into account is the fact that the power output of the mobile phone varies continuously and is controlled by the base station. Most mobile phone networks have a 100:1 operating range for the radiofrequency power of the mobile units and the network reduces the radiofrequency power of each roaming unit at the minimum level compatible with the voice quality required for a phone conversation.

It is clear that the assessment of radiofrequency exposure from using mobile phones is extremely complicated. Billing records are relatively easy to obtain but are probably a poor reflection of exposure, as they do not record incoming calls, do not specify who is using the phone, and do not contain any information on the power levels during the call. Software-modified phones have been developed by some manufacturers to record data including power output during phone calls, call duration, left- or right-hand use, positioning of phone at the face, and phone model. The use of such phones is likely to provide useful data related to radiofrequency exposure, especially when validating information from questionnaires or interviews on frequency and duration of use of mobile phones. A number of such validation studies are currently being carried out in centres participating in the INTERPHONE study.

17.6 Future developments

Mobile phones of the 1980s relied on analogue technologies, where the radio signal was not significantly different in nature from TV and radio broadcasts. With the advent of digital (GSM) technologies in the 1990s, the nature of the exposure changed: GSM phones produce exposures with a very distinctive pulse-modulation, which is quite different from any previous source of exposure. There has been debate about whether this pulse modulation may have any significance for health, but it is certainly an aspect of exposure that must be considered in epidemiological studies.

The pace of technological change is increasing in the twenty-first century, and we are seeing the emergence of new communications technologies. It is likely that so-called third-generation phones, with a different modulation regime than GSM phones, will be available soon. This may or may not have consequences for health, but will certainly need to be considered in epidemiological studies. There are parallel changes in other communications technologies that reflect the ways in which the mobile phone is evolving into a multimedia device. Personal organizers and cameras are already integrated into phones, and further developments will allow the devices to interact with each other and with other technologies in ways we cannot yet foresee. The convergence of multimedia, personal organizers, and wireless connections is likely to lead to increased exposures of the body from higher-power devices in the pocket or hand, possibly accompanied by lower exposures to the head.

There are other communications technologies that can produce radiofrequency exposures similar to GSM phones. TETRA radio is a pan-European trunked radio system that is intended as a digital alternative to the VHF radios used by emergency services and the private mobile radios used by public utilities and, for example, taxi companies. TETRA has much higher security than analogue VHF radio and can be used, like GSM, to carry data. TETRA operates at lower frequency than GSM—around 400 MHz—and has a pulse modulation frequency of around 17 Hz rather than the 217 Hz modulation of GSM. There are few published studies on the health effects of TETRA, and it has been argued that because of its different emission characteristics the published data from GSM health investigations may not be directly applicable.

In any further epidemiological studies of occupational and general populations, close attention must be paid to quality and validity of the assessment of exposure. Suitable equipment will need to be developed that will be able to detect low levels of exposure for various frequency ranges including low frequency modulation effects. Personal dosimeters are available for occupational situations with relatively high radiofrequency exposures, and these need to be adapted to be more sensitive so that radiofrequency exposures for children and their parents living or going to schools near mobile phones base stations can be investigated. Further data need to be gathered on the determinants of exposure from mobile phones by using software-modified phones. In addition, information from complex computational modelling and laboratory work using physical models (phantoms) should be linked with information on patterns of use to develop more accurate and realistic exposure estimates.

References

Allen, S. G., Blackwell, R. P., Chadwick, P. J., Driscoll, C. M. H., Pearson, A. J., Unsworth, C., and Whillock, M. J. (1994). *Review of occupational exposure to optical radiation and electric and magnetic fields with regard to the proposed CEC physical agents directive.* NRPB-R265. National Radiological Protection Board, Chilton, Didcot. ISBN 0 85951 368 8.

Auvinen, A., Hietanen, M., Luukkonen, R., and Koskela, R.-S. (2002). Brain tumours and salivary gland cancers among cellular telephone users. *Epidemiology*, **13**, 356–9.

Balzano, Q. (1999). Exposure metrics for RF epidemiology: cellular phone handsets. *Radiation Protection Dosimetry*, **83**, 165–9.

Bergqvist, U. (2001). *Exposure to radiofrequency fields and mobile phone telephony.* X2001, Gothenburg, June 2001.

Borbely, A. A., Huber, R., Graf, T., Fuchs, B., Gallmann, E., and Achermann, P. (1999). Pulsed high-frequency electromagnetic field affects human sleep and sleep electroencephalogram. *Neuroscience Letters*, **275**, 207–10.

Cantor, K., Stewart, P., Brinton, L., and Dosemeci, M. (1995). Occupational exposures and female breast cancer mortality in the United States. *Journal of Occupational and Environmental Medicine*, **37**, 336–48.

Cardis, E. and Kilkenny, M. (1999). International case–control study of adult brain, head and neck tumours: results of the feasibility study. *Radiation Protection and Dosimetry*, **83**, 179–83.

CENELEC (2001). EN50630/1:2001: Basic and product standards to demonstrate the compliance of handheld mobile phones with the basic restrictions related to human exposure to radio frequency electromagnetic fields.

Dahme, M. (1999). Residential RF exposure. *Radiation Protection Dosimetry*, **83**, 113–18.

Davis, R. L. and Mostofi, F. K. (1993). Cluster of testicular cancer in police officers exposed to hand-held radar. *American Journal of Industrial Medicine*, **24**, 231–3.

Demers, P. A., Thomas, D. B., and Rosenblatt, K. A. (1991). Occupational exposure to electromagnetic fields and breast cancer in men. *American Journal of Epidemiology*, **134**, 340–7.

Dimbylow, P. J. and Mann, S. M. (1999). Characterisation of energy deposition in the head from cellular phones. *Radiation Protection Dosimetry*, **83**, 139–41.

Dolk, H., Shaddick, G., Wallis, P., Grundy, C., Thakrar, B., Kleinschmidt, L., and Elliott, P. (1997a). Cancer incidence near radio and television transmitters in Great Britain. I. Sutton Coldfield transmitter. *American Journal of Epidemiology*, **145**, 1–9.

Dolk, H., Elliott, P., Shaddick, G., Walls, P., and Thakrar, B. (1997b). Cancer incidence near radio and television transmitters in Great Britain. II. All high power transmitters. *American Journal of Epidemiology*, **145**, 10–17.

Dreyer, N. A., Loughlin, J. E., and Rothman, K. J. (1999). Cause-specific mortality in cellular phone users. *Journal of the American Medical Association*, **282**, 1814–16.

Grayson, J. K. (1996). Radiation exposure, socio-economic status and brain tumour risk in US Air Force: a nested case–control study. *American Journal of Epidemiology*, **143**, 480–6.

Groves, F. D., Page, W. F., Gridley, G., Lisimaque, L., Stewart, P. A., Tarone, R. E., Gail, M. H., Boice, J. D., and Beebe, G. W. (2002). Cancer in Korean war navy technicians: mortality survey after 40 years. *American Journal of Epidemiology*, **155**, 810–18.

Hallberg, O. and Johansson, O. (2002). Melanoma incidence and frequency modulation (FM) broadcasting. *Archives of Environmental Health*, **57**, 32–40.

Hardell, L., Nasman, A., Phalson, A., Hallquist, A., and Hansson Mild, K. (1999). Use of cellular telephones and the risk for brain tumours: a case–control study. *International Journal of Oncology*, **15**, 113–16.

Hardell, L., Hallquist, A., Hansson Mild, K., Carlberg, M., Pahson, A., and Lilja, A. (2002). Cellular and cordless telephones and the risk for brain tumours. *European Journal of Cancer Prevention*, **11**, 377–86.

Hayes, R. B., Morris Brown, L., Pottern, L. M., Gomez, M., Kardaun, J. W. P. F., Hoover, R. N., O'Connell, K. J., Sutzman, R. E., and Javadpour, N. (1990). Occupation and risk for testicular cancer: a case–control study. *International Journal of Epidemiology*, **19**, 825–31.

Hocking, B., Gordon, I. R., Grain, H. L., and Hatfield, G. E. (1996). Cancer incidence and mortality and proximity to TV towers. *Medical Journal of Australia*, **165**, 601–5.

IARC (2001). *Static and extremely low-frequency electric and magnetic fields*. IARC Monographs Vol. 80, Lyon, France.

ICNIRP (1998). Guidelines for limiting exposure to time-varying electric, magnetic, and electromagnetic fields (up to 300 GHz). *Health Physics*, **74**, 494–522. (http://www.icnirp.org/documents/emfgdl.pdf)

IEGMP (2000). *Mobile phones and health*. National Radiological Protection Board, Didcot, UK. (http://www.iegmp.org.uk/report/index.htm)

Inskip, P. D., Tarone, R. E., Hatch, E. E., Wilcosky, T. C., Shapiro, W. R., Selker, R. G., Fine, H. A., Black, P. M., Loeffler, J. S., and Linet, M. S. (2001). Cellular telephone use and brain tumours. *The New England Journal of Medicine*, **344**, 79–86.

Johansen, C., Boice, J. D., McLaughlin, J. K., and Olsen, J. H. (2001). Cellular telephones and cancer—a nationwide cohort study in Denmark. *Journal of the National Cancer Institute*, **93**, 203–7.

Jokela, K. and Puranen, L. (1999). Occupational RF exposures. *Radiation Protection Dosimetry*, **83**, 119–24.

Koivisto, M., Revonsuo, A., Krause, C. M., Haarala, C., Sillanmäki, L., Laine, M., and Hämäläinen, H. (2000). Effects of 902 MHz electromagnetic field emitted by cellular telephones on response times in humans. *Neuroreport*, **11**, 413–15.

Krause, C. M., Sillanmäki, L., Koivisto, M., Häggqvist, A., Saarela, C., Revonsuo, A., Laine, M., and Hämäläinen, H. (2000). Effects of electromagnetic field emitted by cellular phones on the EEG during a memory task. *Neuroreport*, **11**, 761–4.

Lagorio, S., Rossi, S., Vecchia, P., De Santis, M., Bastianini, L., Fusilli, M., Ferrucci, E., and Comba, P. (1997). Mortality of plastic ware workers exposed to radiofrequencies. *Bioelectromagnetics*, **18**, 418–21.

Lai, H. and Singh, N. P. (1995). Acute low-intensity microwave exposure increases DNA single strand breaks in rat brain cells. *Bioelectromagnetics*, **16**, 207.

Lai, H. and Singh, N. P. (1996). Single- and double-strand DNA breaks in rat brain cells after acute exposure to radiofrequency electromagnetic radiation. *International Journal of Radiation Biology*, **69**, 513–21.

Malyapa, R. S., Ahern, E. W., Straube, W. L., Moros, E. G., Pickard, W. F., and Roti-Roti, J. L. (1997*a*). Measurement of DNA damage after exposure to 2450 MHz electromagnetic radiation. *Radiation Research*, **148**, 608–17.

Malyapa, R. S., Ahern, E. W., Straube, W. L., Moros, E. G., Pickard, W. F., and Roti-Roti, J. L. (1997*b*). Measurement of DNA damage after exposure to electromagnetic radiation in the cellular phone communication frequency band (835.62 and 847.74 MHz). *Radiation Research*, **148**, 618–27.

Malyapa, R. S., Ahern, E. W., Bi, C., Straube, W. L., LaRegina, M., Pickard, W. F., and Roti-Roti, J. L. (1998). DNA damage in rat brain cells after *in vivo* exposure to 2450 MHz electromagnetic radiation and various methods of Euthanasia. *Radiation Research*, **149**, 637–45.

Mann, S. M., Cooper, T. G., Allen, S. G., Blackwell, R. P., and Lowe, A. J. (2000). *Exposure to radio waves near mobile phone base stations*. NRPB-R321. National Radiological Protection Board. Chilton, Didcot UK. ISBN 0 85951 455 2.

Mann, K. and Roschke, J. (1996). Effects of pulsed high-frequency electromagnetic fields on human sleep. *Neuropsychobiology*, **33**, 41.

Mantiply, E. D., Pohl, K. R., Poppell, S. W., and Murphy, J. A. (1997). Summary of measured radiofrequency electric and magnetic fields (10 kHz to 30 GHz) in the general and work environment. *Bioelectromagnetics*, **18**, 563–77.

McKenzie, D. R., Yin, Y., and Morrell, S. (1998). Childhood incidence of acute lymphoblastic leukemia and exposure to broadcast radiation in Sydney—a second look. *Australian & New Zealand Journal of Public Health*, **22**, 360–7.

Michelozzi, P., Capon, A., Kirchmayer, U., Forastiere, F., Biggeri, A., Barca, A., and Perucci, C. A. (2002). Adult and childhood leukemia near a high-power radio station in Rome, Italy. *American Journal of Epidemiology*, **155**, 1096–103.

Milham, S. (1982). Mortality from leukemia in workers exposed to electrical and magnetic fields. *New England Journal of Medicine*, **307**, 249.

Milham, S. (1988). Increased mortality in amateur radio operators due to lymphatic and hematopoietic malignancies. *American Journal of Epidemiology*, **127**, 50–4.

Morgan, R. W., Kelsh, M. A., Zhao, K., Exuzides, K. A., Heringer, S., and Negrete, W. (2000). Radiofrequency exposure and mortality from cancer of the brain and lymphatic/hematopoietic systems. *Epidemiology*, **13**, 118–27.

Muscat, J. E., Malkin, M. G., Thompson, S., Shore, R. E., Stellman, S. D., McRee, D., Neugut, A. I., and Wynder, E. L. (2000). Handheld cellular telephone use and risk of brain cancer. *Journal of the American Medical Association*, **284**, 3001–7.

Muscat, J. E., Malkin, M. G., Shore, R. E., Thompson, S., Neugut, A. I., Stellman, S. D., and Bruce, J. (2002). Handheld cellular phones and risk of acoustic neuroma. *Neurology*, **58**, 1304–6.

NRPB (2001). *ELF electromagnetic fields and the risk of cancer: report of an advisory group on non-ionising radiation*. Documents of the NRPB: Vol. 12, No. 1. Didcot, UK.

Preece, A. W., Iwi, G., Davies-Smith, A., Wesner, K., Butler, S., Lim, E., and Varey, A. (1999). Effect of a 915 MHz simulated mobile phone signal on cognitive function in man. *International Journal of Radiation Biology*, **75**, 447–56.

Repacholi, M. H., Basten, A., Gebski, V., Noonan, D., Finnie, J., and Harris, A. W. (1997). Lymphomas in Eμ-Pim1 transgenic mice exposed to pulsed 900 MHz electromagnetic fields. *Radiation Research*, **147**, 631–40.

Robinette, C. D., Silverman, C., and Jablon, S. (1980). Effects upon health of occupational exposure to microwave radiation (Radar). *American Journal of Epidemiology*, **112**, 39–53.

Rothman, K. J., Loughlin, J. E., Funch, D. P., and Dreyer, N. A. (1996). Overall mortality of cellular telephone costumers. *Epidemiology*, **7**, 303–5.

Royal Society of Canada (1999). *A review of the potential health risks of radiofrequency fields from wireless telecommunication devices*. The Royal Society of Canada.

Schüz, J. and Mann, S. (2000). A discussion of potential exposure metrics for use in epidemiological studies on human exposure to radiowaves from mobile phone base stations. *Journal of Exposure Analysis and Environmental Epidemiology*, **10**, 600–5.

Swerdlow, A. J. (1999). Measurement of radiofrequency radiation exposure in epidemiological studies. *Radiation Protection Dosimetry*, **83**, 149–53.

Szmigielski, S. (1996). Cancer morbidity in subjects occupationally exposed to high frequency (radiofrequency and microwave) electromagnetic radiation. *Science of the Total Environment*, **18**, 9–17.

Thomas, T. L., Stolley, P. D., Stemhagen, A., Fontham, E. T. H., Bleecker, M. L., Stewart, P. A., and Hooever, R. N. (1987). Brain tumor mortality risk among men with electrical and electronics jobs: a case–control study. *Journal of National Cancer Institute*, **789**, 233–8.

Tynes, T., Andersen, A., and Langmark, F. (1992). Incidence of cancer in Norwegian workers potentially exposed to electromagnetic fields. *American Journal of Epidemiology*, **136**, 81–8.

Tynes, T., Hannevik, M., Andersen, A., Vistnes, A. I., and Haldorsen, T. (1996). Incidence of breast cancer in Norwegian female radio and telegraph operators. *Cancer Causes Control*, **7**, 197–204.

Utteridge, T. D., Gebski, V., Finnie, J. W., Vernon-Roberst, B., and Kuchel, T. R. (2002). Long-term exposure of Eµ-*Pim1* transgenic mice to 898.4 MHz microwaves does not increase lymphoma incidence. *Radiation Research*, **158**, 357–64.

Wertheimer, N. and Leeper, E. (1979). Electrical wiring configurations and childhood cancer. *American Journal of Epidemiology*, **109**, 273–84.

Zmirou (2001). *Mobile telephones, base stations and health: current state-of-knowledge and recommendations*. A report to the General Director of Health of France. Translated by MCL (www.mcluk.org).

Index

absorption *see* dermal absorption
accuracy 17, 114
acetaldehyde 238
acrylates 134
active sampling 76–7
advection 44
aeroallergens
  flour 14, 74–6
  mouse urinary proteins 209
  rat urinary proteins 209, 214
  see also allergen exposure
aids to recall 33–4
air pollution 61–2
aldehydes 238
allergen exposure 203–19
  allergen standards 207–8
  antibody sources 207
  exposure routes 208–10
  measurement of allergen levels 206–8
  sampling 204–6
  validation and standardization 208
  see also aeroallergens
ambient levels 80–2
American Conference of Governmental
    Industrial Hygienists 134
ammonia 8
α-amylase 14–15, 207
analysis of variance 86–9
  nested 88
ANOVA *see* analysis of variance
antibodies 207
area-under-the curve (AUC) 158
arithmetic mean 10
arsenic 39, 178
  emissions 48–50
  hair and nails 172
  house dust 179
  soil 179
  urine 179
asbestos 8
autocorrelation 175–6
average sampling 78–9

baker's asthma 74
bakery workers 14–15, 74–6, 212, 215
  ANOVA model of flour dust exposure 89–91

  see also flour aeroallergen
bayesian analysis 161–2
benzene 133
  exhaled breath 172
  urine sampling 168
Berkson error 182–3, 194–5
bias 17, 198
biological measurements 107–8
biological monitoring 167–80
  autocorrelation 175–6
  damping of exposure variability 176
  half-life 173–5
  models and determinants 177–9
  quality control 179
  types of samples 168–73
    blood 170–1
    breast milk 172–3
    exhaled breath 171–2
    fat 172
    hair and nails 172
    urine 168–70
  variability 176–7
biologically relevant dose 6
biomarkers 108
biomonitoring 13–14, 36, 140
  chlorination disinfection 239–40
blood samples 170–1
body fat samples 172
bootstrapping 100
box models 44, 66–7
breast milk samples 172–3
bromochloroacetonitrile 238
bromodichloromethane 237, 238
bromoform 52, 237, 238

cadmium, half-life 173
cancer
  pesticides 251–62
  radiofrequency exposure 263–75
carbaryl 133
carbon monoxide 5–6, 39, 78–9
  exhaled breath 172
  half-life 173
  personal exposure monitoring 78–9
carbon tetrachloride 133
  exhaled breath 172